A SHORT TEXTBOOK OF PSYCHIATRY

Every effort has been made to ensure that drug dosage schedules in this book are accurate and conform to the standards accepted at the time of publication. However, as treatment recommendations vary in the light of continuing research and clinical experience, the reader is advised to verify drug dosage schedules contained in the product information sheets included in the package of each drug, before the drug is administered. It is the responsibility of the treating physician, relying on experience and knowledge of the patient, to determine the dosages and the best treatment for the patient. Neither the publisher nor the author assumes any responsibility for any untoward consequences.

A SHORT TEXTBOOK OF PSYCHIATRY

FIFTH EDITION

NIRAJ AHUJA, MD
Associate Professor (Psychiatry)
GB Pant Hospital and
Associated Maulana Azad Medical College (MAMC) and
Lok Nayak Hospital, New Delhi

Previously at
Department of Psychiatry,
Jawaharlal Institute of Postgraduate Medical Education and Research (JIPMER), Pondicherry
Lady Hardinge Medical College (LHMC) and Smt. SK Hospital, New Delhi, and
All India Institute of Medical Sciences (AIIMS), New Delhi

Contributing Editor
DR. S. AHUJA

JAYPEE BROTHERS
MEDICAL PUBLISHERS (P) LTD.
NEW DELHI

Published by

Jitendar P Vij
Jaypee Brothers Medical Publishers (P) Ltd
EMCA House, 23/23B Ansari Road, Daryaganj
New Delhi 110 002, India
Phones: 23272143, 23272703, 2328202, 23245672, 23245683
Fax: 011-23276490 e-mail: jpmedpub@del2.vsnl.net.in
Visit our website: http://www.jpbros.20m.com

Branches

- 202 Batavia Chambers, 8 Kumara Kruppa Road, Kumara Park East, **Bangalore** 560 001, Phones: 2285971, 2382956 Tele Fax: 2281761
  e-mail: jaypeebc@bgl.vsnl.net.in
- 282 IIIrd Floor, Khaleel Shirazi Estate, Fountain Plaza
  Pantheon Road, **Chennai** 600 008, Phone: 28262665 Fax: 28262331
  e-mail: jpmedpub@md3.vsnl.net.in
- 4-2-1067/1-3, Ist Floor, Balaji Building, Ramkote, Cross Road
  Hyderabad 500095, Phone: 55610020, 24758498 Fax: 24758499
  e-mail: jpmedpub@rediffmail.com
- 1A Indian Mirror Street, Wellington Square
  Kolkata 700 013, Phone: 22451926 Fax: 22456075
  e-mail: jpbcal@cal.vsnl.net.in
- 106 Amit Industrial Estate, 61 Dr SS Rao Road, Near MGM Hospital
  Parel, **Mumbai** 400 012 , Phones: 24124863, 24104532 Fax: 24160828
  e-mail: jpmedpub@bom7.vsnl.net.in

A Short Textbook of Psychiatry

First Edition: 1990
Second Edition: 1992
Third Edition: 1995
Fourth Edition: 1999
Fifth Edition: 2002
Reprint: 2005

ISBN 81-7179-987-6

Typeset at JPBMP typesetting unit
Printed at Gopsons Papers Ltd., Sector 60, Noida

To

My Daughters

Manisha

and

Neha

Preface to the Fifth Edition

In last twelve and a half years, the *Short Textbook of Psychiatry* has enjoyed a wide distribution among undergraduate medical students, interns, junior residents, nursing students, psychology and psychiatric social work students, occupational therapy and physiotherapy students, general medical practitioners, other physicians and health professionals in India and other countries. I am indebted to the many readers who have provided constructive feed-back as well as encouraging comments regarding the existing format and the contents of the book.

The fifth edition of the *Short Textbook of Psychiatry* has been once again extensively revised and updated. One of the prominent additions of the fourth edition continues to stay in this book, namely the inclusion of the International Classification of Diseases, 10th Revision, 1992 (ICD-10), World Health Organization, throughout the book.

Significant changes have been made in almost all the chapters, especially in chapters on diagnosis and classification, psychoactive substance use disorders, psychopharmacology, community psychiatry, and child psychiatry. Shaded boxes have been added at various places in the text to highlight important points in tables and figures. The chapter on psychiatric history and examination now contains a resume of laboratory tests in psychiatry, in addition to other significant changes. The appendices have also been revised and now contain a glossary of common psychiatric terms.

The *Short Textbook of Psychiatry* sincerely hopes to retain its original aim of providing a brief yet comprehensive account of the psychiatric disorders and their allied aspects in a 'user-friendly' and 'easy-to-follow' manner.

I am very grateful to Mr. Jitendar P. Vij, Managing Director, JPB Medical Publishing House for his exquisite control over the production and distribution of the Short Textbook of Psychiatry. I also deeply appreciate the advise received from Dr. RK Yadav (Editorial Consultant).

I welcome critical comments and constructive suggestions from the readers.

June, 2002

NIRAJ AHUJA MD

Preface to the First Edition

Psychiatry, as a branch of Medicine, has been cold-shouldered by physicians for a long time. There are various reasons for such an attitude. But, the most important exposition is an unfamiliarity with the psychiatric disorders and their treatment. This is easy to understand in the light of the fact that an easily comprehensible, non-intimidating and concise text on psychiatry was not earlier available.

Recently too, the various postgraduate entrance examinations have laid an increasing emphasis on psychiatry and its related branches. Keeping this in mind, the *MEDICAL EXAMINATION REVIEW–PSYCHIATRY* (Multiple Choice Questions with Explanatory Answers) was written, the new edition of which appears this year. Its tremendous success during the last four years and encouraging suggestions from the readers have been a source of stimulation for drafting this text.

The *Short Textbook of Psychiatry* aims to provide a brief yet comprehensive account of psychiatric disorders and their allied aspects. While striving to make the book simple and easy to follow, an attempt has been made to keep the book aligned to the most recent developments in classification, terminology and treatment methods.

The *Short Textbook* is addressed to medical students, interested physicians & other health professionals. A postgraduate student in psychiatry will find the text elementary and basic, although a first year postgraduate will find it useful for a broad introduction to the subject.

I will like to put on record my deep appreciation for Mr. Jitendar Vij, Managing Director; Mr. Pawaninder Vij, Production Manager and their efficient staff at the JPB Publishing House, Delhi for bringing out this volume in a short time.

I welcome critical comments and constructive suggestions from the readers.

January, 1990

NIRAJ AHUJA MD

Contents

1 Diagnosis and Classification in Psychiatry

Classification is a process by which the complex phenomena are organized into categories, classes or ranks so as to bring together those things that most resemble each other, and to separate those that differ.

Any classification of psychiatric disorders, like that of medical illnesses, should ideally be based on etiology. For a large majority of psychiatric disorders, no distinct etiology is known at present, although there are many attractive probabilities for each.

Hence, the only rational way to classify is *syndromal*. A *syndrome* is defined as a group of symptoms and signs that often occur together, and delineate a recognizable clinical condition.

This approach of classifying psychiatric disorders on the basis of their clinical signs and symptoms is very similar to the approach of classifying medical illnesses about a century back, when etiology of a majority of medical illnesses was obscure.

There are three major purposes of classification:

1. To enable *communication*, regarding the diagnosis.
2. To facilitate *comprehension*, of the underlying causes.
3. To aid *prediction* of the prognosis.

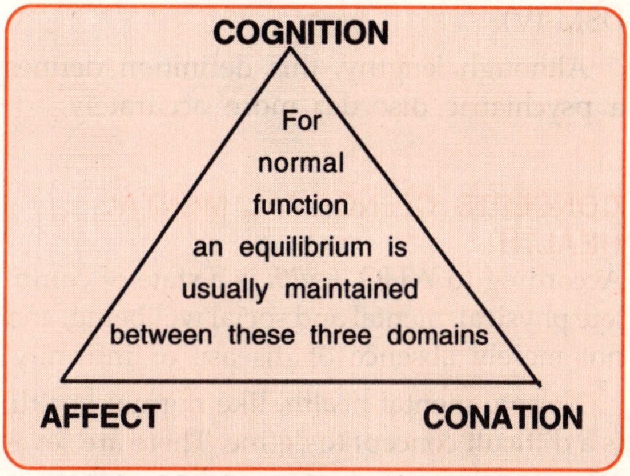

FIG. 1.1. PSYCHIATRIC DOMAINS

This syndromal approach of classification, in the absence of known etiologies, fulfils these purposes reasonably well. Before proceeding to classify psychiatric disorders, it is important to define what is a psychiatric disorder.

DEFINITION OF A PSYCHIATRIC DISORDER

The simplest way to conceptualize a psychiatric disorder is as a disturbance of

i. Cognition (i.e. thought), or
ii. Conation (i.e. action), or
iii. Affect (i.e. feeling), or

any disequilibrium between the three.

Another way to define a *psychiatric disorder* is as a clinically significant psychological or behavioral syndrome that causes significant distress (subjective symptomatology), disability (objective symptomatology), or loss of freedom; and which is not merely a socially deviant behavior or an expected response to a stressful life event (e.g. loss of a loved one). Conflicts between society and the individual are not mental disorders. A mental disorder should be a manifestation of behavioral, psychological, and/or biological dysfunction in that person (Definition modified after DSM-IV).

Although lengthy, this definition defines a psychiatric disorder more accurately.

CONCEPTS OF NORMAL MENTAL HEALTH

According to WHO, *health* is a state of complete physical, mental and social wellbeing, and not merely absence of disease or infirmity.

Normal mental health, like normal health, is a difficult concept to define. There are several models for understanding what is '*normality*'.

1. ***Medical Model (Normality as Health)***: Normal mental health is conceptualized as absence of (psychiatric) disease or psychopathology.
2. ***Statistical Model (Normality as an Average)***: Statistically normal mental health falls with in two standard deviations (SDs) of the normal distribution curve.
3. ***Utopian Model (Normality as Utopia)***: In this model, the focus in defining normality is on 'optimal functioning'.
4. ***Subjective Model***: According to this model, normality is viewed as an absence of distress, or disability, or help-seeking behavior thereof. This definition is similar to the medical model.
5. ***Social Model***: A normal person, according to this definition, is expected to behave in a socially permissive behavior.
6. ***Process Model (Normality as a Process)***: This model views normality as a dynamic and changing process, rather than as a static concept. This model can be combined with any other model mentioned here.
7. ***Continuum Model (Normality as a Continuum)***: This model describes normality and mental disorder as falling at the two ends of a continuum, rather than being disparate entities.

Although, normality is not an easy concept to define, the following traits are more commonly found in normal individuals.

1. Reality orientation.
2. Self-awareness and self-knowledge.
3. Self-esteem and self-acceptance.
4. Ability to exercise voluntary control over behavior.
5. Ability to form affectionate relationships.
6. Pursuance of productive, goal-directive activities.

CLASSIFICATION IN PSYCHIATRY

Like any growing branch of medicine, Psychiatry has seen rapid changes in classification to keep up with a conglomeration of growing research data dealing with epidemiology, symptomatology, prognostic factors, treatment methods and new theories for causation of psychiatric disorders.

Although the first attempts to classify madness or mental illnesses can be traced back

TABLE 1.1. SOME VERSIONS OF ICD-10

1. Clinical Descriptions and Diagnostic Guidelines (CDDG)
2. Diagnostic Criteria for Research (DCR)
3. Multi-axial Classification Version
4. Primary Care Version

to Ayurveda, Plato (4th century BC) and Asclepiades (1st century BC), classification in Psychiatry has come far ever since.

At present, there are two major classifications in Psychiatry, namely ICD-10 (1992) and DSM-IV-TR (2000).

1. ***ICD-10*** (*International Classification of Diseases*—10th Revision, 1992) is WHO's classification for all diseases and related health problems. Chapter 'F' classifies psychiatric disorders as *mental and behavioral disorders* and codes them on an alphanumeric system from F00 to F99. ICD-10 is now available in several versions, the most important of which are listed in the accompanying box:
2. ***DSM-IV-TR*** (*Diagnostic and Statistical Manual of Mental Disorders* - IV Edition, Text Revision, 2000) is APA's (American Psychiatric Association's) classification of mental disorders. DSM-IV-TR is a minor revision of the DSM-IV (1994).

For the purpose of this book, it is intended to follow the ICD-10 classification, as it is easy to follow, has been tested extensively all over the world (51 countries; 195 clinical centers), and has been found to be generally applicable across the globe. At some places, DSM-IV-TR is also discussed whenever appropriate.

The earlier classifications were based on *hierarchies* of diagnosis (presence of a diagnosis higher in the hierarchy ruling out a diagnosis lower in the hierarchy), but the current classifications encourage recording of multiple diagnoses in a given patient (*co-morbidity*) regardless of hierarchy.

MENTAL AND BEHAVIORAL DISORDERS (ICD-10)

F00-F09 Organic, Including Symptomatic, Mental Disorders

This group includes mental and behavioral disorders due to demonstrable cerebral disease or disorder, either primary (primary brain pathology) or secondary (brain dysfunction due to systemic diseases). The use of term *organic* here does not imply that other psychiatric disorders are 'non-organic' in the sense of having no biological basis. It simply means that the disorders listed in this section have a demonstrable and independently diagnosable cerebral disease or disorder.

The disorders in this section include delirium, dementia, organic amnestic syndrome, and other organic mental disorders.

F10-F19 Mental and Behavioral Disorders due to Psychoactive Substance Use

This group includes mental and behavioral disorders due to the use of one or more psycho-active substances.

The disorders in this section include acute intoxication, harmful use, dependence syndrome, withdrawal state, amnestic syndrome, and psychotic disorders due to psycho-active substance use.

F20-F29 Schizophrenia, Schizotypal and Delusional Disorders

This group includes mental and behavioral disorders characterized by prominent disturbances of thought, perception, affect, and/or behavior.

The disorders in this section include schizophrenia, schizotypal disorder, persistent delusional disorders, acute and transient psychotic disorders, induced delusional disorder, and schizo-affective disorders.

F31-F39 Mood (Affective) Disorders

This group includes mental and behavioral disorders characterized by a prominent disturbance of mood.

The disorders in this section include manic episode, depressive episode, bipolar affective disorder, recurrent depressive disorder, and persistent mood disorder.

F40-F48 Neurotic, Stress-related and Somatoform Disorders

(There is no category with code number F49)

This group includes mental and behavioral disorders that were earlier labeled as neurotic disorders, with an emphasis on psychological causation.

The disorders in this section include anxiety disorders, phobic anxiety disorders, obsessive-compulsive disorder, dissociative (conversion) disorders, somatoform disorders, reaction to stress, and adjustment disorders, and other neurotic disorders.

F50-F59 Behavioral Syndromes Associated with Physiological Disturbances and Physical Factors

This group includes mental and behavioral disorders that were earlier called psychosomatic disorders. The term psychosomatic is no longer used because its use implied that the association between the psychological factors and physical disorder is etiological. Also it presumed that the psychological factors are not important in other medical illnesses and physical disorders.

The disorders in this section include eating disorders, non-organic sleep disorders, sexual dysfunctions (not caused by organic disorder or disease), mental and behavioral disorders associated with puerperium, and abuse of non-dependence-producing substances.

F60-F69 Disorders of Adult Personality and Behavior

This group includes mental and behavioral disorders that are the persistent expression of an individual's characteristic lifestyle and mode of relating to self and others.

TABLE 1.2. THE FIVE AXES OF DSM-IV

AXIS I:	Clinical Psychiatric Diagnosis
AXIS II:	Personality Disorders and Mental Retardation
AXIS III:	General Medical Conditions
AXIS IV:	Psychosocial and Environmental Problems
AXIS V:	Global Assessment of Functioning: Current and in past one year (rated on a scale)

The disorders in this section include specific personality disorders, enduring personality changes, habit and impulse disorders, gender-identity disorders, disorders of sexual preference, and psychological and behavioral disorders associated with sexual development and orientation.

F70-F79 Mental Retardation

This group includes disorders with arrested or incomplete development of the intellectual abilities and adaptive behavior, which may or may not be associated with other physical or mental disorder.

The disorders in this section include mild, moderate, severe, and profound mental retardation.

F80-F89 Disorders of Psychological Development

This group includes mental and behavioral disorders with an onset during infancy or childhood and characterized by an impairment or delay in the development of functions that are strongly related to biological maturation of the central nervous system.

The disorders in this section include specific developmental disorders of speech and language, specific developmental disorders of scholastic skills, specific developmental disorders of motor function, mixed specific developmental disorders, and pervasive developmental disorders.

F90-F98 Behavioral and Emotional Disorders with Onset Usually Occurring in Childhood and Adolescence

This group includes miscellaneous mental and behavioral disorders that have an onset in childhood and adolescence.

The disorders in this section include hyperkinetic disorders, conduct disorders, mixed disorders of conduct and emotions, tic disorders, and other disorders.

F99 Unspecified Mental Disorder

Multi-Axial Classification

Labeling the patient with a diagnosis is not enough. This degrades the individual to just another case and does not direct attention to the whole individual.

Recently, there has been an upsurge of interest in multi-axial systems for achieving a more complete diagnosis. The pattern adopted by DSM-IV is a good example. In this system, an individual patient is diagnosed on five separate axes (Table 1.2).

This method helps in a more holistic assessment of an individual patient. Recently, ICD-10 has also brought out its own multi-axial classification version (Table 1.1).

2 Psychiatric History and Examination

Familiarity with the technique of *psychiatric assessment* is important not only for the psychiatrist but also for a medical specialist or practitioner, since a large percentage (more than one-third) of medical patients have psychiatric disorders.

INTERVIEW TECHNIQUE

In no other branch of medicine is the history taking interview as important as in psychiatry. Most physicians also have to talk with (or at least to) patients and they are never taught how to talk with them. Skillful interview results in obtaining better information, making a more accurate diagnosis, establishing a better rapport, and ensuring greater compliance with treatment.

Psychiatric interview is different from routine medical interview in several ways (Table 2.1). Certain important points regarding the interview technique are mentioned below. These serve as pointers towards a technique which has to be mastered over a period of time with repeated examinations.

1. A *consistent scheme* should be used each time for recording the interview, although the interview need not follow a fixed and rigid method. The interview technique should have flexibility, varying according to the varying clinical circumstances.
2. Whenever possible, the patient should be seen first. When the account of present (or past) history given by the patient and the informant(s) is different, *record* both of them *separately*.
3. During the interview, the patient should be put at ease and a warm, *empathic relationship* should be established whenever possible.
4. In psychiatric assessment, history taking interview and mental status examination should not be always conducted separately (although, they must be recorded separately). During the history taking session, the interviewer must observe the abnormalities in verbal and non-verbal communication and make a note of them.
5. It is helpful to record the patient's responses *verbatim*, rather than naming them (e.g. rather than writing delusion of persecution, it is better to write verbatim: "my brother and my nephew are trying to poison me with arsenic"). It is best done in the patient's own spoken language, whenever possible.
6. It is useful to ask *open-ended* and *non-directive questions* (e.g. 'how are you feeling today'?) rather than asking direct, leading questions (e.g. 'are you feeling sad at present'?).
7. The most important interviewing skill is *listening* and showing that you are

TABLE 2.1. PSYCHIATRIC VS. MEDICAL INTERVIEW

A *psychiatric interview* is different from a medical interview in several ways, some of which are:

1. Presence of disturbances in thinking and behavior, interfering with meaningful communication
2. Need for information from *significant others*
3. More important to obtain information regarding personal history and premorbid personality
4. More need for astute observation of patient
5. Difficulty in establishing rapport may be encountered more often
6. Patient may lack insight into his illness and have poor judgement
7. More important to elicit information regarding stressors

interested in listening and attending to the patient. Remember, listening is an active, and not a passive, process.

8. *Confidentiality* must always be observed. However, in cases of suicidal/homicidal risk and child abuse, an exception may have to be made.

A complete psychiatric interview may often require more than one session.

The psychiatric assessment can be discussed under the following headings.

IDENTIFICATION DATA

It is best to start the interview by obtaining the identification data, i.e. Name (including aliases and pet name), Age, Sex, Marital status, Education, Occupation, Income, Residential and Office Address(es), Religion, and Socio-economic background. It is useful to also record the source of referral of the patient. In medico-legal cases, in addition, two identification marks should also be recorded.

INFORMANTS

Since sometimes the history provided by a psychiatric patient may be incomplete, due to factors like absent insight or uncooperative-ness, it is important to take the history from the patient's relatives or friends who are acting as informants.

Their identification data should be recorded along with their *relationship* to the patient, whether they stay with the patient or not, and the duration of stay together.

Finally, a comment should be made regarding the *reliability of the information* provided. The reliability of the information provided by the informants should be assessed on the following parameters:

1. Relationship with patient,
2. Intellectual and observational ability,
3. Familiarity with the patient and length of stay with the patient,
4. Degree of concern regarding the patient.

The *source of referral* may also provide valuable information regarding the patient's condition.

PRESENTING CHIEF COMPLAINTS

Presenting complaints and/or reasons for consultation should be recorded. Both the patient's and the informant's *version* should be recorded separately. If the patient says that he has no complaints, this should also be recorded.

Use the patient's own words and note the *duration* of each presenting complaint. Additional points to be noted are:

1. Onset of present illness.
2. Duration of present illness.
3. Course.
4. Precipitating factors (include life stressors, if any).
5. Aggravating, maintaining, and/or relieving factors, if any.

HISTORY OF PRESENT ILLNESS

1. When the patient was last well (or asymptomatic) should be noted.

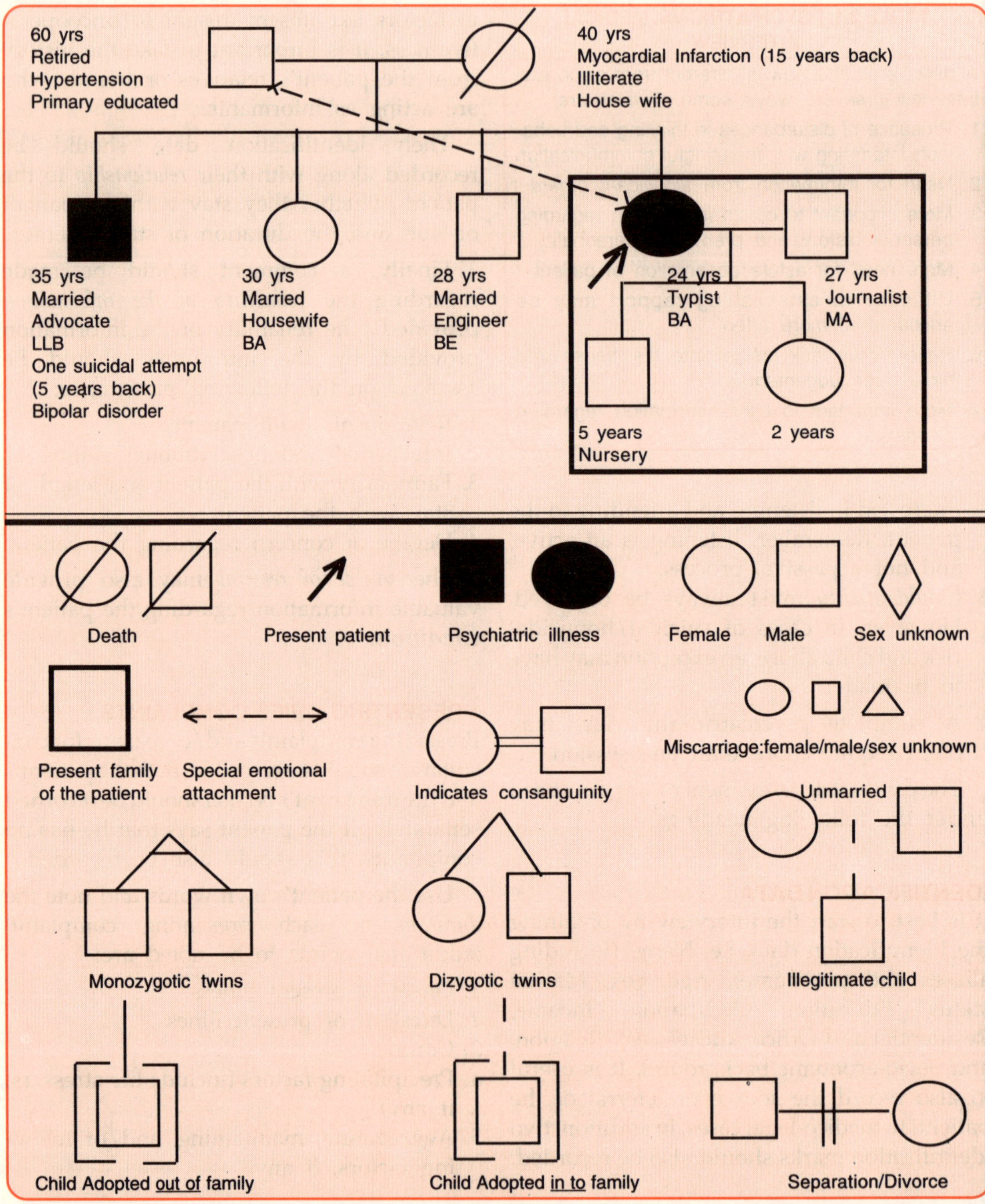

FIG. 2.1. A TYPICAL FAMILY TREE AND COMMON PEDIGREE SYMBOLS

2. The time of onset should be established.
3. The symptoms of the illness from the earliest time at which a change was noticed until the present time should be narrated *chronologically*, in a coherent manner.
4. The presenting chief complaints should be expanded.
5. In particular, any disturbances in the physiological functions like sleep, appetite, and sexual functioning should be inquired.
6. Always enquire about the presence of suicidal ideation.
7. Important negative history should be recorded (e.g. no history of head injury before the onset of illness).
8. A *life chart* provides a valuable display of the course of illness and episodic sequence, polarity (if any), severity, frequency, and relationship (if any) to stressors and response to treatment.

PAST PSYCHIATRIC AND MEDICAL HISTORY

History of similar or any other psychiatric illness in the past, if present, should be obtained. Past history of psychotropic medication, alcohol and drug abuse or dependence and psychiatric hospitalization should be asked for.

Past history of any serious medical, neurological or surgical illness, surgical procedure, accident and hospitalization should be obtained. The nature of treatment received, if any, should be ascertained. Past history of head injury, convulsions, unconsciousness, diabetes mellitus, hypertension, coronary artery disease, acute intermittent porphyria, syphilis and HIV positivity (or AIDS) should be particularly looked for.

TREATMENT HISTORY

Details of the treatment given in the present episode and the previous episodes should be asked along with the response to treatment.

FAMILY HISTORY

Family history usually includes the *'family of origin'* (i.e. the patient's parents, siblings, grandparents, uncles, etc.). However, the *'family of procreation'* (i.e. the patient's spouse, children and grandchildren) can also be recorded here instead of under personal history. Family history is recorded under the following headings:

1. *Family Structure*: Drawing of a 'family tree' (*pedigree chart*) helps in recording all the relevant information in very little space and is easily readable. An example of a typical family tree is given in Fig. 2.1.
   It should be noted whether the family is nuclear or extended nuclear (or joint) family. If consanginous relationship is present, it should be recorded. Age and cause of death (if any) of the family members should be asked.
2. *Family history of* similar or other psychiatric illnesses, major medical illnesses, alcohol or drug dependence and suicide (and suicidal attempts) should be recorded.
3. *Current social situation*: Home circumstances, per-capita income, socio-economic status, leader of the family (nominal as well as functional) and current attitude of the family members towards the patient's illness should be noted.
   The communication patterns in the family, range of affectivity, cultural and religious values and social support system should be inquired about, when relevant.

PERSONAL HISTORY

The younger the patient, it is possible to give more attention to details. In older patients, there may be considerable retrospective falsification. Parents, if alive, can often provide much additional information regarding the past personal history.

Personal history can be recorded under the following headings:

1. Perinatal History

Any febrile illness; medications, drugs and/or alcohol use; trauma to abdomen and any physical or psychiatric illness during pregnancy (particularly in the first three months of gestation) should be asked. Other relevant questions are: whether the patient was a wanted or unwanted child; date of birth; whether normal or abnormal delivery; any instrumentation; where born (hospital or home); any perinatal complications (cyanosis, convulsions, jaundice); APGAR score (if available); birth cry (immediate or delayed); any birth defects; any prematurity.

2. Childhood History

Whether the patient was brought up by mother or someone else; breast-feeding; weaning; any history suggestive of maternal deprivation, should be asked.

The age of passing each important developmental milestone should be noted. The age and ease of toilet training should be asked.

The occurrence of neurotic traits should be noted. These include stuttering, stammering, tics, enuresis, encopresis, night terrors, thumb sucking, nail biting, head banging, body rocking, morbid fears or phobias, somnambulism, temper tantrums, and food fads.

3. Educational History

The age of beginning and finishing formal education, academic achievements and relationships with peers and teachers, should be asked.

Any school phobia, non-attendance, truancy, any learning difficulties and reasons for termination of studies (if occurs prematurely) should be noted.

4. Play History

The questions to be asked are, what games were played at what stage, with whom and where. Relationships with peers, particularly the opposite sex, should be recorded.

5. Puberty

The age at menarche, and reaction to menarche (in females), the age at appearance of secondary sexual characteristics, nocturnal emissions (in males), masturbation and any anxiety related to puberty changes should be asked.

6. Menstrual and Obstetric History

The regularity and duration of menses, the length of each cycle, any abnormalities, the last menstrual period, the number of children born, termination of pregnancy if any, should be asked for.

7. Occupational History

The age at starting work; jobs held in chronological order; reasons for changes; job satisfactions; ambitions; relationships with authorities, peers and subordinates; present income; and whether the job is appropriate to the educational and family background, should be asked.

8. Sexual and Marital History

Sexual information, how acquired and of what kind; masturbation (fantasy and activity); sex play, if any; adolescent sexual activity; premarital and extramarital sexual relationships, if any; sexual practices (normal and abnormal); and any gender identity disorder, are the areas to be inquired about.

The duration of marriage; time known the partner before marriage; marriage arranged by parents with or without consent, or by self-choice with or without parental consent; number of marriages, divorces or separations; role in marriage; interpersonal and sexual relations; contraceptive measures used; sexual satisfaction; mode and frequency of sexual intercourse; and psychosexual dysfunction (if any) should be asked.

Although conventionally the details of the *'family of procreation'* are recorded here, they can also be recorded in the family tree.

9. Premorbid Personality (PMP)

It is important to elicit details regarding the personality of the individual (*temperament*, if the age is less than 16 years). Rather than giving labels like schizoid or histrionic, it is more useful to describe the personality in some detail. The following subheadings are often used for the description.

i. *Interpersonal relationship*

Interpersonal relationship with family members, friends, work-mates and superiors; introverted/extraverted; ease of making and keeping social relations.

ii. *Use of leisure time*

Hobbies; interests; intellectual activities; critical faculty; energetic/sedentary.

iii. *Predominant mood*

Optimistic/pessimistic; stable/prone to anxiety; cheerful/despondent; reaction to stressful life events.

iv. *Attitude to self and others*

Self-confidence level; self-criticism; self-consciousness; selfish/thoughtful of others; self-appraisal of abilities, achievements and failures.

v. *Attitude to work and responsibility*

Decision making; acceptance of responsibility; flexibility; perseverance; foresight.

vi. *Religious beliefs and moral attitudes*

Religious beliefs; toleration of others' standards and beliefs; conscience; altruism.

vii. *Fantasy life*

Sexual and nonsexual fantasies; daydreaming-frequency and content; recurrent or favorite daydreams; dreams.

viii. *Habits*

Food fads; alcohol; tobacco; drugs; sleep.

The most reliable method of premorbid personality assessment is, interviewing an informant familiar with the patient prior to the onset of illness.

PHYSICAL EXAMINATION

A detailed general physical examination (GPE) and systemic examination is a must in

TABLE 2.2. MENTAL STATUS EXAMINATION

1. General Appearance and Behavior
- i. General Appearance
- ii. Attitude towards Examiner
- iii. Comprehension
- iv. Gait and Posture
- v. Motor Activity
- vi. Social Manner
- vii. Rapport

2. Speech
- i. Rate and Quantity
- ii. Volume and Tone
- iii. Flow and Rhythm

3. Mood and Affect

4. Thought
- i. Stream and Form
- ii. Content

5. Perception

6. Cognition (Higher Mental Functions)
- i. Consciousness
- ii. Orientation
- iii. Attention
- iv. Concentration
- v. Memory
- vi. Intelligence
- vii. Abstract thinking

7. Insight

8. Judgement

every patient. Physical disease which is etiologically important (for causing the psychiatric symptomatology), accidentally co-existent, or secondarily caused by the psychiatric condition, is often present and can be detected by a good physical examination.

MENTAL STATUS EXAMINATION (MSE)*

Mental status examination is a standardized format in which the clinician records the psychiatric signs and symptoms present at the time of the interview.

MSE should describe all areas of mental functioning. Some areas, however, may deserve more emphasis according to the clinical impressions that may arise from the history, e.g. mood and affect in depression, cognitive functions in delirium and dementia.

* *The definition of some MSE terms is given in Appendix III.*

1. General Appearance and Behavior

A rich deal of information can be elicited from the examination of general appearance and behavior. While examining, it is important to remember the socio-cultural background and personality of the patient.

Understandably, general appearance and behavior needs to be given more emphasis in the examination of an uncooperative patient.

i. *General Appearance*

The points to be noted are:

Physique and body habitus (build) and physical appearance (approximate height, weight, and appearance),
Looks comfortable / uncomfortable,
Physical health,
Grooming, Hygiene, Self care,
Dressing (adequate, appropriate, any peculiarities),
Facies (non-verbal expression of mood),
Effeminate / masculine.

ii. *Attitude Towards The Examiner*

Cooperation / guardedness / evasiveness / hostility / combativeness / haughtiness,
Attentiveness,
Appears interested / disinterested / apathetic,
Any ingratiating behavior,
Perplexity.

iii. *Comprehension*

Intact / impaired (partially / fully).

iv. *Gait and Posture*

Normal or abnormal (way of sitting, standing, walking, lying).

v. *Motor Activity*

Increased / decreased,
Excitement / stupor,
Abnormal involuntary movements (AIMs) like tics, tremors, akathisia,
Restlessness / ill at ease,
Catatonic signs (mannerisms, stereotypies, posturing, waxy flexibility, negativism, ambitendency, automatic obedience, stupor, echopraxia, psychological pillow, forced grasping) (see Chapter 5 for details),
Conversion and dissociative signs (pseudoseizures, possession states),
Social withdrawal, autism,
Compulsive acts, rituals or habits (e.g. nail biting),
Reaction time.

vi. *Social Manner and non-verbal behavior*

Increased, decreased, or inappropriate.
Eye contact (gaze aversion, staring vacantly, staring at the examiner, hesitant eye contact, or normal eye contact).

vii. *Rapport*

Whether a *working and empathic relationship* can be established with the patient, should be mentioned.

viii. *Hallucinatory Behavior*

Smiling or crying without reason, muttering or talking to self (non-social speech) and odd gesturing in response to auditory or visual hallucinations.

2. Speech

Speech can be examined under the following headings:

i. *Rate and Quantity of Speech*

Whether speech is present or absent (mutism),
If present, whether it is spontaneous,
Productivity is increased or decreased,
Rate is rapid or slow (its appropriateness),
Pressure of speech or poverty of speech.

ii. *Volume and Tone of Speech*

Increased/decreased (its appropriateness),
Low/high/normal pitch.

iii. *Flow and Rhythm of Speech*

Smooth/hesitant, Blocking (sudden),
Dysprosody, stuttering/stammering/clutte-ring, any accent,
Circumstantiality, tangentiality,
Verbigeration, stereotypies (verbal),
Flight of ideas, clang associations.

3. Mood and Affect

Mood is the pervasive feeling tone which is *sustained* (lasts for some length of time) and colors the total experience of the person. *Affect*, on the other hand, is the outward expression (objective) of the immediate (*cross-sectional)* experience of emotion at a given time.

The assessment of mood includes testing the *quality of mood,* which is assessed subjectively ('how do you feel') and objectively (by examination). The other components are *stability of mood* (over a period of time), *reactivity of mood* (variation in mood with stimuli), and *persistence of mood* (length of time the mood lasts).

The *affect* is similarly described under *quality of affect, range of affect* (of emotional changes displayed over time), *depth* or *intensity of affect* (normal, increased or blunted) and *appropriateness of affect* (in relation to thought and surrounding environment).

Mood is described as general warmth, euphoria (mild happiness), elation, exaltation and/or ecstasy (seen in severe mania) in *mania*; anxious and restless in *anxiety* and *depression;* sad, irritable, angry and/or despaired in *depression;* shallow, blunted, indifferent, restricted, inappropriate and/or labile in *schizophrenia.*

Anhedonia may occur in both *schizophrenia* and *depression.*

4. Thought

Normal thinking is a goal directed flow of ideas, symbols and associations initiated by a problem or a task, characterized by rational connections between successive ideas or thoughts, and leading towards a reality oriented conclusion. Therefore, thought process that is not goal-directed, or not logical, or does not lead to a realistic solution to the problem at hand, is not normal.

Traditionally, in the clinical examination, thought is assessed (by the content of speech) under the four headings of *stream, form, content* and *possession* of thought. However, since there is widespread disagreement regarding this subdivision, 'thought' is discussed here under the following two headings of '*stream and form*', and of '*content*':

i. *Stream and Form of Thought*

'Stream of thought' overlaps with examination of 'speech'. Spontaneity, productivity, flight of ideas, prolixity, poverty of content of speech, and thought block should be mentioned here.

Continuity of thought is assessed. Whether the thought processes are relevant to the questions asked. Any loosening of associations, tangentiality, circumstantiality, illogical thinking, perseveration, or verbigeration is noted.

ii. *Content of Thought*

Any preoccupations;
Obsessions (recurrent, irrational, intrusive, ego-dystonic, ego-alien ideas);
Contents of phobias (irrational fears);
Delusions (false, unshakeable beliefs) or over-valued ideas;
Explore for delusions / ideas of persecution, reference, grandeur, love, jealousy (infidelity), guilt, nihilism, poverty, somatic (hypochondriacal) symptoms, hopelessness, helplessness, worthlessness, and suicidal ideation.
Delusions of control, thought insertion, thought withdrawal, thought broadcasting are Schneiderian first rank symptoms (SFRS). The presence of neologisms should be recorded here.

5. Perception

Perception is the process of being aware of a sensory experience and being able to recognize it by comparing it with previous experiences.

Perception is assessed under the following headings:

i. *Hallucinations*

The presence of hallucinations should be noted. Whether hallucinations are auditory, visual, olfactory, gustatory or tactile should be asked.

Auditory hallucinations are commonest type of hallucinations in non-organic psychiatric disorders. Clarify whether they are elementary (only sounds are heard) or complex (voices heard). It should be further inquired what was heard, how many voices were heard, in which part of the day, male or female voices, how interpreted and whether second person or third person hallucinations (i.e., whether the voices were addressing the patient or were discussing him in third person); enquire about *command* (*imperative*) *hallucinations*.

Enquire whether the hallucinations occurred during wakefulness, or were they hypnagogic (occurring while going to sleep) and / or hypnopompic (occurring while getting up from sleep) hallucinations.

ii. *Illusions and Misinterpretations*

Whether visual, auditory, or in other sensory fields; whether occur in clear consciousness or not; whether any steps taken to check the reality of distorted perceptions.

iii. *Depersonalization/Derealization*

Depersonalization and derealization are abnormalities in the perception of a person's reality.

TABLE 2.3. CLINICAL RATING OF INSIGHT

Insight is rated on a 6-point scale from one to six.

1. Complete denial of illness.
2. Slight awareness of being sick and needing help, but denying it at the same time.
3. Awareness of being sick, but it is attributed to external or physical factors.
4. Awareness of being sick, due to something unknown in self.
5. *Intellectual Insight*: Awareness of being ill and that the symptoms/failures in social adjustment are due to own particular irrational feelings/thoughts; yet does not apply this knowledge to the current/future experiences.
6. *True Emotional Insight*: It is different from intellectual insight in that the awareness leads to significant basic changes in the future behavior and personality.

TABLE 2.4. SOME INVESTIGATIONS IN PSYCHIATRY

I. BIOLOGICAL INVESTIGATIONS

A. Medical Screen: Some of the following tests may be useful in screening for the medical disorders causing the psychiatric symptoms. The examples of indications are mentioned in front of the tests.

Hemoglobin: Routine screen.

Total and differential leucocyte counts (TLC, DLC): Routine screen, Treatment with antipsychotics (e.g. clozapine), lithium, carbamazepine.

Mean Corpuscular Volume (MCV): Alcohol dependence (increased).

Urinalysis: Routine screen. Drug screening.

Peripheral smear.

Renal function tests: Treatment with lithium.

Liver function tests: Treatment with carbamazepine, valproate, benzodiazepines. Alcohol dependence.

Serum electrolytes: Dehydration, SIADH, Treatment with carbamazepine, antipsychotics, lithium.

Blood glucose: Routine screen (age > 35 years).

Thyroid function tests: Refractory depression, rapid cycling mood disorder. Treatment with lithium, carbamazepine.

Electrocardiogram (EKG): Age > 35 years, Treatment with lithium, antidepressants, ECT, antipsychotics.

HIV testing: Intravenous drug users, suggestive sexual history, AIDS dementia.

VDRL: Suggestive sexual history.

X-ray Chest: Age > 35 years, Treatment with ECT.

X-ray Skull.

Serum CPK: Neuroleptic malignant syndrome (markedly increased levels).

B. Toxicology Screen

Useful when substance use is suspected, e.g. alcohol, cocaine, opiates, cannabis, phencyclidine, benzodiazepines, barbiturates.

C. Drug Levels

Drug levels are indicated to test for therapeutic blood levels, for toxic blood levels, and for testing drug compliance. Examples are lithium (0.6-1.6 meq/L), carbamazepine (6-12 mg/ml), valproate (50-100 mg/ml), haloperidol (8-18 ng/ml), tricyclic antidepressants (nortriptyline 50-150 ng/ml; imipramine 200-250 ng/ml), benzodiazepines, barbiturates.

D. Electrophysiological Tests

EEG (Electroencephalogram): Seizures, dementia, pseudoseizures vs. seizures, episodic abnormal behavior.

BEAM (Brain electrical activity mapping): Provides topographic imaging of EEG data.

Video-telemetry EEG.

Evoked potentials (e.g. p 300): Research tool.

Polysomnography/Sleep studies: Sleep disorders, seizures (occurring in sleep). The various components in sleep studies include EEG, EKG, EOG, EMG, airflow measurement, penile tumescence, oxygen saturation, body temperature, GSR (Galvanic skin response), and body movement.

Holter EKG: Panic disorder.

E. Brain Imaging Tests (Cranial)

Computed Tomography (CT) Scan: Dementia, delirium, seizures, first episode psychosis.

Magnetic Resonance Imaging (MRI) Scan: Dementia. Higher resolution than CT scan.

Positron Emission Tomography (PET) Scan: Research tool for study of brain function and physiology.

Single Photon Emission Computed Tomography (SPECT) Scan: Research tool.

Magnetic Resonance (MR) Angiography.

Magnetic Resonance (MR) Spectroscopy: Cerebral Angiography.

F. Neuro-Endocrine Tests

Dexamethasone Suppression Test (DST): Research tool in depression (response to antidepressants or ECT). If plasma cortisol is more than 5 mg/100ml following administration of dexamethasone (1 mg, given at 11 PM the night before and plasma cortisol taken at 4 PM and 11 PM the next day).

Contd...

TABLE 2.4. *Contd...*

TRH Stimulation Test: Lithium-induced hypothyroidism, refractory depression. If the serum TSH is more than 35 mIU/ml (following 500 mg of TRH given IV), the test is positive.

Serum Prolactin Levels: Seizures vs. pseudoseizures, galactorrhea with antipsychotics.

Serum 17-hydroxycorticosteroid: Organic mood (depression) disorder.

Serum Melatonin Levels: Seasonal mood disorders.

G. Biochemical Tests

5-HIAA: Research tool (depression, suicidal and/or aggressive behavior).

MHPG: Research tool (depression).

Platelet MAO: Research tool (depression).

Catecholamine levels: Organic anxiety disorder (e.g. pheochromocytoma).

H. Genetic Tests

Cytogenetic work-up is useful in some cases of mental retardation.

I. Sexual Disorder Investigations

Papaverine test: Male erectile disorder (intracavernosal injection of papaverine is sometimes used to differentiate organic from non-organic male erectile disorder).

Nocturnal penile tumescence: Male erectile disorder.

Serum testosterone: Sexual desire disorders, Male erectile disorder.

Penile Doppler: Male erectile disorder.

J. Miscellaneous Tests

Lactate provocation test: Panic disorders (In about 70% of patients with panic disorders, sodium lactate infusion can provoke a panic attack).

Drug assisted interview (Amytal interview): Useful in catatonia, unexplained mutism, and dissociative stupor. Discussed in Chapter 18.

CSF examination: Meningitis.

II. <u>PSYCHOLOGICAL INVESTIGATIONS</u>

A. Objective Tests

These are pen-and paper, objective tests, which are employed to test the various aspects of personality and intelligence in a person.

Objective personality tests: Some examples of objective personality tests are MMPI (Minnesota multiple personality inventory) and 16-PF (16 personality factors).

Intelligence tests: Some commonly used tests of intelligence are *WAIS* (*Wechsler adult intelligence scale*), *Stanford-Binet test* and *Bhatia's battery of intelligence tests.*

B. Projective Tests

In projective tests, ambiguous stimuli are used which are not clear to the person immediately. Some commonly used projective tests of personality are *Rorschach inkblot test, TAT* (Thematic apperception test), *DAPT* (Draw-a-person test), and *sentence completion test.*

C. Neuropsychological Tests

Some of the commonly used neuropsychological tests are *Wisconsin card sorting test*, *Wechsler memory scale*, *PGI memory scale*, *BG test* (Bender Gestalt test), *BVRT* (Benton visual retention test), *Luria-Nabraska neuropsychological test battery*, *Halstead-Reitan neuropsychological test battery*, and *PGI battery of brain dysfunction.*

D. Rating Scales

Several rating scales are used in Psychiatry to quantify the psychopathology observed. Some of the commonly used scales are *BPRS* (Brief psychiatric rating scale), *SANS* (Scale for assessment of negative symptoms), *SAPS* (Scale for assessment of positive symptoms), *HARS* (Hamilton's anxiety rating scale), *HDRS* (Hamilton's depression rating scale), and *YBOCS* (Yale Brown obsessive-compulsive scale).

E. Diagnostic Standardized Interviews

These instruments make the diagnostic assessment more standardized. These include *PSE* (Present state examination), *SCAN* (Schedules for Clinical Assessment in Neuropsychiatry), *SCID* (Structured Clinical Interview for DSM-IV), and *IPDE* (International Personality Disorder Examination), among many others.

iv. *Somatic Passivity Phenomenon*

Somatic passivity is the presence of strange sensations described by the patient as being imposed on the body by 'some external agency', with the patient being a passive recipient. It is one of the Schneider's first rank symptoms.

v. *Others*

Autoscopy, abnormal vestibular sensations, sense of presence should be noted here.

6. Cognition (Neuropsychiatric) Assessment

Cognitive or Higher mental functions are an important part of the MSE. Their significant disturbance commonly points to the presence of an organic psychiatric disorder.

i. *Consciousness*

The intensity of stimulation needed to arouse the patient should be indicated to demonstrate the level of alertness, e.g. by calling patient's name in a normal voice, calling in a loud voice, light touch on the arm, vigorous shaking of the arm, or painful stimulus.

Grade the level of consciousness; whether conscious/confusion/somnolence/clouding/delirium/stupor/coma. Any disturbance in the level of consciousness should ideally be rated on Glasgow Coma Scale, where a numeric value is given to the best response in each of the three categories (eye opening, verbal, motor).

ii. *Orientation*

Whether the patient is well oriented to *time* (test by asking the time, date, day, month, year, season, and the time spent in hospital), *place* (test by asking the present location, building, and city) and *person* (test by asking his own name, and can he identify people around him and their role in that setting). Disorientation in time usually precedes disorientation in place and person.

iii. *Attention*

Is the attention easily aroused and sustained; Ask the patient to repeat digits forwards and backwards (*digit span test; digit forward and backward test*), one at a time (e.g. patient may be able to repeat 5 digits forward and 3 digits backwards). Start with two digit numbers, increasing gradually up to eight digit numbers or till failure occurs on three consecutive occasions.

iv. *Concentration*

Can the patient concentrate; Is he easily distractible; Ask to subtract serial sevens from hundred (*100-7 test*), or serial threes from forty (*40-3 test*), or to count backwards from 20, or enumerate the names of the months (or days of the week) in the reverse order.

Note down the answers and the time taken to perform the tests.

v. *Memory*

a. *Immediate Retention and Recall (IR and R)*

Use the *digit span test* to assess the immediate memory; *digit forwards* and *digit backwards subtests* (also used for testing attention; are described under attention).

b. *Recent Memory*

Ask how did the patient come to the room/hospital; what he ate for dinner the day before or for breakfast the same morning.

Give an address to be memorized and ask it to be recalled 15 minutes later or at the end of the interview.

c. *Remote Memory*

Ask for the date and place of marriage, name and birthdays of children, any other relevant questions from the person's past.

Note any amnesia (anterograde/retrograde), or confabulation, if present.

vi. *Intelligence*

Intelligence is the ability to think logically, act rationally, and deal effectively with the environment.

Ask questions about general information, keeping in mind the patient's educational and social background, his experiences and interests, e.g. ask about the current and the past prime ministers and presidents of India, the capital of India, and the name of the various states.

Test for reading and writing. Give simple tests of calculation.

vii. *Abstract Thinking*

Abstract thinking is characterized by the ability to:

a. assume a mental set voluntarily,
b. shift voluntarily from one aspect of a situation to another,
c. keep in mind simultaneously the various aspects of a situation,
d. grasp the essentials of a 'whole' (e.g. situation or concept), and
e. to break a 'whole' into its parts.

Abstract thinking testing assesses patient's concept formation. The methods used are:

a. Proverb Testing: The meaning of simple proverbs (at least 3) should be asked.

b. Similarities (and also the differences) between familiar objects should be asked, like: table/chair; banana/orange; dog/lion; eye/ear.

The answers may be overly concrete or abstract. Appropriateness of answers is judged. Concretization of responses or inappropriate answers may occur in schizophrenia.

7. Insight

Insight is the degree of awareness and understanding that the patient has regarding his illness.

Ask the patient's attitude towards his present state; whether there is an illness or not; if yes, which kind of illness (physical, psychiatric or both); is any treatment needed; is there hope for recovery; what is the cause of illness. Depending on the patient's responses, grade the insight (Table 2.3).

8. Judgement

Judgement is the ability to assess a situation correctly and act appropriately with in that situation. Both social and test judgement are assessed.

i. *Social judgement* is observed during the hospital stay and during the interview session. It includes evaluation of personal judgement.
ii. *Test judgement* is assessed by asking the patient what he would do in certain test situations, like 'a house on fire', or 'a man lying on the road', or 'a sealed, stamped, addressed envelope lying on a street'.

Judgement is rated as Good/Intact/Normal or Poor/Impaired/Abnormal.

INVESTIGATIONS

After a detailed history and examination, *investigations* (laboratory tests, diagnostic standardized interviews, family interviews, and/or psychological tests) are carried out based on the diagnostic and etiological possibilities. Some of these investigations are discussed in Table 2.4.

FORMULATION

After complete psychiatric assessment, a *diagnostic formulation* summarizes the detailed positive (and important negative) information regarding the patient under the focus of care, before listing a *differential diagnosis, prognostic factors,* and a *management plan*.

Thus, psychiatric assessment is an initial step towards diagnosis and management of psychiatric disorders.

SPECIAL INTERVIEWS

There are different formats available for detailed evaluation of special populations, e.g. uncooperative patients, hostile and aggressive patients (Chapter 19), suicidal patients (Chapter 19), and children. These formats should be used whenever appropriate.

3

Organic (Including Symptomatic) Mental Disorders

It is assumed that all psychological and behavioral processes, whether normal or abnormal, are a result of normal or deranged brain function. A rational corollary would be that all psychiatric disorders are due to abnormal brain functioning, i.e. are organic. But, this would be a gross oversimplification.

According to our present knowledge, there are three types of psychiatric disorders:

1. Those due to a known organic cause.
2. Those in whose causation an organic factor has not yet been found or proven.
3. Those that are primarily due to psychosocial factors.

Only the disorders of first type are called *organic mental disorders*. Thus, organic mental disorders are behavioral or psychological disorders associated with transient or permanent brain dysfunction and include only those mental and behavioral disorders that are due to *demonstrable* cerebral disease or disorder, either *primary* (primary brain pathology) or *secondary* (brain dysfunction due to systemic diseases).

The use of term '*organic*' here does not imply that other psychiatric disorders are 'non-organic' in the sense of having no biological basis. It simply means that the organic mental disorders have a *demonstrable* and *independently diagnosable* cerebral disease or disorder.

Since organic brain illness can mimic any psychiatric disorder, especially in the initial stages, *organic mental disorder should be the first consideration in evaluating a patient with any psychological or behavioral clinical syndrome.*

Presence of the following features requires a high index of suspicion for the presence of '*organicity*' (organic mental disorder):

1. First episode.
2. Sudden onset.
3. Older age of onset.
4. History of drug or alcohol use disorder.
5. Concurrent medical or neurological illness.
6. Neurological symptoms or signs, like seizures, impairment of consciousness, head injury, sensory or motor disturbance.
7. Presence of confusion, disorientation, memory impairment or soft neurological signs.
8. Prominent visual or other non-auditory hallucinations.

These disorders can be subcategorized into the following categories:

1. Delirium,
2. Dementia,
3. Organic amnestic syndrome, and
4. Other organic mental disorders.

DELIRIUM

Delirium is the commonest organic disorder seen in clinical practice. 5-15% of all patients in medical and surgical inpatient units are estimated to develop delirium. This percentage is higher in the post-operative patients.

Delirium is the most appropriate substitute for a variety of names used in the past like acute confusional states, acute brain syndrome, acute organic reaction, toxic psychosis, metabolic (and other acute) encephalopathies and the like.

Clinical Features

Delirium is characterized by the following features: a relatively acute onset; clouding of consciousness (characterized by a decreased awareness of surroundings and a decreased ability to respond to environmental stimuli); and disorientation (most commonly in time, then in place and rarely in person), associated with a decreased attention span and distractibility. Marked perceptual disturbances (most commonly visual, although other types also occur) like illusions, misinterpretations, and hallucinations also occur.

There is a disturbance of the sleep-wake cycle, most commonly insomnia at night with daytime drowsiness. Diurnal variation is marked, usually worsening of symptoms in evening and night (called *sun downing*). There is an impairment of registration and retention of new memories. Psychomotor disturbance (usually in form of agitation and occasionally retardation) is present. Autonomic dysfunction is generalized. Speech and thought disturbances like slurring of speech, incoherence, dysarthria, and fleeting delusions are present.

Motor symptoms include asterixis (flapping tremor), multifocal myoclonus, *carphologia/floccillation* (picking movements at coversheets/clothes), and *occupational delirium* (elaborate pantomimes as if continuing the usual occupation in a hospital bed), tone and reflex abnormalities. Lability of affect is usually present. Motor and verbal perseveration, dysnomia, agraphia and impaired comprehension are also seen.

Diagnosis

The diagnosis of delirium is often missed, as the possibility is often overlooked in the medical/surgical setting. It is important to recognize delirium at the earliest possible, as delirium often has an underlying etiology which may be correctable. Any delay in diagnosis, and thus starting treatment, may lead to permanent deficits which are irreversible.

The diagnosis of delirium is mainly clinical. No ancillary laboratory test is diagnostic, although it may help in finding the etiology.

According to the ICD-10 (CDDG), for a definite diagnosis of delirium, symptoms, mild or severe, should be present in each one of the following areas:

1. Impairment of consciousness and attention (on a continuum from clouding to coma; reduced ability to direct, focus, sustain, and shift attention);
2. Global disturbance of cognition (perceptual distortions, illusions and hallucinations - most often visual; impairment of abstract thinking and comprehension, with or without transient delusions, but typically with some degree of incoherence; impairment of immediate recall and of recent memory but with relatively intact remote memory; disorientation for time as well as, in more severe cases, for place and person);
3. Psychomotor disturbances (hypo- or hyperactivity and unpredictable shifts from one to the other; increased reaction time; increased or decreased flow of speech; enhanced startle reaction);
4. Disturbance of sleep-wake cycle (insomnia or, in severe cases total sleep loss or

TABLE 3.1. DELIRIUM: IMPORTANT CAUSES

A. Metabolic causes
- i. Hypoxia, carbon dioxide narcosis.
- ii. Hypoglycemia.
- iii. Hepatic encephalopathy, uremic encephalopathy.
- iv. Cardiac failure, cardiac arrhythmias, cardiac arrest.
- v. Water and electrolyte imbalance (water, Na^+, K^+, Mg^{++}, Ca^{++}).
- vi. Metabolic acidosis or alkalosis.
- vii. Fever, anemia, hypovolemic shock.
- viii. Carcinoid syndrome, porphyria.

B. Endocrine causes
- i. Hypo- and hyper-pituitarism.
- ii. Hypo- and hyper-thyroidism.
- iii. Hypo- and hyper-parathyroidism.
- iv. Hypo- and hyper-adrenalism.

C. Drugs (both ingestion and withdrawal can cause delirium) and poisons
- i. Digitalis, quinidine, antihypertensi-ves.
- ii. Alcohol, sedatives, hypnotics (especially barbiturates).
- iii. Tricyclic antidepressants, antipsy-chotics, anticholinergics, disulfiram.
- iv. Anticonvulsants, L-dopa, opiates.
- v. Salicylates, steroids, penicillin, insulin.
- vi. Methyl alcohol, heavy metals, biocides.

D. Nutritional deficiencies
- i. Thiamin, niacin, pyridoxine, folic acid, B_{12}.
- ii. Proteins.

E. Systemic infections
- i. Acute and chronic, e.g. septicemia, pneumonia, endocarditis.

F. Intracranial causes
- i. Epilepsy (including post-ictal states).
- ii. Head injury, subarachnoid hemorrhage, subdural hematoma.
- iii. Intracranial infections, e.g. meningitis, encephalitis, cerebral malaria.
- iv. Migraine.
- v. Stroke (acute phase), hypertensive encephalopathy.
- vi. Focal lesions, e.g. right parietal lesions (like abscess, neoplasm).

G. Miscellaneous
- i. Postoperative states (including ICU delirium).
- ii. Sleep deprivation.
- iii. Heat, electricity, radiation.

TABLE 3.2. PREDISPOSING FACTORS IN DELIRIUM

1. Pre-existing brain damage or dementia.
2. Extremes of age (very old and very young).
3. Previous history of delirium.
4. Alcohol or drug dependence.
5. Generalized or focal cerebral lesion.
6. Chronic medical illness.
7. Surgical procedure and post-operative period.
8. Severe psychological symptoms, like fear.
9. Treatment with psychotropic medicines.
10. History of head injury.
11. Individual susceptibility to delirium.

reversal of the sleep-wake cycle; daytime drowsiness; nocturnal worsening of symptoms; disturbing dreams or nightmares, which may continue as hallucinations after awakening);

5. Emotional disturbances, e.g. depression, anxiety or fear, irritability, euphoria, apathy, or wondering perplexity.

The onset is usually rapid, the course diurnally fluctuating, and the total duration of the condition less than 6 months. The above clinical picture is so characteristic that a fairly confident diagnosis of delirium can be made even if the underlying cause is not clearly established. History of an underlying physical or brain disease, and/or evidence of cerebral dysfunction (e.g. an abnormal EEG, usually but not always, showing slowing of the background activity) help in the diagnosis.

TABLE 3.3. DELIRIUM AND DEMENTIA

Features	Delirium	Dementia
1. Onset	Usually acute	Usually insidious
2. Course	Usually recover in 1 week May take upto 1 month	Usually protracted, Although may be reversible
3. Clinical features		
i. Consciousness	Clouded	Usually normal
ii. Orientation	Grossly disturbed	Usually normal Disturbed only in late stages
iii. Memory	Immediate retention and recall disturbed Recent memory disturbed	Immediate retention and recall normal Recent memory disturbed Remote memory disturbed only in late stages.
iv. Comprehension	Impaired	Impaired only in late stages
v. Sleep-wake cycle	Grossly disturbed	Usually normal
vi. Attention and Concentration	Grossly disturbed	Usually normal
vii. Diurnal variation	Marked. Sundowning present	Usually absent
viii. Perception	Visual illusions and hallucinations very common	Hallucinations may occur
ix. Other features	Asterixis, Multifocal myoclonus	Catastrophic reaction Perseveration

Predisposing Factors

The presence of certain predisposing factors lower the threshold for the development of delirium (Table 3.2).

Etiology

The list of possible causes of delirium is virtually endless. Any factor which disturbs the metabolism of brain sufficiently can cause delirium.

The causation of delirium demonstrates a *threshold phenomenon*, with a combination of factors adding up to cross a threshold for causing delirium, which is different for each individual.

One of the important causes of delirium, namely post-cardiac surgery delirium, is discussed in Chapter 12. The most important causes are listed in Table 3.1.

Management

1. In cases, where a cause is not obvious (or other contributory causes are suspected), the following investigations should be done, e.g. CBC, urinalysis, blood glucose, blood urea, serum electrolytes, liver and renal function tests, arterial pO_2 and pCO_2, thyroid function tests, serum B_{12} and folate levels, X-ray chest, EKG, CSF examination, urine for porphyrins, drug screens, VDRL, HIV testing, EEG, and cranial CT scan or MRI scan.
2. Identification of cause and its immediate correction, e.g. 50 mg. of 50% dextrose IV for hypoglycemia, O_2 for hypoxia, 100 mg of B_1 IV for thiamin deficiency, IV fluids for fluid and electrolyte imbalance.
3. *Symptomatic measures:* as many patients are agitated, emergency psychiatric treatment may be needed.

Benzodiazepines (10 mg diazepam or 2 mg lorazepam IV) or antipsychotics (5 mg haloperidol or 50 mg chlorpromazine IM) may be given.

Maintenance treatment is with oral haloperidol or lorazepam, till recovery occurs (usually within a week's time).

4. Supportive medical and nursing care.

DEMENTIA

Dementia is a chronic organic mental disorder characterized by the following features: impairment of *intellectual functions,* impairment of *memory* (predominantly of recent memory, especially in early stages), deterioration of *personality* with lack of personal care. Impairment of all functions occurs globally, causing interference with day-to-day activities and interpersonal relationships. There is impairment of judgement and impulse control, and impairment of abstract thinking. There is no impairment of consciousness. The course of dementia can be progressive, stationary or reversible.

Additional features may also be present. These include:

1. Emotional *lability* (marked variation in emotional expression).
2. *Catastrophic reaction* (when confronted with an assignment which is beyond the residual intellectual capacity, patient may go into a sudden rage).
3. Thought abnormalities, e.g. delusions, perseveration.
4. Urinary and fecal incontinence may develop in late stages.
5. Disorientation in time; disorientation in place and person may also develop in late stages.
6. Neurological signs may or may not be present depending on the underlying cause.

TABLE 3.4. DEMENTIA VS. PSEUDODEMENTIA

Dementia	Pseudodementia (Depressive)
1. Patient rarely complains of the cognitive impairment	Patient usually always complains about the impairment
2. Patient emphasizes achievements	Patient emphasizes disability
3. Patient appears unconcerned	Patient communicates distress
4. Usually labile affect	Severe depression
5. Patient makes mistakes on examination	'Don't know' answers are frequent
6. Recent memory impairment found on examination	Recent memory rarely found on examination
7. Confabulation may be present	Confabulation very rare
8. Consistently poor performance on similar tests	Marked variability in performance on similar tests
9. History of depression uncommon	Past history of manic/depressive episodes may be present

Diagnosis

Like delirium, the diagnosis of dementia is clinical. Although ancillary laboratory investigations may help in elucidating the etiology, they do not help in diagnosing dementia per se.

According to the ICD-10 (CDDG), the following features are required for the diagnosis:

1. Evidence of decline in both memory and thinking, sufficient enough to impair personal activities of daily living.
2. Memory impairment typically affects the registration, storage, and retrieval of new information (recent memory), but previously learned material (remote memory) may also be lost, particularly in later stages.

3. Thinking is impaired, the flow of ideas is reduced, and the reasoning capacity is also impaired.
4. Presence of clear consciousness (Consciousness can be impaired if delirium is also present).
5. Duration of at least 6 months.

The following conditions must be kept in mind in the *differential diagnosis* of dementia.

1. *Normal aging process:* Although impairment of memory and intellect are common in old, they do not justify a diagnosis of dementia. Dementia is diagnosed only when there is demonstrable evidence of memory and other intellectual function impairment which is of sufficient severity to interfere with social or occupational functioning. The normal memory impairment in old age is called as *benign senescent forgetfulness.*
2. *Delirium* (Table 3.3): Syndromes of delirium and dementia may overlap.
3. *Depressive pseudodementia:* Depression in elderly patients may present as dementia clinically. It is called *depressive pseudodementia* (Table 3.4). The identification of depression is very important as it is far more easily treatable than dementia. Depressive patients them-selves complain of memory impairment, difficulty in sustaining attention and concentration and reduced intellectual capacity.

   In contrast, a patient of dementia does not complain of these disturbances. In fact when confronted with the evidence of memory impairment, he often confabulates.

   As depression may often be superimposed on dementia, it is at times necessary to give a therapeutic trial with antidepressants.

It is useful to differentiate dementia in to cortical and subcortical subtypes (Table 3.6).

TABLE 3.5. SOME IMPORTANT CAUSES OF DEMENTIA

A. Parenchymatous brain disease
Alzheimer's disease, Pick's disease, Parkinson's disease, Huntington's chorea, Steel Richardson syndrome (progressive supranuclear palsy)

B. Vascular dementia
Multi-Infarct dementia, sub-cortical vascular dementia (Binswanger's disease)

C. Toxic dementias
Bromide intoxication, drugs, heavy metals, alcohol, carbon monoxide, analgesics, anticonvulsants, benzodiazepines, psychotropic drugs

D. Metabolic dementias
Chronic hepatic or uremic encephalo-pathy, dialysis dementia, Wilson's disease

E. Endocrine causes
Thyroid, parathyroid, pituitary, adrenal dysfunction

F. Deficiency dementias
Pernicious anemia, pellagra, folic acid deficiency, thiamine deficiency

G. Dementias due to infections
Creutzfeldt-Jacob disease, neurosyphilis, chronic meningitis, viral encephalitis, AIDS dementia, other HIV-related disorders, subacute sclerosing panencephalitis

H. Neoplastic dementias
Neoplasms and other intracranial space-occupying lesions

I. Traumatic dementias
Chronic subdural hematoma, head injury

J. Hydrocephalic dementia
Normal pressure hydrocephalus

Etiology

The number of conditions which can cause dementia is large (Table 3.5). But a majority of cases are due to a few common causes, namely Alzheimer's disease, multi-infarct dementia, and hypothyroidism.

TABLE 3.6. CORTICAL AND SUBCORTICAL DEMENTIA

Features	Cortical Dementia	Subcortical Dementia
1. Site of lesion	Cortex (Frontal and temporo-parieto-occipital association areas, and hippocampus)	Subcortical grey matter (Thalamus, basal ganglia, and rostral brain stem)
2. Examples	Alzheimer's disease Pick's disease	Huntington' chorea Parkinson's disease Progressive supranuclear palsy, Wilson's disease
3. Severity	Severe	Mild to moderate
4. Motor system	Usually normal	Dysarthria, flexed/extended posture, tremors, dystonia, chorea, ataxia, rigidity
5. Other features	Simple delusions; Depression uncommon Severe aphasia, amnesia, agnosia, apraxia, acalculia; slowed cognitive speed (*bradyphrenia*)	Complex delusions; Depression common; Rarely mania
6. Memory deficit (Short term)	Recall helped very little by cues	Recall partially helped by cues and recognition tasks

Four clinically important types of dementia are briefly discussed here.

1. Alzheimer's Dementia (Dementia of Alzheimer's Type- DAT)

This is the commonest cause of dementia, seen in about 70% of all cases of dementia in USA. It is more commonly seen in women. Earlier it was differentiated into two forms: a presenile form and a senile form. Now it is known that these two forms represent the same disease clinically and pathologically. There is some evidence to suggest that Alzheimer's disease may have a genetic basis.

The diagnosis of DAT is by exclusion of all other causes of dementia, as there are no distinct diagnostic clinical features or laboratory investigations.

Autopsy shows enlarged cerebral ventricles, widened cerebral sulci and shrinkage of cerebral cortex (macroscopically); and senile plaques, neurofibrillary tangles, cortical nerve cell loss and granulovacuolar degeneration (microscopically). These changes are only quantitatively (not qualitatively) different from normal aged brain. Neurochemically, there is a marked decrease in brain choline acetyl-transferase (CAT) with a similar decrease in brain acetyl cholinesterase (AchE).

At present, DAT is not a treatable disorder. However, recently new drugs like rivastigmine ,donepezil, galantamine and tacrine have been introduced. These elevate Ach (acetylcholine) concentration in the cerebral cortex by slowing the degradation of Ach released by still intact cholinergic neurons in Alzheimer's disease. Both rivastigmine (1.5 mg twice a day to 6 mg twice a day) and donepezil (5-10 mg/day) are available in the Indian market.

2. Multi-Infarct Dementia (MID)

MID is the second commonest cause of dementia, seen in 10-15% of all cases, though some studies indicate that MID is probably far more common in India . It is also one of the important treatable causes of dementia.

Multiple cerebral infarction can lead to progressive disruption of brain function, finally leading to dementia. The most typical form is characterized by an abrupt onset, acute exacerbations (due to repeated infarctions), stepwise deterioration (*step-ladder pattern*), a fluctuating course, presence of hypertension (most commonly) or any other significant cardio-vascular disease, and history of previous stroke or transient ischemic attacks (TIAs).

Focal neurological signs are common. Insight into the illness, is usually present and emotional lability is very common. EEG (showing focal area of slowing) and CT Brain (showing multiple infarcts) help in diagnosis.

The treatment of the underlying cause (usually hypertension) can prevent further deterioration.

3. Hypothyroid Dementia

This is one of the most important treatable and reversible causes of dementia, second only to toxic dementias. Although it accounts for less than 1% of dementias, hypothyroidism should be suspected in every patient of dementia.

Since clinical diagnosis may be difficult, laboratory tests have to be resorted to for correct diagnosis. Prompt treatment can reverse the dementing process and can lead to complete recovery if the treatment is started within two years of the onset of dementia.

4. AIDS Dementia Complex

About 50-70% of patients suffering from AIDS exhibit a triad of cognitive, behavioral and motoric deficits of *subcortical dementia* type, known as the AIDS-Dementia complex (ADC). Dementia can be an initial presentation in about 25% cases of AIDS.

As the AIDS virus (a lenti-virus, a type of retro-virus) is highly neurotropic and the virus crosses the blood-brain barrier early in the course of the disease, cognitive impairment is nearly ubiquitous in AIDS.

The diagnosis is established by ELISA (enzyme-linked immuno-sorbent assay) showing anti-HIV antibodies, and Western Blot test (blotting of antibody specificities to HIV-specific proteins). Cranial CT scan shows cortical atrophy 1-4 months before the onset of clinical dementia while MRI scan detects the white matter lesions.

Management

1. Basic Investigations

CBC, urinalysis, blood glucose, serum electrolytes, renal function tests, thyroid function tests, serum B_{12} and folate levels, serological tests for syphilis, arterial pO_2 and pCO_2, X-ray chest, EKG, X-ray skull, EEG, lumbar puncture, CT scan / MRI scan of brain, psychological tests, and drug screens. Diagnostic tests are of great importance in finding the cause, or to exclude all other causes before diagnosing dementia of Alzheimer's type (DAT).

2. Treatment of the underlying cause, if treatable

For example, the management of hypertension in multi-infarct dementia, thyroid replacement in hypothyroid dementia, shunting in hydrocephalic dementia, levodopa in parkinsonism, and removal of the toxic agent in toxic dementia.

3. Symptomatic Management

i. Environmental manipulation to reduce stress in day-to-day activities.
ii. Treatment of medical complications.

iii. Care of food and hygiene; and supportive care for the patient and family.
iv. Anxiety can be treated with short acting benzodiazepines (lorazepam and oxazepam) in low doses.
v. Depression can be treated with low doses of citalopram, sertraline or tianeptine (as these agents have low anticholinergic activity and low cardiac toxicity. Agents with high anticholinergic activity can cause confusion or frank delirium).
vi. Psychotic symptoms and disruptive behaviors can be treated with low doses of antipsychotics. Haloperidol and risperidone are preferred as they are less sedative and have low cardiac toxicity. However, if sleep induction is also needed, olanzapine and chlorpromazine can be used in low doses.
vii. Short term hospitalization.
viii. Institutionalization may be necessary in late stages.
ix. Specific drug treatment, e.g. donepezil or rivastigmine in Alzheimer's disease.

ORGANIC AMNESTIC SYNDROME

Organic amnestic syndrome is characterized by the following clinical features: impairment of memory due to an underlying organic cause, no disturbance of consciousness and attention (unlike delirium), and no disturbance of global intellectual function, abstract thinking, or personality (unlike dementia).

The *impairment of memory* is characterized by a severe impairment of recent memory or short-term memory (inability to learn new material). This is associated with impaired remote memory or long-term memory (inability to recall previously learnt material). There is no impairment of immediate memory (i.e. immediate retention and recall).

As recent memory is more severely disturbed, very remote events are better remembered, especially in the initial stages. Recent memory impairment also leads to disorientation in time and place. To fill in the memory gaps, patient uses imaginary events in the early phase of illness (*confabulation*). With the progression of the disease, confabulation disappears.

Diagnosis

According to the ICD-10 (CDDG), the following features are required for the diagnosis:

1. Recent memory impairment; anterograde and retrograde amnesia.
2. No impairment of immediate retention and recall, attention, consciousness, and global intellectual functioning.
3. Historical or objective evidence of brain disease or injury (especially with bilateral involvement of diencephalic and medial temporal structures).

Differential Diagnosis

Amnestic syndrome should be differentiated from delirium, dementia, non-organic mental disorders and transient global amnesia. Differentiation from the first three is relatively easy on the basis of pattern of memory loss.

Transient global amnesia

A rare disorder with an abrupt onset, it resembles the amnestic syndrome closely. Differentiation is made on the basis of abrupt onset and patient's severe distress because of loss of memory in transient global amnesia. This syndrome is probably caused by temporary cerebral ischemia in the distribution of posterior cerebral circulation.

Etiology

1. *Thiamin deficiency:* The most common cause is chronic alcoholism (alcohol dependence). It is also called as *Wernicke-Korsakoff syndrome*. Wernicke's encephalopathy is the acute phase of delirium preceding the

amnestic syndrome, while Korsakoff's syndrome is the chronic phase of amnestic syndrome.

2. *Any other lesion involving bilaterally the inner core of limbic system* (i.e. mammillary bodies, fornix, hippocampus and para-hippocampal structures of medial temporal lobe, posterior hypothalamus and dorso-medial thalamic nuclei), like
   i. Head trauma.
   ii. Surgical procedure (bilateral temporal lobectomy).
   iii. Hypoxia.
   iv. Posterior cerebral artery stroke (bilateral).
   v. Herpes simplex encephalitis.
   vi. Space occupying lesions in the region of III ventricle (e.g. neoplasms).

Management

1. Treatment of the underlying cause, e.g. thiamin (high doses) in Wernicke-Korsakoff syndrome. But, usually the treatment is of not much use. The prognosis is often poor.
2. Supportive care for general condition and the associated medical illness.

OTHER ORGANIC MENTAL DISORDERS (DUE TO BRAIN DAMAGE AND DYSFUNCTION, AND TO PHYSICAL DISEASES)

This group includes miscellaneous mental disorders which are causally related to brain dysfunction due to primary cerebral disease, systemic disease (secondary), or toxic substances.

According to the ICD-10 (CDDG), the following features are required for the diagnosis:

1. Evidence of cerebral disease, damage or dysfunction, or of systemic physical disease, known to be associated with one of the listed syndromes;
2. A temporal relationship (weeks or a few months) between the development of the underlying disease and the onset of the mental syndrome;
3. Recovery from the mental disorder following removal or improvement of the underlying presumed cause;
4. Absence of evidence to suggest an alternative cause of the mental syndrome (such as a strong family history or precipitating stress).

If conditions 1 and 2 are present, a provisional diagnosis can be made; if all four are present, the certainty of diagnostic classification is significantly increased.

The following conditions are known to be associated with an increased risk for these other organic mental disorders:

1. *Primary cerebral diseases*

Epilepsy, limbic encephalitis, Huntington's disease, head trauma, brain neoplasms, vascular cerebral disease, cerebral malformations.

2. *Systemic diseases*

Extracranial neoplasms (e.g. carcinoma pancreas), collagen diseases (e.g. systemic lupus erythematosis), endocrine disease (e.g. hypothyroidism, hyperthyroidism, Cushing's disease), metabolic disorders (e.g. hypoglycemia, porphyria, hypoxia); infectious diseases (e.g. trypanosomiasis).

3. *Drugs*

Steroids, propranolol, levodopa, methyldopa, antihypertensives, anti-malarials, alcohol and psychoactive substances.

ORGANIC HALLUCINOSIS

According to the ICD-10 (CDDG), the following features are required for the diagnosis of organic hallucinosis, in addition to the general guidelines for the diagnosis of other organic mental disorders, described earlier:

1. Persistent or recurrent hallucinations due to an underlying organic cause. The hallucinations can occur in any sensory modality but are usually *visual* (most common) or auditory in nature. In many cases, they depend on the underlying cause. These *hallucinations* can range from very simple and unformed, to very complex and well-organized.
   Usually the patients realize that the hallucinations are not real but sometimes there may be a delusional elaboration of hallucinations.
2. No major disturbance of consciousness, intelligence, memory, mood or thought.

Etiology

1. *Drugs*: Hallucinogens (LSD, psilocybin, mescaline), cocaine, cannabis, phencyclidine (PCP), levodopa, bromocriptine, amantadine, ephedrine, propranolol, pentazocine, methylphenidate, imipramine, anticholinergics, bromide.
2. *Alcohol (alcoholic hallucinosis):* Here auditory hallucinations are more common.
3. *Sensory deprivation.*
4. *'Release' hallucinations* due to sensory pathway disease, e.g. bilateral cataracts, otosclerosis, optic neuritis.
5. *Migraine.*
6. *Epilepsy:* Complex partial seizures.
7. *Intracranial space occupying lesions.*
8. *Temporal arteritis.*
9. *Brain stem lesions* (peduncular hallucinosis).

Management

1. Treatment of the underlying cause, if treatable.
2. Symptomatic treatment with antipsychotics (e.g. haloperidol, risperidone) may be needed.

ORGANIC CATATONIC DISORDER

According to the ICD-10 (CDDG), the following features are required for the diagnosis of organic catatonic disorder, in addition to the general guidelines for the diagnosis of other organic mental disorders, described earlier:

1. *Stupor* (diminution or complete absence of spontaneous movement with partial or complete mutism, negativism, and rigid posturing);
2. *Excitement* (gross hypermotility with or without a tendency to assaultiveness);
3. *Mixed* (shifting rapidly and unpredictably from hypo- to hyper-activity).

The presence of other catatonic phenomena increases the confidence in the diagnosis. The catatonic symptoms and signs are described in detail in Chapter 5.

Etiology

The etiology and management of organic catatonic disorder is described in detail in Chapter 19.

Management

1. Treatment of the underlying cause, if amenable to treatment.
2. Symptomatic treatment with antipsychotics (e.g. risperidone, haloperidol) and electroconvulsive therapy (if needed).

ORGANIC DELUSIONAL (SCHIZOPHRENIA-LIKE) DISORDER

According to the ICD-10 (CDDG), the following features are required for the diagnosis of organic delusional disorder, in addition to the general guidelines for the diagnosis of other organic mental disorders, described earlier:

1. Predominant delusions which are persistent or recurrent, caused by an underlying organic cause.
2. No major disturbance of consciousness, orientation, memory or mood.

The *delusions* are variable and their type depends on the underlying etiology. The most common delusions are *persecutory* in nature. Hallucinations (*visual* more common than auditory) may accompany the delusions. Schneider's first rank symptoms (SFRS) are not usually seen in organic delusional disorder, in contrast to schizophrenia.

Diagnosis

Organic delusional disorder secondary to amphetamine use may be difficult to differentiate from paranoid schizophrenia. The differentiating points are an acute onset, history of amphetamine use prior to the onset, predominant visual hallucinations which may be fleeting, absence of formal thought disorder and a more "appropriate" affect.

Etiology

1. *Drugs:* Amphetamines, hallucinogens, cannabis, clonazepam, disulfiram, propranolol.
2. *Complex partial seizures* (temporal lobe epilepsy).
3. *Huntington's chorea* (initial stages), *Parkinson's disease, Wilson's disease,* and *ideopathic basal ganglia calcification.*
4. *Right parietal lobe lesions,* especially vascular lesions.
5. Lesions involving limbic system (e.g. tumors).
6. *Spinocerebellar degeneration.*
7. *Cerebral malaria.*
8. *Herpes simplex encephalitis.*
9. *Nutritional deficiencies* (Vitamin B_{12}, iron)
10. *Demyelinating disorders* (e.g. multiple sclerosis, metachromatic leucodystrophy)

Management

1. Treatment of the underlying cause, e.g. removal of toxic agent in amphetamine psychosis.
2. Symptomatic management with antipsychotics (e.g. risperidone, haloperidol) may be needed.

ORGANIC MOOD (AFFECTIVE) DISORDER

According to the ICD-10 (CDDG)*, the following features are required for the diagnosis of organic mood disorder, in addition to the general guidelines for the diagnosis of other organic mental disorders, described earlier:

1. Prominent and persistent mood disturbance, caused by an underlying organic cause.
2. No major disturbance of consciousness, orientation, or memory.

The *mood disturbance* can be a major depressive episode, a manic episode, or a mixed affective disorder. The severity may vary from mild to severe.

Etiology

Some of the causes of organic mood disorder are listed below:

1. *Drugs:* Any drug a depressed person is taking should be considered a potential factor in the causation of depression.
   Mania: INH, levodopa, bromide, LSD, corticosteroids (hypomania), hallucinogens, tricyclic antidepressants, cocaine, baclofen, amphetamines, bromocriptine, cimetidine, procyclidine.
   Depression: Reserpine, ethanol, clonidine, methyldopa, propranolol, corticosteroids, antipsychotics, cimetidine, anticancer chemotherapy, oral contraceptives.
2. *Endocrine disorders:*
   Mania: Hyperthyroidism.
   Depression: Hypothyroidism, Cushing's syndrome, Addison's disease, hyper- and hypo- parathyroidism .
3. *CNS disorders:* Parkinsonism, Huntington's chorea, PSP (progressive supranuclear

TABLE 3.4. ORGANIC PERSONALITY DISORDERS

Organic Personality Disorder	Clinical Features
1. Frontal Lobe Syndrome (Types)	
a. Orbito-frontal syndrome *(Pseudo-psychopathic)*	Disinhibition, jocularity, impulsivity, impaired insight and judgement
b. Frontal convexity type *(Pseudo-depressive)*	Apathy, lack of initiative, retardation, perseveration
c. Medial frontal syndrome *(Akinetic)*	Akinesis, incontinence, poor verbal output
2. Temporal Lobe Syndrome	Egocentricity, explosive affect, perseveration, excessive religiosity, obsessional traits
3. Bilateral temporal lobe or limbic system lesions	Emotional placcidity, hyper-orality, altered sexual behavior, excessive exploration of environment (*hyper-metamorphosis*).

palsy; depression more likely), CVAs (cerebro-vascular accidents; left sided anterior lesions and right sided posterior lesions cause depression in stroke), cerebral tumors, epilepsy (complex partial), neurosyphilis (GPI), head injury (mania more likely), multiple sclerosis.
4. *Post-viral illnesses:* Influenza, infectious mononucleosis, viral pneumonia, infectious hepatitis.
5. *Deficiencies*: Pellagra, deficiency of thiamine, folate, niacin, folate, B_{12}.
6. *Others:* Carcinoma pancreas (depression), systemic lupus erythematosis (SLE), pernicious anemia, temporal arteritis (depression), carcinoid syndrome (mania).

Management

1. Management of the underlying organic cause, if treatable.
2. Symptomatic management, if the episodes are severe. For example, for a *manic episode*, low dose antipsychotics (e.g. risperidone, haloperidol) and/or lithium; and for a *depressive episode*, low dose antidepressants (e.g. sertraline) and/or electroconvulsive therapy.

ORGANIC ANXIETY DISORDER

According to the ICD-10 (CDDG), the following features are required for the diagnosis of organic anxiety disorder, in addition to the general guidelines for the diagnosis of other organic mental disorders, described earlier:

1. Prominent and persistent generalized anxiety, or prominent and recurrent panic attacks caused by an underlying organic cause.
2. No major disturbance of consciousness, orientation, memory, personality, thought, perception, or mood.

Etiology

1. *Drugs and toxins:* Cocaine, caffeine, amphetamines and other sympathomimetics, alcohol and drug withdrawal, heavy metals, penicillin.
2. *Endocrine disorders:* Thyroid, pituitary, parathyroid, or adrenal dysfunction; pheochromocytoma; fasting hypoglycemia, carcinoid syndrome.
3. *Systemic diseases:* Cardiac arrhythmias, mitral valve prolapse syndrome, chronic obstructive pulmonary disease, coronary artery disease, pulmonary embolism, anemia, fever, deficiency diseases.
4. *CNS diseases:* Cerebral tumors, epilepsy (especially complex partial seizures of temporal lobe origin), cerebrovascular disease, postconcussional syndrome.

Management

1. Treatment of the underlying organic cause, if treatable.

2. Symptomatic treatment with benzodiazepines, β-blockers (propranolol), behavior therapy, relaxation techniques and psychotherapy may be needed.

ORGANIC PERSONALITY DISORDER (PERSONALITY AND BEHAVIORAL DISORDERS DUE TO BRAIN DISEASE, DAMAGE, AND DYSFUNCTION)

The organic personality disorder is characterized by significant alteration of the premorbid personality caused by an underlying organic cause without major disturbance of consciousness, orientation, memory or perception. The *personality change* may be characterized by poor impulse control, emotional lability, apathy, accentuation of earlier personality traits, or hostility.

According to the ICD-10 (CDDG), the following features are required for the diagnosis of organic personality disorder, in addition to the general guidelines for the diagnosis of other organic mental disorders, described earlier:

In addition to an established history or other evidence of brain disease, damage, or dysfunction, a definitive diagnosis requires the presence of two or more of the following features:

1. Consistently reduced ability to persevere with goal-directed activities, especially those involving longer periods of time and postponed gratification;
2. Altered emotional behavior, characterized by emotional lability, shallow and unwarranted cheerfulness (euphoria, inappropriate jocularity), and easy change to irritability or short-lived outbursts of anger and aggression; in some instances apathy may be a more prominent feature;
3. Expression of needs and impulses without consideration of consequences or social convention (the patient may engage in dissocial acts, such as stealing, inappropriate sexual advances, or voracious eating, or may exhibit disregard for personal hygiene);
4. Cognitive disturbances, in the form of suspiciousness or paranoid ideation, and/or excessive preoccupation with a single, usually abstract, theme (e.g. religion, 'right and wrong');
5. Marked alteration of the rate and flow of language production, with features such as circumstantiality, over-inclusiveness, viscosity, and hypergraphia;
6. Altered sexual behavior (hyposexuality or change of sexual preference).

Etiology

1. *Temporal lobe epilepsy* (complex partial seizures) causing temporal lobe (personality) syndrome (see Table 3.4).
2. *Concussion* (post-concussional syndrome).
3. *Encephalitis* (post-encephalitis syndrome).
4. *Multiple sclerosis* (early).
5. *Cerebral neoplasms,* especially in frontal lobe (frontal lobe syndromes) and parietal lobe (see Table 3.4).
6. *Cerebrovascular disease.*
7. *Psychoactive drugs* (rarely).

Management

1. Treatment of the underlying cause, if treatable.
2. Symptomatic treatment, with lithium, carbamazepine for aggressive behavior and impulse dyscontrol, and/or antipsychotics (occasionally) for violent behavior may be needed.

MISCELLANEOUS ORGANIC MENTAL DISORDERS

Other organic mental disorders described in ICD-10 include organic dissociative disorder, organic emotionally labile (asthenic) disorder, and mild cognitive disorder.

4 Psychoactive Substance Use Disorders

Drug is defined (WHO) as any substance that, when taken into the living organism, may modify one or more of its functions. This definition conceptualizes 'drug' in a very broad way, including not only the medications but also the other pharmacologically active substances.

The words 'drug addiction' and 'drug addict' were dropped from scientific use due to their derogatory connotation. Instead 'drug abuse', 'drug dependence', 'harmful use', and 'psychoactive substance use disorders' are the terms used in the current nomenclature. A *psychoactive drug* is one that is capable of altering the mental functioning.

There are four important patterns of drug use disorders, which may overlap with each other.

1. Acute intoxication,
2. Withdrawal state,
3. Dependence syndrome, and
4. Harmful use.

1. Acute intoxication

According to the ICD-10 (CDDG), acute intoxication is a transient condition following the administration of alcohol or other psychoactive substance, resulting in disturbances in level of consciousness, cognition, perception, affect or behavior, or other psychophysiological functions and responses. This is usually associated with high blood levels of the drug. However, in certain cases, where threshold is low (e.g. in chronic renal failure) or idiosyncratic sensitivity is present, even a low dose may lead to intoxication.

The intensity of intoxication lessens with time, and effects eventually disappear in the absence of further use of the substance. The recovery is therefore complete except where tissue damage or another complication has arisen.

The following codes may be used to indicate whether the acute intoxication was associated with any complications:

i. *uncomplicated* (symptoms of varying severity, usually dose-dependent, particularly at high dose levels);
ii. *with trauma or other bodily injury;*
iii. *with other medical complications* (such as hematemesis, inhalation of vomitus);
iv. *with delirium;*
v. *with perceptual distortions;*
vi. *with coma;*
vii. *with convulsions;* and
viii. *pathological intoxication* (only for alcohol).

2. Withdrawal state

This is characterized by a cluster of symptoms, often specific to the drug used, which develop on total or partial withdrawal of a drug, usually after repeated and / or high-dose use. This, too, is a short-lasting syndrome with usual duration of few hours to few days. Typically, the patient reports that withdrawal symptoms are relieved by further substance use.

The withdrawal state is further classified as

i. *uncomplicated;*
ii. *with convulsions;* and
iii. *with delirium.*

3. Dependence syndrome

According to the ICD-10 (CDDG), the dependence syndrome is a cluster of physiological, behavioral, and cognitive phenomena in which the use of a substance or a class of substances takes on a much higher priority for a given individual than other behaviors that once had greater value.

A central descriptive characteristic of the dependence syndrome is the desire (often strong, sometimes overpowering) to take psychoactive drugs (which may or may not have been medically prescribed), alcohol, or tobacco. There may be evidence that return to substance use after a period of abstinence leads to a more rapid reappearance of other features of the syndrome than occurs with non-dependent individuals.

A definite diagnosis of dependence should usually be made only if at least three of the following have been experienced or exhibited at some time during the previous year:

1. A strong *desire* or sense of *compulsion* to take the substance.
2. *Difficulties in controlling* substance-taking behavior in terms of its onset, termination, or levels of use.
3. A physiological *withdrawal state* when substance use has ceased or been reduced, as evidenced by the characteristic withdrawal syndrome for the substance; or use of the same (or a closely related) substance with the intention of relieving or avoiding withdrawal symptoms.
4. Evidence of *tolerance,* such that increased doses of the psychoactive substance are required in order to achieve effects originally produced by lower doses (clear examples of this are found in alcohol- and opiate-dependent individuals who may take daily doses sufficient to incapacitate or kill non-tolerant users).
5. Progressive *neglect* of alternative pleasures or interests because of psychoactive substance use, increased amount of time necessary to obtain or take the substance or to recover from its effects.
6. *Persisting* with substance use despite clear evidence of overtly harmful consequences, such as harm to the liver through excessive drinking, depressive mood states consequent to periods of heavy substance use, or drug-related impairment of cognitive functioning; efforts should be made to determine that the user was actually, or could be expected to be, aware of the nature and extent of the harm.

Narrowing of the personal repertoire of patterns of psychoactive substance use has also been described as a characteristic feature (e.g. a tendency to drink in the same way on weekdays and weekends, regardless of social constraints that determine appropriate drinking behavior).

It can be further coded as

i. *currently abstinent;*
ii. *currently abstinent, but in a protected environment* (e.g. in hospital, in a therapeutic community, in prison, etc.);
iii. *currently on a clinically supervised maintenance or replacement regime* (controlled dependence, e.g. with methadone; nicotine gum or nicotine patch);
iv. *currently abstinent, but receiving treatment with aversive or blocking drugs* (e.g. naltrexone or disulfiram);
v. *currently using the substance* (active dependence);

TABLE 4.1. PSYCHOACTIVE SUBSTANCE USE DISORDERS

Drug	Usual Route of Administration	Physical Dependence	Psychic Dependence	Tolerance
1. Alcohol	Oral	+ +	+ +	+
2. Opioids	Oral, Parenteral, Smoking	+ + +	+ + +	+ + +
3. Cannabis (Marihuana)	Smoking, Oral	±	+ +	+
4. Cocaine	Inhalation, Oral, Smoking Parenteral	±	+ +	—
5. Amphetamines	Oral, Parenteral	+ +	+ +	+ + +
6. Lysergic acid diethylamide (LSD)	Oral	—	+	+
7. Barbiturates	Oral, Parenteral	+ +	+ +	+ + +
8. Benzodiazepines	Oral, Parenteral	+	+	+
9. Volatile solvents	Inhalation	±	+ +	+
10. Phencyclidine (PCP)	Smoking, Inhalation, Parenteral, Oral	±	+	+
11. Caffeine	Oral	+	++	+
12. Nicotine	Oral, Smoking	+	++	+

— = None; ± = Probable/Little; + = Some/Mild; ++ = Moderate; +++ = Severe.

vi. *continuous use*; and
vii. *episodic use* (*dipsomania*).

The dependence can be either *psychic*, or *physical*, or both.

4. Harmful use

Harmful use is characterized by:

1. Continued drug use despite awareness of harmful medical and/or social effect of the drug being used, and/or
2. A pattern of physically hazardous use of drug (e.g. driving during intoxication).

The diagnosis requires that actual damage should have been caused to the mental or physical health of the user.

Harmful use is not diagnosed, if dependence syndrome is present. DSM-IV uses the term *substance abuse*, with minor variations.

The other syndromes associated with the psychoactive substance use in ICD-10 include psychotic disorder, amnesic syndrome, and residual and late-onset (delayed onset) psychotic disorder.

Psychoactive Substances

The major dependence producing drugs are:

1. Alcohol
2. Opioids
3. Cannabinoids, e.g. cannabis
4. Cocaine
5. Amphetamine and other sympathomimetics
6. Hallucinogens, e.g. LSD, phencyclidine
7. Sedatives and hypnotics, e.g. barbiturates
8. Inhalants, e.g. volatile solvents
9. Nicotine
10. Other stimulants (e.g. caffeine).

The various psychoactive substances are summarized in Table 4.1.

TABLE 4.2. ETIOLOGICAL FACTORS IN SUBSTANCE USE DISORDERS

1. **Biological Factors**
   - i. Genetic vulnerability (family history of substance use disorder, e.g. in type II alcoholism)
   - ii. Co-morbid psychiatric disorder or personality disorder
   - iii. Co-morbid medical disorders
   - iv. Reinforcing effects of drugs (explains continuation of drug use)
   - v. Withdrawal effects and craving (explains continuation of drug use)
   - vi. Biochemical factors (e.g. role of dopamine and norepinephrine in cocaine, ethanol and opioid dependence)
2. **Psychological Factors**
   - i. Curiosity; need for novelty seeking
   - ii. General rebelliousness and social non-conformity
   - iii. Early initiation of alcohol and tobacco
   - iv. Poor impulse control
   - v. Sensation-seeking (high)
   - vi. Low self-esteem (anomie)
   - vii. Concerns regarding personal autonomy
   - viii. Poor stress management skills
   - ix. Childhood trauma or loss
   - x. Relief from fatigue and/or boredom
   - xi. Escape from reality
   - xii. Lack of interest in conventional goals
   - xiii. Psychological distress
3. **Social Factors**
   - i. Peer pressure (often more important than parental factors)
   - ii. Modeling (imitating behavior of important others)
   - iii. Ease of availability of alcohol and drugs
   - iv. Strictness of drug law enforcement
   - v. Intrafamilial conflicts
   - vi. Religious reasons
   - vii. Poor social/familial support
   - viii. 'Perceived distance' within the family
   - ix. Permissive social attitudes
   - x. Rapid urbanization.

Etiology

The various etiological factors in substance use disorders are briefly summarized in Table 4.2.

ALCOHOL USE DISORDERS

Alcohol dependence was earlier called as *alcoholism*. This term, like 'addiction', has been dropped due to its derogatory meaning.

According to Jellinek, there are five 'species' of alcohol dependence ('*alcoholism*') on the basis of patterns of use (and not on the basis of severity).

A. Alpha (α) Alcoholism

i. Excessive and inappropriate drinking to relieve physical and/or emotional pain.
ii. No loss of control.
iii. Ability to abstain present.

B. Beta (β) Alcoholism

i. Excessive and inappropriate drinking.

TABLE 4.3. CLASSIFICATION OF ALCOHOLISM

Factors	Type I	Type II
Synonym	Milieu-limited	Male-limited
Sex	Both sexes	Mostly in males
Age of onset	> 25 years	< 25 years
Etiological factors	Genetic factors important; strong environmental influences are contributory	Heritable; environmental influences are limited
Family history	May be positive	Parental alcoholism and antisocial behavior usually present
Loss of control	Present	No loss of control
Other features	Psychological dependence; and guilt present	Drinking followed by aggressive behavior; spontaneous alcohol seeking
Pre-morbid personality traits	Harm avoidance; high reward dependence	Novelty-seeking

TABLE 4.4. SOME COMPLICATIONS OF ALCOHOL DEPENDENCE

I. MEDICAL COMPLICATIONS

A. Gastro-intestinal System

i. Fatty liver, cirrhosis of liver, hepatitis, liver cell carcinoma, liver failure
ii. Gastritis, reflux esophagitis, esophageal varices, Mallory-Weiss syndrome, achlorhydria, peptic ulcer, carcinoma stomach and esophagus
iii. Malabsorption syndrome, protein-losing enteropathy
iv. Pancreatitis: acute, chronic, & relapsing

B. Central Nervous System

i. Peripheral neuropathy
ii. Delirium tremens
iii. Rum fits
iv. Alcoholic hallucinosis
v. Alcoholic jealousy
vi. Wernicke-Korsakoff psychosis
vii. Marchiafava-Bignami disease
viii. Alcoholic dementia
ix. Suicide
x. Cerebellar degeneration
xi. Central pontine myelinosis
xii. Head injury and fractures.

C. Miscellaneous

i. Acne rosacea, palmar erythema, rhinophyma, spider nevi, parotid enlargement, ascitis
ii. Fetal alcohol syndrome (cranio-facial anomalies, growth retardation, major organ system malformations)
iii Alcoholic hypoglycemia & ketoacidosis
iv. Cardiomyopathy, cardiac beri-beri
v. Alcoholic myopathy
vi. Anemia, thrombocytopenia, Vit. K factor deficiency, hemolytic anemia
vii. Accidental hypothermia
vii. Pseudo-Cushing's syndrome, hypogonadism, gynecomastia (in men), amenorrhea, infertility, decreased testosterone and increased LH levels
ix. Risk for coronary artery disease
x. Malnutrition, pellagra
xi. Decreased immune function and proneness to infections, like tuberculosis
xii. Sexual dysfunction

II. SOCIAL COMPLICATIONS

i. Accidents
ii. Marital disharmony
iii. Divorce
iv. Occupational problems, with loss of productive man-hours
v. Increased incidence of drug dependence
vi. Criminality, occasionally
vii. Financial difficulties.

ii. Physical complications (e.g. cirrhosis, gastritis and neuritis) due to cultural drinking patterns and poor nutrition.
iii. No dependence.

C. Gamma (γ) Alcoholism

Also called as *malignant alcoholism.*

i. Progressive course.
ii. Physical dependence with tolerance and withdrawal symptoms.
iii. Psychological dependence, with inability to control drinking.

D. Delta (δ) Alcoholism

i. Inability to abstain.
ii. Tolerance.
iii. Withdrawal symptoms.
iv. The amount of alcohol consumed can be controlled.
v. Social disruption is minimal.

E. Epsilon(ε) Alcoholism

i. *Dipsomania* (compulsive-drinking).
ii. Spree-drinking.

Earlier, it was believed that γ-alcoholism is more common in America, while δ-alcoholism is commoner in the wine-drinking countries, like France. Now-a-days, the existence of this pattern of distribution is doubted.

Cloninger has classified alcoholism into two types on the basis of genetic and environmental factors (Table 4.3).

TABLE 4.5. CAGE QUESTIONNAIRE

The CAGE questionnaire consists of four questions:

i. Have you ever had to **C**ut down on alcohol (amount).
ii. Have you ever been **A**nnoyed by people's criticism of alcoholism.
iii. Have you ever felt **G**uilty about drinking.
iv. Have you ever needed **E**ye opener drink (early morning drink).

A score of 2 or more identifies problem drinkers.

Alcohol dependence is more common in males, and has an onset in late second or early third decade. The course is insidious. There is often an associated abuse or dependence of other drugs. If the onset occurs late in life, especially after 40 years of age, underlying mood disorder or brain disease should be looked for.

Certain laboratory markers of alcohol dependence have been suggested. These include:

i. *GGT* (γ-glutyl-transferase) is raised to about 40 IU/L in 80% of alcohol dependent individuals. GGT returns to normal rapidly (with in 48 hours) on abstinence from alcohol. An increase of GGT of more than 50% in an abstinent individual signifies a resumption of heavy drinking.
ii. *MCV* (mean corpuscular volume) is more than 92 fl (normal = 80-90 fl) in 60% of alcohol dependent individuals. MCV takes several weeks to return to normal after abstinence.
iii. *Other lab markers* include alkaline phosphatase, AST, ALT, uric acid, blood triglycerides and CPK.

GGT and MCV together can identify 3 out of 4 problem drinkers. In addition, BAC (blood alcohol concentration) and breath-analyzer can be used for the purpose of identification.

For detection of problem drinkers in the community, several screening instruments are available. MAST (Michigan Alcoholism Screening Test) is frequently used for this purpose, while CAGE questionnaire (Table 4.5) is the easiest to be administered (it takes only about 1-2 minutes).

Complications

Alcohol dependence is often associated with complications, medical and social (Table 4.4).

A. Acute Intoxication

After a brief period of excitation, there is a generalized central nervous system depression. With increasing intoxication, there is increased reaction time, slowed thinking, distractibility and poor motor control. Later, dysarthria, ataxia and incoordination occur. There is progressive loss of self control with frank disinhibited behavior.

TABLE 4.6. BODY FLUID ALCOHOL LEVELS

BAC*	Behavioral Correlates
25-100 mg%	Excitement
80 mg%	Legal limit for driving (in UK)
100-200 mg%	Serious intoxication, slurred speech, incoordination, nystagmus
200-300 mg%	Dangerous
300-350 mg%	Hypothermia, dysarthria, cold sweats
350-400 mg%	Coma, respiratory depression
>400 mg%	Death may occur

Urinary Alcohol Concentration	Diagnostic Use	Equivalent BAC
>120 mg%	Suggestive	80 mg%
>200 mg%	Diagnostic	150 mg%

*BAC - Blood Alcohol Concentration

The duration of intoxication depends on the amount and the rapidity of ingestion of alcohol. Usually the signs of intoxication are obvious with blood levels of 150-200 mg%. With blood alcohol levels of 300-450 mg%, increasing drowsiness followed by coma, and respiratory depression develop. Death occurs with blood alcohol levels between 400 mg% to 800 mg% (Table 4.6).

Occasionally a small dose of alcohol may produce acute intoxication in some persons. It is known as *pathological intoxication*. Another feature, sometimes seen in acute intoxication, is the development of amnesia or *blackouts*.

B. Withdrawal Syndrome

The most common withdrawal syndrome is *hangover* on the next morning. Mild tremors, nausea, vomiting, weakness, irritability, insomnia and anxiety are also common withdrawal symptoms. Sometimes, the withdrawal syndrome may be more severe, characterized by one of the following three disturbances: delirium tremens, alcoholic seizures, and alcoholic hallucinosis.

1. Delirium tremens

Delirium tremens (DT) is the most severe alcohol withdrawal syndrome. It occurs usually within 2-4 days of complete or significant abstinence from heavy alcohol drinking in 5% of patients, as compared to acute tremulousness which occurs in 34% of patients. The course is short, with recovery occurring within 3-7 days. This is an acute organic brain syndrome with the characteristic features of:

i. Clouding of consciousness with disorientation in time and place.
ii. Poor attention span and distractibility.
iii. Visual (and also auditory) hallucinations and illusions, which are often vivid and frightening. Tactile hallucinations of insects crawling over body may occur.
iv. Marked autonomic disturbance with tachycardia, fever, sweating, hypertension and pupillary dilation.
v. Psychomotor agitation and ataxia.
vi. Insomnia, with a reversal of sleep-wake pattern.
vii. Dehydration with electrolyte imbalance.

Death, if occurs, is due to cardiovascular collapse, infection, hyperthermia or self-inflicted injury. Intercurrent medical illnesses like pneumonia, fractures, liver disease and pulmonary tuberculosis may complicate the clinical picture.

2. Alcoholic seizures ('rum fits')

Generalized tonic clonic seizures occur in about 10% of alcohol dependence patients, usually 12-48 hours after a heavy bout of drinking. Usually these patients have been drinking alcohol in large amounts on a regular basis for many years.

Multiple seizures, 2-6 at one time, are more common than single seizures. Sometimes, status epilepticus may be precipitated. In 30% of cases, delirium tremens follows.

3. Alcoholic hallucinosis

This is characterized by the presence of hallucinations (usually auditory) during abstinence, following regular alcohol intake. It occurs in about 2% of patients. These hallucinations persist after the withdrawal syndrome is over, and classically occur in clear consciousness.

Usually recovery occurs within one month and the duration is very rarely more than six months.

C. Neuropsychiatric Complications of Chronic Alcohol Use

1. Wernicke's encephalopathy

This is an acute reaction to severe thiamin deficiency, the commonest cause being chronic alcohol use. Characteristically, the onset occurs after a period of persistent vomiting. The important clinical signs are

i. *Ocular signs:* Coarse nystagmus and ophthalmoplegia with bilateral external rectus paralysis occur early. Pupillary irregularities, retinal hemorrhages and papilledema can occur causing impairment of vision.

ii. *Higher mental function disturbance:* Disorientation, confusion, recent memory disturbances, poor attention span and distractibility are common. Apathy and ataxia are early symptoms.

Peripheral neuropathy and serious malnutrition are often co-existent. Neuropathologically, neuronal degeneration and hemorrhage is seen in thalamus, hypothalamus, mammillary bodies and midbrain.

2. Korsakoff's psychosis

As Korsakoff's psychosis often follows Wernicke's encephalopathy, these are together referred to as Wernicke-Korsakoff syndrome.

Clinically, Korsakoff's psychosis presents as an *amnestic syndrome,* characterized by gross memory disturbances with confabulation. Insight is often impaired.

The neuropathological lesion is usually widespread, but the most consistent changes are seen in bilateral dorsomedial nuclei of thalamus and mammillary bodies. The changes are also seen in periventricular and periaqueductal grey matter, cerebellum and parts of brain stem.

The cause is severe, untreated, thiamin deficiency secondary to chronic alcohol use.

3. Marchiafava-Bignami disease

This is a rare disorder characterized by disorientation, epilepsy, ataxia, dysarthria, hallucinations, spastic limb paralysis, and personality and intellectual deterioration. There is a widespread demyelination of corpus callosum, optic tracts and cerebellar peduncles. The cause is probably some alcohol-related nutritional deficiency.

4. Others

These include:

i. Alcoholic dementia.
ii. Cerebellar degeneration.
iii. Peripheral neuropathy.
iv. Central pontine myelinosis.

Treatment

Before starting any method of treatment, it is important to follow these steps :

i. Ruling out or diagnosing any physical disorder.
ii. Ruling out or diagnosing any psychiatric disorder.
iii. Assessment of motivation for treatment.
iv. Assessment of social support system.
v. Assessment of personality characteristics of the patient.
vi. Current and past social, interpersonal and occupational functioning.

The treatment can be broadly divided into two types, which are often interlinked. These are: detoxification and treatment of alcohol dependence.

1. Detoxification

This is the treatment of alcohol withdrawal symptoms, i.e. symptoms produced by the removal of the 'toxin' (alcohol). The best way to stop alcohol (or any other drug of dependence) is to stop it suddenly. The usual duration of uncomplicated withdrawal syndrome is 7-14 days. The aim of detoxification is the symptomatic management of the emergent withdrawal symptoms.

The drugs of choice are *benzodiazepines.* Chlordiazepoxide (80-200 mg/day in divided doses) and diazepam (40-80 mg/day in divided doses) are the most frequently used benzodiazepines. The higher limit of the normal dose range is used in delirium tremens. Clormethiazole (1-2 g/day) and carbamazepine (600-1600 mg/day) are experimental drugs used in some countries for detoxification. These drugs are used in a standardized protocol with the dosage steadily decreasing every day before being stopped, usually on the tenth day.

In addition, vitamins should be administered. In patients suffering from or likely to suffer from delirium tremens, peripheral neuropathy, Wernicke-Korsakoff syndrome, or other signs of vitamin B deficiency (especially thiamin and nicotinic acid), a preparation of vitamin B containing 100 mg of thiamin should be administered parenterally, twice every day for 3-5 days. This should be followed by oral administration of vitamin B_1 for at least 6 months. The care of *hydration* is another important step. It is extremely important not to give 5% dextrose (or any carbohydrate) in delirium tremens (or even uncomplicated alcohol withdrawal syndro-me) without thiamine.

Although detoxification can be achieved on an outpatient (OPD) basis, some patients do require hospitalization. These patients may present with:

i. Signs of impending delirium tremens (tremor, autonomic hyperactivity, disorientation, or perceptual abnormalities), or
ii. Psychiatric symptoms or disorders (mood disorder, schizophrenia, suicidal ideation and/or attempts, other alcohol-induced neuropsychiatric disorders), or

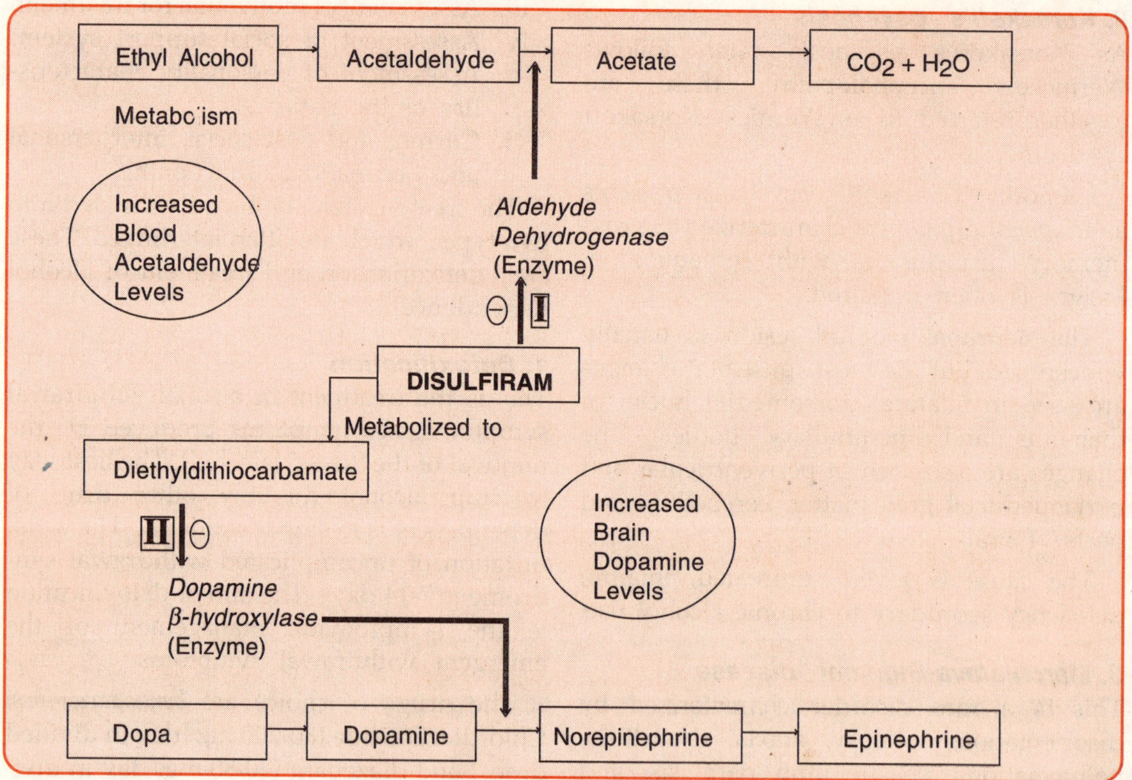

FIG. 4.1. DISULFIRAM: MODE OF ACTION

iii. Physical illness (caused by chronic alcohol use or incidental), or
iv. Inability to stop alcohol in the setting of home.

Detoxification is the first step in treatment of alcohol dependence.

2. Treatment of alcohol dependence

After the step of detoxification is over, there are several methods to choose from, for further management. The important methods include:

i. Behavior therapy

The most commonly used behavior therapy is *aversion therapy*, using either a sub-threshold electric shock or an emetic, like apomorphine. Many other methods (*covert sensitization*, relaxation techniques, assertiveness training, self-control skills, positive reinforcements) have been used alone or in combination with aversion therapy.

ii. Psychotherapy

Supportive psychotherapy and individual psychotherapy have been used. The patient should be educated about the risks of continuing alcohol use, asked to resume personal responsibility for change and given a choice of options for change.

iii. Group therapy

Of particular importance is a voluntary self-help group — AA (Alcoholics Anonymous) —with branches all over the world and a membership in hundreds of thousands. Although the approach is partly religious in nature, many patients derive benefits from group meetings (non-professional in nature).

iv. Deterrent agents

The deterrent agents are also called *alcohol sensitizing drugs*.

Disulfiram (tetraethyl thiuram disulfide) was discovered in 1930s, when it was seen that workers in rubber industry developed unpleasant reactions to alcohol intake, due to accidental absorption of antioxidant disulfiram. The mechanism of action of disulfiram is shown in the Fig. 4.1.

When alcohol is ingested by a person who is on disulfiram, alcohol-derived acetaldehyde can not be oxidized to acetate and this leads to an accumulation of acetaldehyde in blood. This causes the important *disulfiram-ethanol reaction* (DER), characterized by flushing, tachycardia, hypotension, tachypnea, palpitations, headache, sweating, nausea, vomiting, giddiness, and a sense of impending doom associated with severe anxiety.

The onset of the reaction occurs within 30 minutes, becomes full blown within 1 hour, and subsides usually within 2 hours of ingestion of alcohol.

In sensitive patients or in those who have ingested a large amount of alcohol, the DER can be very severe and life threatening due to one or more of the following: shock, myocardial infarction, convulsions, hypoxia, confusion and coma. Therefore, the treatment with disulfiram is begun in an inpatient hospital setting, usually after a *challenge test* with alcohol to demonstrate that unpleasant and dangerous side-effects occur, if alcohol or alcohol-containing eatable/drink is consumed while treatment is continued with disulfiram.

The usual dose of disulfiram is 250-500 mg/day (taken before bedtime to avoid drowsiness in daytime) in the first week and 250 mg/day subsequently for maintenance treatment. The effect begins within 12 hours of first dose and remains for 7-10 days after the last dose. The patient should carry a *warning card* detailing the forbidden alcohol-containing articles, the side-effects and their emergency treatment, along with patient identification.

The *contraindications* of disulfiram use are first trimester of pregnancy, coronary artery disease, liver failure, chronic renal failure, peripheral neuropathy, muscle disease and history of psychosis in past.

In selected patients (e.g. older age group, good motivation for deaddiction, good social support, absent underlying psychopathology and good treatment compliance); the response can be dramatic. In addition to oral preparations, subcutaneous disulfiram implants are also available. However, they provide unpredictable blood levels of disulfiram.

Other deterrent agents

1. Citrated calcium carbimide (CCC): Mechanism of action is similar to disulfiram but onset of action occurs within 1 hour and is reversible. The usual dosage is 100 mg/d in 2 divided doses.
2. Metronidazole.
3. Nitrafezole: It is safer and long-acting.
4. Methyltetrazolethiol.
5. Animal charcoal, a fungus (*Coprinus atramentarius*), sulfonylureas and certain cephalosporins also cause a disulfiram like action.

v. Anti-craving agents

Acamprosate, naltrexone and SSRIs (e.g. fluoxetine) are among the medications tried as anti-craving agents in alcohol dependence.

Acamprosate (the Ca^{++} salt of N-acetyl-homotaurinate) interacts with NMDA receptor-mediated glutamatergic neurotrans-mission in various brain regions and reduces Ca^{++} fluxes through voltage-operated channels.

Naltrexone (opioid receptor antagonist) probably interferes with alcohol-induced reinforcement by blocking opioid receptors.

TABLE 4.7. OPIOID DERIVATIVES

A. Natural Alkaloids of Opium
1. Morphine
2. Codeine
3. Thebaine
4. Noscapine
5. Papaverine.
B. Synthetic Compounds
1. Heroin
2. Nalorphine
3. Hydromorphone
4. Methadone
5. Dextropropoxyphene
6. Meperidine (Pethidine)
7. Cyclazocine
8. Levallorphan
9. Diphenoxylate

Fluoxetine (and other SSRIs) have been occasionally used as anti-craving agents in usual antidepressant doses.

vi. Other medications

A variety of other medicines like benzodiazepines, antidepressants, antipsychotics, lithium, carbamazepine, narcotics have been tried. These should be used only if there is a special indication for their use (e.g. tricyclic antidepressants for underlying depression).

vii. Psychosocial rehabilitation

Rehabilitation is an integral part of multimodal treatment of alcohol dependence.

OPIOID USE DISORDERS

Dried exudate obtained from unripe seed capsules of *Papaver somniferum* has been used and abused for centuries. The natural alkaloids of opium and synthetic preparations are highly dependence producing. These are listed in Table 4.7.

In the last few decades, the use of opioids has increased markedly the world over. India, surrounded on both sides by routes of illicit transport, namely *Golden Triangle* (Burma-Thailand-Laos) and *Golden Crescent* (Iran-Afganistan-Pakistan), is particularly severely affected.

The most important dependence producing derivatives are morphine and heroin. They both, like majority of dependence producing opioids, bind to μ (mu) opioid receptors. The other opioid receptors are *k* (kappa, e.g. for pentazocine), δ (delta, e.g. for a type of enkephalin), σ (sigma e.g. for phencyclidine), ε (epsilon) and λ (lambda). Heroin or diacetyl-morphine is about two times more potent than morphine in injectable form.

Apart from the parenteral mode of administration, heroin can also be smoked or 'chased' (*chasing the dragon*), often in an impure form (called *'smack'* or *'brown sugar'* in India). Heroin is more addicting than morphine and can cause dependence after a short period of exposure. Tolerance to heroin occurs rapidly and can be increased to more than 100 times the first dose needed.

Acute Intoxication

This is characterized by apathy, bradycardia, hypotension, respiratory depression, subnormal core body temperature and pin-point pupils. Later, delayed reflexes, thready pulse and coma may occur in case of a large overdose. In severe intoxication, mydriasis may occur due to hypoxia.

Withdrawal Syndrome

The onset of withdrawal symptoms occurs typically within 12-24 hours, has a peak within 24-72 hours and symptoms subside within 7-10 days of the last dose of opioid. The characteristic symptoms include lacrimation, rhinorrhea, pupillary dilation, sweating, diarrhea, yawning, tachycardia, mild hypertension, insomnia, raised body temperature, muscle cramps, generalized bodyache, severe anxiety, piloerection, nausea, vomiting and anorexia. There are marked individual differences in withdrawal symptoms. The heroin withdrawal syndrome is more severe than the withdrawal syndrome of morphine.

Complications

The important complications of chronic opioid use may include one or more of the following:

1. Complications due to illicit drug (contaminants): Parkinsonism, peripheral neuropathy, degeneration of globus pallidus, transverse myelitis, amblyopia.
2. Complications due to intravenous use: Skin infections, thrombophlebitis, pulmonary embolism, endocarditis, septicemia, AIDS, viral hepatitis, tetanus.
3. Drug peddling and involvement in criminal activities (social complication).

Treatment

Before treatment, a correct diagnosis must be made on the basis of history, examination (pin-point pupils during intoxication or withdrawal symptoms) and laboratory tests. These tests are:

1. Naloxone challenge test (to precipitate the withdrawal symptoms).
2. Urinary opioids testing: with radio-immuno assay (RIA), free radical assay technique (FRAT), thin layer chromatography (TLC), gas-liquid chromatography (GLC), high pressure liquid chromatography (HPLC) or enzyme-multiplied immuno-assay technique (EMIT).

The treatment can be divided into 3 main types:

1. Treatment of overdose.
2. Detoxification.
3. Maintenance therapy.

1. Treatment of Opioid Overdose

An overdose of opioid can be treated with *narcotic antagonists* (e.g. naloxone, naltrexone).

Usually an intravenous injection of 2 mg naloxone followed by a repeat injection in 5-10 minutes causes reversal of overdose. But as naloxone has a short half-life, repeated doses are needed every 1-2 hours. This should be combined with general care and supportive treatment.

2. Detoxification

This is a mode of treatment in which the dependent person is 'taken off' opioids. This is usually done abruptly, followed by management of the withdrawal symptoms. Withdrawal symptoms can be managed by one of the following methods:

i. *Use of substitution drugs*, like methadone (not available in India at present), to ameliorate the withdrawal symptoms. The aim is to gradually taper off the patient from methadone (which is less addicting, has a longer half life, and has a milder withdrawal syndrome). Relapses are common and one dependence is often replaced by another (methadone).

ii. *Clonidine* is an α_2 agonist which acts by inhibiting norepinephrine release at the presynaptic a_2 receptors. The usual dose is 0.3-1.2 mg/day, and is tapered off in 10-14 days. It can be started after stoppage of either the opioid itself or the substitution drug. The important side effects are excessive sedation and postural hypotension. The treatment is started preferably in an inpatient setting.

iii. *Naltrexone with clonidine:* Naltrexone is an orally available narcotic antagonist which, when given to an opioid dependent individual, causes withdrawal symptoms. These symptoms are managed with the addition of clonidine for 10-14 days. After that, clonidine is withdrawn and patient is continued on naltrexone alone. Now if the person takes an opioid, there are no pleasurable experiences as the opioid receptors are blocked by naltrexone. So, this method is a combination of detoxification and maintenance treatment. The usual dose of naltrexone is 100 mg orally, every alternate day.

iv. *Others:* The other detoxification agents include LAAM (levo-alpha-acetyl-methadol), propoxyphene, diphenoxylate, buprenorphine (long acting partial μ-agonist), and lofexidine (α_2 agonist like clonidine).

TABLE 4.8. CANNABIS PREPARATIONS

Cannabis preparation	Portion of plant	THC content(%)	Potency (as compared to 'Bhang')
1. Hashish/ Charas	Resinous exudate from the flowering tops of cultivated plants	8-14%	10
2. Ganja	Small leaves and brackets of inflorescence of highly cultivated plants	1-2%	2
3. Bhang	Dried leaves, flowering shoots and cut tops of uncultivated plants	1%	1
4. Hash oil	Lipid soluble plant extract	15-40%	25

3. Maintenance therapy

After the detoxification phase is over, patient is maintained on one of the following regimens:

i. Methadone maintenance (Agonist substitution therpay)

This a very popular method used widely in the West. 20-50 mg/day of methadone is given to the patient to shift him from 'hard' drugs, thus decreasing IV use and criminal behavior. Its use in India has not been recommended by an expert committee for de-addiction services. Other drugs like LAAM and buprenorphine can be used for maintenance treatment.

ii. Opioid antagonists

Opioid antagonists have been in use for a long time but they were either partial antagonists (nalorphine) or had to be administered parenterally (naloxone). Now with the availability of orally effective and very potent antagonist, naltrexone, the use of opioid antagonists in routine practice has been simplified. The usual maintenance dose is 100 mg on Mondays and Wednesdays, and 150 mg on Fridays. Naltrexone combined with clonidine, as described above, is a very effective method for detoxification as well as for maintenance treatment.

iii. Other methods

These include individual psychotherapy, behavior therapy, interpersonal therapy, cognitive therapy, motivational enhancement therapy, self-control strategies, psychotropic drugs for the associated psychopathology, family therapy, and group therapy (e.g. in therapeutic communities like *Synanon*, self-help groups like *Narcotic Anonymous or NA*). These methods have to be tailored for use in an individual patient.

iv. Psychosocial rehabilitation

This is a very important post-detoxification step, in the absence of which relapse rates are very high. Rehabilitation should be at both the occupational and social levels.

CANNABIS USE DISORDER

Cannabis is derived from the hemp plant, *Cannabis sativa*, which has several varieties named after the region in which it is found (e.g. *sativa indica* in India and Pakistan, and *americana* in America). Cannabis produces more than 400 identifiable chemicals of which about 50 are cannabinoids, the most active being Δ-9-tetrahydrocannabinol (Δ^9-THC). The pistillate form of the female plant is more important in cannabis production (Table 4.8).

Recently, a G_i-protein (inhibitory G-protein) linked cannabinoid receptor has been found (in basal ganglia, hippocampus and cerebellum) which inhibits the adenylate cyclase activity in a dose-dependent manner. Cannabis produces a very mild physical dependence, with a relatively mild withdrawal syndrome characterized by fine tremors, irritability, restlessness, nervousness, insomnia, decreased appetite and craving. This syndrome begins within few hours of stopping cannabis use and lasts for 4 to 5 days. Psychological dependence ranges from mild (occasional 'trips') to marked (compulsive use).

All the active ingredients are called as *marijuana* or *marihuana.*

Acute Intoxication

Mild cannabis intoxication is characterized by mild impairment of consciousness and orientation, lightheadedness, tachycardia, a sense of floating in the air, a euphoric dream-like state, alternation (either an increase or decrease) in psychomotor activity and tremors, in addition to photophobia, lacrimation, tachycardia, reddening of conjunctiva, dry mouth and increased appetite. There is often a curious splitting of consciousness, the user observing his own intoxication as a non-participant observer.

Perceptual disturbances are common and include depersonalization, derealization, *synesthesias* (sensation in one sensory modality caused by a sensation in another sensory modality, e.g. seeing the music) and increased sensitivity to sound. However, hallucinations are seen only in marked to severe intoxication. These are often visual, ranging from elementary flashes of lights and geometrical figures to complex human faces and pictures.

Mild cannabis intoxication releases inhibitions, which is expressed in words and emotions rather than in actions.

'Flashback phenomenon' has been described, characterized by a recurrence of cannabis use experience in the absence of cannabis use.

Complications

The complications of cannabis use include:

1. *Transient or short-lasting psychiatric disorders*: Acute anxiety, paranoid psychosis, hysterical fugue-like states, suicidal ideation, hypomania, schizophrenia-like state (characterized by persecutory delusions, hallucinations and at times catatonic symptoms), acute organic psychosis and, very rarely, depression.
2. *Amotivational syndrome*: Chronic cannabis use is postulated to cause lethargy, apathy, loss of interest, anergia, reduced drive and lack of ambition. The etiological role of cannabis in this disorder is far from proven.
3. *Hemp insanity or cannabis psychosis*: *Indian hemp insanity* was first described by Dhunjibhoy in 1930. Thereafter, several reports appeared in literature from India, Egypt, Morocco and Nigeria. It was described as being similar to acute schizophreniform disorder with disorientation and confusion, and with a good prognosis. The validity of this disorder is currently doubted.
4. *Other complications*: Chronic cannabis use sometimes leads to memory impairment, worsening or relapse in schizophrenia or mood disorder, chronic obstructive airway disease, pulmonary malignancies, alteration in both humoral and cell-mediated immunity, anovulatory cycles, decreased testosterone levels, reversible inhibition of spermatogenesis, blockade of gonadotropin releasing hormone, and increased risk for the developing fetus if taken during pregnancy.

Treatment

As the withdrawal syndrome is very mild, the management consists of supportive and symp-

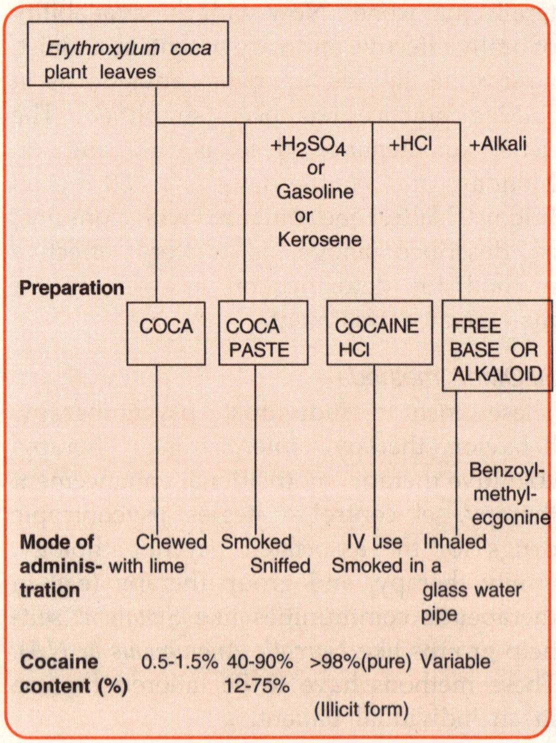

FIG. 4:2. COCAINE PREPARATIONS

TABLE 4.9. PHASES IN COCAINE WITHDRAWAL SYNDROME

Phase	Substage	Duration	Clinical Features
I (Crash phase)	i	9 hours to 4 days after discontinuation	Agitation, depression, anorexia, craving +++
	ii		Fatigue, depression, sleepiness, craving +
	iii		Exhaustion, hypersomnia with intermittent awakening, hyperphagia, craving ±
II	i	4 to 7 days after discontinuation	Normal sleep, improved mood, craving ±
	ii		Anxiety, anergia, anhedonia, craving ++
III (Extinction phase)		After 7-10 days of discontinuation	No withdrawal symptoms, increased vulnerability to relapse

tomatic treatment. The psychiatric symptoms may require proper psychotropic medication and sometimes hospitalization. Psychotherapy and family therapy are important in the management of psychic dependence.

COCAINE USE DISORDER

Cocaine is an alkaloid derived from the coca bush, *Erythroxylum coca*, found in Bolivia and Peru. It was isolated by Albert Neimann in 1860 and was used by Karl Koller (a friend of Freud) in 1884 as the first effective local anesthetic agent.

Cocaine (common street name *Crack*) can be administered orally, intranasally, by smoking *(free basing)* or parenterally, depending on the preparation available (Fig. 4.2). Cocaine HCl is the commonest form used followed by the free base alkaloid. Both intravenous use and free base inhalation produce a 'rush' of pleasurable sensations.

Cocaine is a central stimulant which inhibits the reuptake of dopamine along with that of norepinephrine and serotonin. In animals, cocaine is the most powerful reinforcer of drug taking behavior. A typical pattern of cocaine use is cocaine 'runs' (binges) followed by cocaine 'crashes' (interruption of use). Cocaine is sometimes used in combination with opiates like heroin ('speed ball') or at times amphetamines. Cocaine dependence is relatively uncommon in India.

Acute Intoxication

Acute cocaine intoxication is characterized by pupillary dilatation, tachycardia, hypertension, sweating, and nausea or vomiting. A hypomanic picture with increased psychomotor activity, grandiosity, elation of mood, hypervigilance and increased speech output may be present. Later, judgement is impaired and there is impairment of social or occupational functioning.

Withdrawal Syndrome

Cocaine use produces a very mild physical, but a very strong psychic, dependence. A triphasic withdrawal syndrome follows an abrupt discontinuation of chronic cocaine use (Table 4.9).

Complications

The complications of chronic cocaine use include acute anxiety reaction, uncontrolled compulsive behavior, psychotic episodes (with persecutory delusions, and tactile and other hallucinations), delirium and delusional disorder. High doses of cocaine can induce seizures, respiratory depression, cardiac arrhythmias, coronary artery occlusion, myocardial infarction, lung damage, gastrointestinal necrosis, fetal anoxia and perforation of nasal septum.

Treatment

Before starting treatment, it is essential to diagnose or rule out coexistent psychiatric and/or physical disorder, and assess the motivation for treatment. Cocaine use disorder is commonly associated with mood disorder, particularly major depression and cyclothymia.

1. Treatment of cocaine overdose

The treatment consists of oxygenation, muscle relaxants, and IV thiopentone and/or IV diazepam (for seizures and severe anxiety). IV propranolol, a specific antagonist of cocaine-induced sympa-thomimetic effects, can be used in a dose of 1 mg every minute. Haloperidol or pimozide can be used for the treatment of psychosis as well as for blocking the cardio-stimulatory effects of cocaine.

2. Treatment of chronic cocaine use

The treatment of underlying or co-existent psychopathology is the most important step in the management of chronic cocaine use. The pharmacological treatment includes the use of bromocriptine (a dopaminergic agonist) and amantadine (an antiparkinsonian) in reducing cocaine craving. Other useful drugs are desipramine, imipramine and trazodone (both for reducing craving and for antidepressant effect). The goal of the treatment is total abstinence from cocaine use.

The psychosocial treatment techniques, like supportive psychotherapy and contingent behavior therapy, are useful in the post-withdrawal treatment and in prevention of relapse.

AMPHETAMINE USE DISORDER

Though synthesized by Edleano in 1887, it was introduced in Medicine in 1932 as benzedrine inhaler, for the treatment of coryza, rhinitis and asthma. Later, it was recommended for a variety of conditions like narcolepsy, post-encephalitic parkinsonism, obesity, depression, and even to heighten energy and capacity to work.

Amphetamine refers to a unique chemical which is precisely phenyl-iso-propylamine or methyl-phenethyl-amine. It is a powerful CNS stimulant, with peripheral sympathomimetic effects. The dextro-amphetamine isomer is 3-4 times more potent than the levo-isomer. It acts primarily on norepinephrine release in brain, along with an action on the release of dopamine and serotonin.

Although still clinically indicated for narcolepsy, attention deficit hyperactivity disorder and rarely, for obesity and mild depression, one of the commonest patterns of use is seen amongst students and sportspersons to overcome the need for sleep and fatigue. Tolerance usually develops to the central as well as cardiovascular effects of amphetamines.

Recently, there has been a resurgence of amphetamine use in USA, with the availability of 'designer' amphetamines, like MDMA (3,4-methylenedioxy-amphetamine; street name: *ecstasy* or *XTC*).

Intoxication and Complications

The signs and symptoms of acute amphetamine intoxication are primarily cardiovascular (tachycardia, hypertension, hemorrhage, cardiac failure and cardiovascular shock) and central (seizures, hyperpyrexia, tremors, ataxia, euphoria, pupillary dilatation, tetany and coma). The neuropsychiatric manifestations include anxiety, panic, insomnia, restlessness, irritability, hostility and bruxism.

Acute intoxication may present as a paranoid hallucinatory syndrome which closely mimics paranoid schizophrenia. The distinguishing features include rapidity of onset, prominence of visual hallucinations, absence of thought disorder, appropriateness of affect, fearful emotional reaction and presence of confusion. However, a confident diagnosis requires estimation of urinary amphetamine levels. Amphetamine-induced psychosis usually resolves within seven days of urinary clearance of amphetamines.

Chronic amphetamine intoxication leads to severe, compulsive craving for the drug. A high degree of tolerance is characteristic, with the dependent individual needing upto 15-20 times the initial dose in order to obtain the pleasurable effects. A common pattern of chronic use is a cycle of *runs* (heavy use for several days) followed by *crashes* (stopping the drug use).

Tactile hallucinations in clear consciousness, may sometimes occur in chronic amphetamine intoxication.

Withdrawal Syndrome

The withdrawal syndrome is typically seen on abrupt discontinuation of amphetamines after a period of chronic use. It is characterized by depression (which may be suicidal), marked asthenia, apathy, fatigue, hypersomnia alternating with insomnia, agitation and hyperphagia.

Treatment

1. Treatment of intoxication

Acute intoxication is treated by symptomatic measures, e.g. hyperpyrexia (cold sponging, parenteral antipyretics), seizures (parenteral diazepam), psychotic symptoms (haloperidol), and hypertension (antihypertensives). Acidification of urine (with oral NH_4Cl-500 mg every 4 hours) facilitates the elimination of amphetamines.

2. Treatment of withdrawal symptoms

The presence of severe suicidal depression may necessitate hospitalization. The treatment includes symptomatic management, use of antidepressants and supportive psychotherapy. The management of withdrawal syndrome is usually the first step towards the treatment of amphetamine dependence.

LSD USE DISORDER

Lysergic acid diethylamide, first synthesized by Albert Hoffman in 1938 and popularly known as 'acid', is a powerful hallucinogen. It is related to the psychedelic compounds found in the 'morning glory' seeds, the lysergic acid amides. As little as 100 μg of LSD is sufficient to produce behavioral effects in man. LSD presumably produces its effects by an action on the 5-HT levels in brain.

Although tolerance and psychological dependence occur with LSD use, no physical dependence or withdrawal syndrome is reported. A common pattern of LSD use is *trip* (occasional use followed by a long period of abstinence).

Intoxication

The characteristic features of acute LSD intoxication are perceptual changes occurring in clear consciousness (e.g. depersonalization, derealization, illusions, intensification of perceptions, synesthesias for example colors are heard, sounds are felt and hallucinations) and autonomic hyperactivity (pupillary dilatation, tachycardia, sweating, tremors, incoordination, palpitations, raised temperature, piloerection and giddiness). These changes are usually associated with marked anxiety or depression, though euphoria is more common in small doses. Persecutory and referential ideation may also occur.

Sometimes, acute LSD intoxication presents with an acute panic reaction, known as a *bad trip*, in which the individual experiences a loss of control over his self. The recovery usually occurs within 8-12 hours of the last dose. Rarely, the intoxication is severe enough to produce an acute psychotic episode resembling a schizophreniform psychosis.

Withdrawal Syndrome

No withdrawal syndrome has been described with LSD use.

However, sometimes, there is a spontaneous recurrence of the LSD use experience in a drug free state. Described as a *flashback*, it usually occurs weeks to months after the last experience. Such episodes are often induced by stress, fatigue, alcohol intake, severe physical illness or marihuana intoxication.

Complications

Long term LSD use is not a common phenomenon. The complications of chronic LSD use include psychiatric symptoms (anxiety, depression, psychosis or visual hallucinosis) and occasionally fetal abnormalities.

Treatment

The treatment of acute LSD intoxication consists of symptomatic management with antianxiety, antidepressant or antipsychotic medication, along with supportive psychotherapy.

BARBITURATE USE DISORDER

Barbiturate use disorder is now subsumed under the sedative, hypnotic and anxiolytic use disorders. However, it has been described separately as it has some distinctive features.

Since their introduction in 1903, barbiturates have been used as sedatives, hypnotics, anticonvulsants, anesthetics and tranquilizers. The commonly abused barbiturates are secobarbital, pentobarbital and amobarbital. Their use has recently decreased markedly as benzodiazepines have replaced barbiturates in the majority of their clinical uses.

Barbiturates produce marked physical and psychological dependence. Tolerance (both central and metabolic) develops rapidly and is usually marked. There is also a cross tolerance with alcohol.

Intoxication and Complications

Acute intoxication, typically occurring as an episodic phenomenon, is characterized by irritability, increased productivity of speech, lability of mood, disinhibited behavior, slurring of speech, incoordination, attentional and memory impairment, and ataxia. Mild barbiturate intoxication resembles alcohol intoxication; severe forms may present with diplopia, nystagmus, hypotonia, positive Romberg's sign and suicidal ideation. Drug automatism may sometimes lead to lethal accidents.

Intravenous use can lead to skin abscesses, cellulitis, infections, embolism and hypersensitivity reactions.

Withdrawal Syndrome

The barbiturate withdrawal syndrome can be very severe. It usually occurs in individuals who are taking more than 600-800 mg/day of secobarbital equivalent for more than one month. It is characterized by marked restlessness, tremors, hypertension, seizures and, in severe cases, a psychosis resembling delirium tremens. The withdrawal syndrome is at its worst about 72 hours after the last dose. Coma, followed by death, can occur in some cases.

Treatment

The barbiturate intoxication should be treated symptomatically. If the patient is conscious, induction of vomiting and use of activated charcoal can reduce the absorption. If coma ensues, intensive care measures should be employed on emergency basis.

The treatment of withdrawal syndrome is usually conservative. However, pentobarbital substitution therapy has been suggested for the treatment of withdrawal from short-acting barbiturates. After the detoxification phase is over, follow-up supportive treatment and treatment of associated psychiatric disorder, usually depression, are important to prevent relapses.

BENZODIAZEPINES AND OTHER SEDATIVE-HYPNOTIC USE DISORDER

Since the discovery of chlordiazepoxide in 1957 by Sternbach, benzodiazepines have replaced other sedative-hypnotics in the treatment of insomnia and anxiety. These are currently one of the most often prescribed drugs.

Benzodiazepines produce their effects by acting on benzodiazepine receptors (GABA-benzodiazepine receptor complex), thereby indirectly increasing the action of GABA.

Benzodiazepine or sedative-hypnotic use disorder can be either iatrogenic or originating with illicit drug use. Dependence, both physical and psychic, occurs and tolerance is moderate.

Intoxication and Complications

Acute intoxication resembles alcohol intoxication, while chronic intoxication causes tolerance, especially to the sedative and anticonvulsant actions. Excessive doses can lead to respiratory depression, coma and death while chronic use has been reported to cause amnestic syndrome.

Withdrawal Syndrome

A typical withdrawal syndrome, after cessation of prolonged use (> 4-6 weeks) in moderate to heavy doses (> 60-80 mg/day of diazepam), is characterized by marked anxiety, irritability, tremors, insomnia, vomiting, weakness, autonomic hyperactivity with postural hypotension, and seizures.

Depression, transient psychotic episodes, suicidal ideation, perceptual disturbances and, rarely, delirium have also been reported in the withdrawsl period.

Treatment

The treatment of benzodiazepine intoxication is usually symptomatic. However, in cases of coma caused by benzodiazepine overdose, flumazenil (a benzodiazepine receptor antagonist) can be used in a dose of 0.3-1.0 mg IV over 1-2 min.

The treatment of low dose dependence syndrome (~15 mg/day of diazepam) is abrupt withdrawal and symptomatic management of withdrawal symptoms. However, moderate to high dose dependence is best managed by gradual withdrawal in a step-wise manner (a reduction of ~10% of the dose every day).

After the detoxification phase, follow-up supportive treatment is essential to prevent relapses.

INHALANTS OR VOLATILE SOLVENT USE DISORDER

The commonly used volatile solvents include gasoline (petrol), glues, aerosols (spray paints), thinners, varnish remover and industrial solvents. The active ingredients usually include toluene, benzene, acetone and halogenated hydrocarbons. It is more common in early adolescence as a group activity, particularly in low socio-economic status groups (e.g. rag-pickers in Mumbai and Delhi).

Intoxication and Complications

Inhalation of a volatile solvent leads to euphoria, excitement, belligerence, dizziness, slurring of speech, apathy, impaired judgement and neurological signs (like decreased reflexes, ataxia, nystagmus, incoordination and coma). Death can occur due to respiratory depression, cardiac arrhythmias, or asphyxia.

The complications include irreversible damage to liver and kidneys, peripheral neuropathy, perceptual disturbances and brain damage.

There appears to be no specific treatment of inhalant use disorder. There is often an associated psychiatric disorder (usually schizophrenia or personality disorder, particularly in solitary sniffers), or there is a history of criminal background. The prognosis is usually guarded.

PHENCYCLIDINE USE DISORDER

Phencyclidine (PCP) was introduced as a dissociative anesthetic agent (similar to ketamine) in 1950s. However, its use was soon restricted to veterinary anesthesia as the human subjects developed delirium while emerging from anesthesia. Classified as an atypical hallucinogen (street name: *angel dust*), PCP selectively antagonizes the neuronal action of NMDA (N-methyl-D-aspartate).

PCP is usually taken either occasionally or in binges (called as *runs*); however some individuals do take PCP in a regular manner. It can be administered orally, intravenously or by snorting.

Intoxication and Complications

Acute PCP intoxication produces euphoria in small doses; higher doses produce dysphoria. Other features may include impulsiveness, agitation, impaired social judgement, assaultiveness, feeling of numbness and inability to move. PCP intoxication can sometimes present with psychiatric syndromes (catatonic syndrome, delirium, stupor, paranoid hallucinatory psychosis, mania or depression) and/or neurological symptoms (nystagmus, ataxia, dysarthria, rigidity, seizures or coma).

Withdrawal Syndrome

Although no clear-cut withdrawal syndrome has been described, craving, social withdrawal, anxiety, depression and impairment in cognitive functions have been reported.

Treatment

The treatment of PCP intoxication is symptomatic and usually involves gastric lavage, isolation, and the use of anticonvulsants (if seizures occur) and antipsychotics (for PCP induced psychosis).

There is no specific treatment for PCP withdrawal syndrome.

OTHER USE DISORDERS

Caffeine and nicotine are among the most widely used substances. Both can cause intoxication, dependence, tolerance, and withdrawal syndrome.

5 Schizophrenia

Schizophrenia has puzzled physicians, philosophers, and general public for centuries. The systematic study of schizophrenia, however, is but a century old. A clinical syndrome with a profound influence on public health, schizophrenia has been called "arguably the worst disease affecting mankind, even AIDS not excepted" (Nature 1988).

To understand what schizophrenia is, it is important to have a brief look at the history of evolution of the concept of schizophrenia.

HISTORICAL BACKGROUND

Although earlier descriptions of schizophrenia-like illness are recorded in literature (e.g. in Ayurveda; Morel's description of *demence precoce*; Kahlbaum's description of *catatonia*; Hecker's description of *hebephrenia*), the scientific study of the disorder began with the description by Emil Kraepelin.

Emil Kraepelin

In 1896, Emil Kraepelin differentiated the major psychiatric illnesses into two clinical types:

1. Dementia precox, and
2. Manic depressive psychosis.

Under dementia precox, he brought together the various psychiatric illnesses which were earlier thought to be distinct illnesses. The emphasis in diagnosis of dementia precox was on an early onset and a poor outcome (*dementia*: deterioration; *precox*: early onset).

TABLE 5.1. EUGEN BLEULER'S FUNDAMENTAL SYMPTOMS OF SCHIZOPHRENIA

(Also called as 4 A's of Bleuler)

1. **Ambivalence**: Marked inability to decide for or against.
2. **Autism**: Withdrawal into self.
3. **Affect disturbances**: For example, inappropriate affect.
4. **Association disturbances**: Loosening of associations; thought disorder.

He recognized the characteristic features of dementia precox, e.g. delusions, hallucinations, disturbances of affect and motor disturbances.

Eugen Bleuler

Eugen Bleuler (1911), while renaming dementia precox as *schizophrenia* (meaning mental splitting), recognized that this disorder did not always have a poor prognosis as described by Kraepelin. Bleuler also recognized that schizo-phrenia consisted of a group of disorders rather than being a distinct entity; hence he used the term *a group of schizophrenias.*

Bleuler described the characteristic symptoms (*fundamental symptoms*) which were then thought to be diagnostic of schizophrenia (Table 5.1). He also described *accessory symptoms* of schizophrenia (thought to be secondary to the fundamental symptoms). These accessory symptoms included delusions, hallucinations and negativism.

TABLE 5.2. FIRST RANK SYMPTOMS (SFRS) OF SCHIZOPHRENIA

A. Hallucinations

1. Audible thoughts: Voices speaking out thoughts aloud or 'thought echo'.
2. Voices heard arguing: Two or more hallucinatory voices discussing the subject in third person.
3. Voices commenting on one's action.

B. Thought Alienation Phenomena

4. Thought withdrawal: Thoughts cease and subject experiences them as removed by external force.
5. Thought insertion: Subject experiences thoughts imposed by some external force on his passive mind.
6. Thought diffusion or broadcasting: Subject experiences that his thoughts are escaping the confines of his self and are being experienced by others around.

C. Passivity Phenomena

7. 'Made' feelings or affect.
8. 'Made' impulses.
9. 'Made' volition or acts.
   In 'made' affect, impulses and volitions, the subject experiences feelings, impulses or acts which are imposed by some external force. In 'made' volition, one's own acts are experienced as being under the control of some external force, the subject being like a robot.
10. Somatic passivity: Bodily sensations, especially sensory symptoms, are experienced as imposed on body by some external force.

D. Delusional Perception

11. Delusional perception: Normal perception has a private and illogical meaning.

Kurt Schneider

Kurt Schneider (1959) described symptoms which, though not specific of schizophrenia, were of great help in making a clinical diagnosis. These are popularly called as *Schneider's first rank symptoms* (*FRS* or *SFRS*) of schizophrenia (Table 5.2). He also described the *second rank symptoms* of schizophrenia (considered less important for diagnosis of schizophrenia), like other forms of hallucinations, perplexity, and affect disturbances.

These symptoms (SFRS) have been described in some detail here as they have very often been used for diagnosis of schizophrenia and have significantly influenced the diagnosis and classification of schizophrenia and related disorders. As mentioned earlier, they are not specific for schizophrenia and may be seen in other psychiatric disorders like mood disorders and organic psychiatric disorders.

EPIDEMIOLOGY

According to the World (Mental) Health Report 2001, 24 million people worldwide suffer from schizophrenia.

The point prevalence of schizophrenia is about 0.5-1%. Schizophrenia is prevalent across racial, socio-cultural and national boundaries, with a few exceptions in the prevalence rates in some isolated communities.

The incidence of schizophrenia is currently about 0.5 per 1000. The onset of schizophrenia occurs usually later in females and often runs a more benign course, as compared to males.

CLINICAL FEATURES

Schizophrenia is characterized by disturbances in thought and verbal behavior, perception, affect, motor behavior and relationship to the external world. The diagnosis is entirely clinical and is based on the following clinical features, none of which are pathognomonic alone.

I. Thought and Speech Disorders

Autistic thinking is one of the most important features of schizophrenia. Here the thinking is governed by private and illogical rules. The patient may consider two things identical because they have identical predicates or properties (*von Domarus Law*); e.g. Lord Rama was a Hindu, I am a Hindu; So, I am Lord Rama.

Loosening of associations is a pattern of spontaneous speech in which things said in juxtaposi-tion lack a meaningful relationship or there is idiosyncratic shifting from one frame of reference to another. The speech is often described as being 'disjointed'. If loosening becomes very severe, speech becomes virtually incomprehensible. This is known as *incoherence*.

Thought blocking is a characteristic feature of schizophrenia, although it can also be seen in complex partial seizures (temporal lobe epilepsy). There is a sudden interruption of stream of speech before the thought is completed. After a pause, the subject can not recall what he had meant to say. This may be associated with thought withdrawal.

Neologisms are newly formed words or phrases whose derivation can not be understood. These are created to express a concept for which the subject has no dictionary word. Sometimes, normal words are used in an unconventional or distorted way but the derivation can be understood, even if bizarre. These are called *word approximations* or *paraphasias*; e.g. describing stomach as a 'food vessel'.

A schizophrenic patient may show complete *mutism* (with no speech production), *poverty of speech* (decreased speech production), *poverty of ideation* (speech amount is adequate but content conveys little information), *echolalia* (repetition or echo by patient of the words or phrases of examiner), *perseveration* (persistent repetition of words beyond their relevance), or *verbigeration* (senseless repetition of same words or phrases over and over again). These are disorders of verbal behavior or speech.

Delusions are false unshakable beliefs which are not in keeping with patient's socio-cultural and educational background. These are of two types: primary and secondary.

1. *Primary delusions* arise de novo and can not be explained on the basis of other experiences or perceptions. Also known as *autochthonous delusions*, these are characteristic of schizophrenia and are usually seen in early stages.
2. *Secondary delusions* are the commonest delusions seen in clinical practice and are not diagnostic of schizophrenia as these can be seen in other psychoses too. Secondary delusions can be explained as arising from other abnormal experiences.

The commonly seen delusions in schizophrenia include:

i. Delusions of persecution (being persecuted against, e.g. 'people are against me').
ii. Delusions of reference (being referred to by others; e.g. 'people talking about me').
iii. Delusions of grandeur (exaggerated self importance).
iv. Delusions of control (being controlled by an external force, known or unknown).
v. Somatic (or hypochondriacal) delusions.

The other clinical features of schizophrenic thought disorder include: *overinclusion* (tending to include irrelevant items in speech), *impaired abstraction* (loss of ability to generalize), *concreteness* (due to impaired abstraction), *perplexity* and *ambivalence*.

The Schneider's first rank symptoms (e.g. thought insertion, thought withdrawal, thought broadcasting, 'made' feeling, 'made' impulses and 'made' volitions) have already been discussed earlier.

II. Disorders of Perception

Hallucinations (perceptions without stimuli) are common in schizophrenia. *Auditory hallucinations* are by far the most frequent. These can be:

i. Elementary auditory hallucinations (i.e. hearing simple sounds rather than voices)
ii. 'Thought echo' ('audible thoughts')
iii. 'Third person hallucinations' ('voices heard arguing', discussing the patient in third person)
iv. 'Voices commenting on one's action'.

Only the 'third person hallucinations' are characteristic of schizophrenia.

Visual hallucinations can also occur, usually along with auditory hallucinations. Tactile, gustatory and olfactory types are less common.

III. Disorders of Affect

These include apathy, emotional blunting, emotional shallowness, anhedonia (incapability of experiencing pleasure) and inappropriate emotional response (emotional response inappropriate to thought).

The incapacity of schizophrenic patient to establish emotional contact with other individuals leads to a *lack of rapport* with the physician.

IV. Disorders of Motor Behavior

There can be either a decrease in psychomotor activity (decreased spontaneity, inertia, stupor) or an increase (excitement, aggressiveness, restlessness, agitation).

Mannerisms, grimacing, *stereotypies* (repetitive strange behavior), decreased self care, and poor grooming are common features. *Catatonic features* are commonly seen in catatonic schizophrenia (and are discussed in detail under that heading).

V. Negative Symptoms

The prominent negative symptoms of schizophrenia include *affective flattening* or *blunting*, *attentional impairment*, *avolition-apathy* (lack of initiative), *anhedonia* (inability to experience pleasure), *asociality* (social withdrawal), and *alogia* (lack of speech output).

VI. Other Features

1. Decreased functioning in work, social relations and self-care, as compared to earlier levels.
2. Loss of ego boundaries (feeling of blurring of boundaries of self with the environment; uncertainty and perplexity regarding own identity and meaning of existence).
3. Multiple somatic symptoms, especially in the early stages.
4. Insight (into the illness) is absent and judgement is usually poor.
5. Suicide can occur in schizophrenia due to several reasons, which include the presence of associated depression, command hallucinations (commanding the patient to commit suicide), impulsive behavior, anhedonia, or return of insight in the illness.
6. There is usually no disturbance of consciousness, orientation, attention, memory and intelligence.
7. There is usually a marked 'variability' in symptomatology over time.
8. There is no underlying organic cause.
9. There is no prominent mood disorder of depressive or manic type.

DIAGNOSIS

According to ICD-10 (CDDG), for the diagnosis of schizophrenia, a minimum of 1 very clear symptom (and usually 2 or more if less clear cut) belonging to any one of the groups referred to as (a) to (d) below, or symptoms from at least 2 of the groups referred to as (e) to (h), should have been clearly present for most of the time *during a period of 1 month or more* (DSM-IV-TR on the other hand requires a minimum period of 6 months). If the duration is less than 1 month, then a diagnosis of acute schizophrenia-like psychotic disorder should be made.

a. Thought echo, thought insertion or withdrawal, or thought broadcasting;
b. Delusions of control, influence, or passivity, clearly referred to body or limb movements or specific thoughts, actions, or sensations; Delusional perception;
c. Hallucinatory voices giving a running commentary on the patient's behavior or discussing the patient among themselves, or other types of hallucinatory voices coming from some part of the body;
d. Persistent delusions of other kinds that are culturally inappropriate and completely impossible (e.g. being able to control the weather, or being in communication with aliens from another world);
e. Persistent hallucinations in any modality, when accompanied by fleeting or half-formed delusions without clear affective content, or by persistent over-valued ideas, or when occurring every day for weeks or months on end;
f. Breaks, or interpolations in the train of thought, resulting in coherence or irrelevant speech, or Neologisms;
g. Catatonic behavior, such as excitement, posturing or waxy flexibility, negativism, mutism, and stupor;
h. 'Negative symptoms', such as marked apathy, paucity of speech, and blunting or incongruity of emotional responses, usually resulting in social withdrawal and lowering of social performance; it must be clear that these are not due to depression or to neuroleptic medication;
i. A significant and consistent change in the overall quality of some aspects of personal behavior, manifest as loss of interest, aimlessness, idleness, a self-absorbed attitude, and social withdrawal.

If the patient also meets criteria for manic episode or depressive episode, the guidelines mentioned above must have been met *before* the disturbance of mood developed. The disorder is not diagnosed in the presence of overt brain disease, or alcohol- or drug-related intoxication, dependence, or withdrawal.

CLINICAL TYPES

Schizophrenia can be classified into the following subtypes:

1. Paranoid
2. Hebephrenic
3. Catatonic
4. Residual
5. Undifferentiated
6. Simple
7. Post-schizophrenic depression
8. Others.

The catatonic and hebephrenic schizophrenias together are called as *nuclear schizophrenia*, as they present with typical symptomatology of schizophrenia and most frequently end in personality deterioration over time.

I. Paranoid Schizophrenia

Paranoid schizophrenia is characterized by the following features, in addition to the general guidelines of schizophrenia described earlier:

1. Delusions of persecution, reference, grandeur (or 'grandiosity'), control, or infidelity (or 'jealousy'). The delusions are usually well-systematized (i.e. thematically well connected with each other).
2. The hallucinations usually have a persecutory or grandiose content.
3. Disturbances of affect, volition, speech, and motor behavior.

The personality deterioration is much less than in other types of schizophrenias. Patients may be apprehensive (due to delusions and hallucinations), evasive and guarded on mental status examination.

The onset of paranoid schizophrenia is usually insidious, occurs later in life (i.e., late 3rd and early 4th decade) as compared to the other types of schizophrenias. The course is usually progressive and complete recovery usually does not occur. There may be frequent remissions and relapses. At times, the functional capability may be only slightly impaired. Differential diagnosis is from delusional (paranoid) disorders and paranoid personality disorders.

TABLE 5.3. SOME IMPORTANT CLINICAL FEATURES OF RETARDED CATATONIA

- i. **Mutism**: Complete absence of speech
- ii. **Rigidity**: Maintenance of a rigid posture against efforts to be moved
- iii. **Negativism**: An apparently motiveless resistance to all commands and attempts to be moved, or doing just the opposite
- iv. **Posturing**: Voluntary assumption of an inappropriate and often bizarre posture for long periods of time
- v. **Stupor**: Akinesis (no movement) with mutism but with evidence of relative preservation of conscious awareness
- vi. **Echolalia**: Repetition, echo or mimicking of phrases or words heard
- vii. **Echopraxia**: Repetition, echo or mimicking of actions observed
- viii. **Waxy flexibility**: Parts of body can be placed in positions that will be maintained for long periods of time, even if very uncomfortable; flexible like wax
- ix. **Ambitendency**: Due to ambivalence, conflicting impulses, tentative actions are made, but no goal directed action occurs, e.g. on asking to take out tongue, tongue is slightly protruded but taken back again
- x. **Other Signs**: Like *mannerisms*, *stereotypies* (verbal and behavioral), *automatic obedience* (commands are followed automatically, irrespective of their nature) and *verbigeration* (incomprehensible speech).

II. Disorganized (or Hebephrenic) Schizophrenia

Disorganized schizophrenia is characterized by the following features, in addition to the general guidelines of schizophrenia described earlier:

1. Marked thought disorder, incoherence and severe loosening of associations. Delusions and hallucinations are fragmentary and changeable.
2. Emotional disturbances (inappropriate affect, blunted affect, or senseless giggling), mannerisms, 'mirror-gazing' (for long periods of time), disinhibited behavior, poor self care and hygiene, markedly impaired social and occupational functioning, extreme social withdrawal and other oddities of behavior.

ICD-10 (CDDG) recommends a period of 2 or 3 months of continuous observation for a confident diagnosis of hebephrenic schizophrenia to be made.

The onset is insidious, usually in the early 2nd decade. The course is progressive and downhill. The recovery from the episode classically never occurs. Severe deterioration, without (significant) remissions, usually occurs over time. Hebephrenic schizophrenia has one of the worst prognosis among the subtypes of schizophrenia.

III. Catatonic Schizophrenia

Catatonic schizophrenia is characterized by marked disturbance of motor behavior, in addition to the general guidelines of schizophrenia described earlier. (*Cata:* disturbed, *tonic:* tone). It can present in three clinical forms: excited catatonia, stuporous catatonia, and catatonia alternating between excitement and stupor.

1. Excited Catatonia

This is characterized by the following features:

i. Increase in psychomotor activity, ranging from restlessness, agitation, excitement, aggressiveness to, at times, violent behavior (*furor*).
ii. Increase in speech production, with increased spontaneity, pressure of speech, loosening of associations and frank incoherence.

The excitement has no relationship with the environment; instead inner stimuli (e.g. thought and impulses) influence the excited behavior. So, the excitement is not goal-directed. Sometimes the excitement can become very severe, and is accompanied by rigidity, hyperthermia and dehydration, finally culminating in death. It is then known as *acute lethal catatonia or pernicious catatonia.* Fortunately, with availability of anti-psychotics, and early diagnosis and treatment, *lethal catatonia* is becoming increasingly rare.

2. Stuporous (or Retarded) Catatonia

This is characterized by extreme retardation of psychomotor function. Characteristic catatonic signs (Table 5.3) are usually observed. Delusions and hallucinations may be present but are not prominent. Not all the features are present at the same time.

3. Catatonia Alternating between Excitement and Stupor

This clinical picture is very common. The features of both excited catatonia and stuporous catatonia are alternatingly present.

The onset of catatonic schizophrenia is usually acute, usually in the late 2nd and early 3rd decade. The course is often episodic and recovery form the episode is usually complete. However, residual features are present after two or more episodes. Differential diagnosis is from other causes of stupor and catatonia. (This is discussed in detail in Chapter 19).

IV. Residual and Latent Schizophrenia

Residual schizophrenia is similar to *latent schizophrenia* and symptoms are similar to prodromal symptoms of schizophrenia. The only difference is that residual schizophrenia is diagnosed after at least one episode has occurred.

According to ICD-10 (CDDG), it is characterized by the following features, in addition to the general guidelines of schizophrenia described earlier:

1. Prominent 'negative' schizophrenic symptoms, i.e. psychomotor slowing, underactivity, blunting of affect, passivity and lack of initiative, poverty of quantity or content of speech, poor nonverbal communication by facial expression, eye contact, voice modulation, and posture, poor self-care and social performance;
2. Evidence in the past of at least one clear-cut psychotic episode meeting the diagnostic criteria for schizophrenia;
3. A period of at least 1 year during which the intensity and frequency of florid symptoms such as delusions and hallucinations have been minimal or substantially reduced and the 'negative' schizophrenic syndrome has been present;
4. Absence of dementia or other organic brain disease or disorder, and of chronic depression or institutionalism sufficient to explain the negative impairments.

V. Undifferentiated Schizophrenia

This is a very common type of schizophrenia and is diagnosed either when features of no subtype are fully present or features of more than one subtype are exhibited. though general criteria for diagnosis of schizophrenia are met.

VI. Simple Schizophrenia

Although called simple, it is one of the subtypes most difficult to diagnose. It is characterized by an early onset (early 2nd decade), very insidious and progressive course, presence of characteristic 'negative symptoms' of residual schizophrenia (like marked social withdrawal, shallow emotional response, with loss of initiative and drive), vague hypochondriacal features, a drift down the social ladder, and living shabbily and wandering aimlessly. Delusions and hallucinations are usually absent, and if present they are short lasting and poorly systematized.

The prognosis is usually very poor.

VII. Post-Schizophrenic Depression

Some schizophrenic patients develop depressive features within 12 months of an acute episode of schizophrenia. The depressive features develop in the presence of residual or active features of schizophrenia and are associated with an increased risk of suicide. Depressive features can occur due to side-effect of antipsychotics, regaining insight after recovery, or just be an integral part of schizophrenia.

It is important to distinguish the depressive features from negative symptoms of schizophrenia and "extrapyramidal" side-effects of antipsychotic medication.

VIII. Other Subtypes

Historically, there are many other subtypes of schizophrenia described, but a majority of them would easily fit in one of the above-mentioned seven subtypes. A few are briefly mentioned due to their historical interest and their popular names; while others are important in their own right.

A. Pseudoneurotic Schizophrenia

Pseudoneurotic schizophrenia was described by Hoch and Polatin. In initial phases, there are predominant neurotic symptoms that last for years and show poor response to treatment.

Three classical features are *pan-anxiety* (diffuse, free-floating anxiety which hardly ever subsides), *pan-neurosis* (almost all neurotic symptoms may be present). and *pan-sexuality* (constant preoccupation with sexual problems).

Now-a-days, this subtype is subsumed under *borderline personality disorder*.

B. Schizophreniform Disorder

This is a diagnostic category in DSM-IV-TR with features of schizophrenia as diagnostic

TABLE 5:4. TYPE I AND TYPE II SCHIZOPHRENIA

Features	Type I	Type II
1. Characteristic symptoms	Positive symptoms, e.g. delusions, hallucinations and thought disorder	Negative symptoms, e.g. affective flattening, alogia, anhedonia-asociality, avolition-apathy, and attentional impairment
2. Type of illness	Acute	Chronic (Defect state)
3. Response to neuroleptics	Good	Poor
4. Outcome	Reversible	Probably irreversible
5. Intellectual impairment	Absent	Sometimes present
6. Postulated pathological process	Increased DA receptors	Cell loss and brain changes
7. CT Scan Brain	Normal	Dilated lateral ventricles

TABLE 5.5. PROGNOSTIC FACTORS IN SCHIZOPHRENIA

Good Prognostic Factors	Poor Prognostic Factors
1. Acute or abrupt onset	1. Insidious onset
2. Onset > 35 years of age (late onset)	2. Onset < 20 years of age (early onset)
3. Presence of precipitating stressor	3. Absence of stressor
4. Good premorbid adjustment	4. Poor premorbid adjustment
5. Catatonic subtype (Paranoid subtype has an intermediate prognosis)	5. Disorganized, simple, undifferentiated, or chronic catatonic subtypes
6. Short duration (< 6 months)	6. Chronic course (> 2 years)
7. Presence of depression	7. Absence of depression
8. Predominance of positive symptoms	8. Predominance of negative symptoms
9. Family history of mood disorder	9. Family history of schizophrenia
10. First episode	10. Past history of schizophrenia
11. Pyknic (fat) physique	11. Asthenic (thin) physique
12. Female sex	12. Male sex
13. Good social support	13. Poor social support or unmarried
14. Presence of confusion, perplexity, or disorientation in the acute phase	14. Flat or blunted affect
15. Proper treatment, good treatment compliance, and good response to treatment	15. Absence of proper treatment or poor response to treatment
16. Outpatient treatment	16. Institutionalization (long term hospitalization)
17. Normal cranial CT scan	17. Evidence of ventricular enlargement on cranial CT scan

criteria. The only difference is that the duration is less than 6 months and prognosis is usually better than that of schizophrenia. This term was originally introduced by Langfeldt (1961) to designate good prognosis cases, distinct from "true" schizophrenia.

A similar condition in ICD-10 is called *acute schizophrenia-like psychotic disorder* (see Chapter 7).

C. Oneiroid Schizophrenia

Described by Mayer-Gross, This is a subtype of schizophrenia with acute onset, clouding of consciousness, disorientation, dream-like states (*oneiroid* means 'dream'), and perceptual disturbances with rapid shifting.

The episode is usually brief.

D. Van Gogh Syndrome

Dramatic self-mutilation occurring in schizophrenia has been also called as *Van Gogh syndrome*, after the name of the famous painter Van Gogh who had cut his ear during the active phase of illness.

E. Late Paraphrenia

Described by Sir Martin Roth, this is a disorder which occurs late in life, usually in the sixth decade. It is more common in women, especially unmarried or widowed women. Delusions of persecution are seen, with bizarre and fantastic contents like being raped or gassed or strangers entering their rooms and interfering.

Hallucinations of all kinds (visual, auditory, tactile, gustatory and olfactory) can be present. Intelligence and judgement outside the area of persecutory delusions are normal. Approximately 25-40% of patients have some defect of sight or hearing.

Presently, this syndrome is placed under paranoid schizophrenia, late onset type.

F. Pfropf Schizophrenia

This is a syndrome of schizophrenia occurring in the presence of mental retardation. It differs from schizophrenia in only that there is poverty of ideation and delusions are not very well-systematized. The behavioral disturbances are more prominent than thought disorder.

G. Type I and Type II Schizophrenia

T. J. Crow has divided schizophrenia into two subtypes, namely type I and II schizophrenias (Table 5.4).

Although a useful concept theoretically, it has not been found to be really valid in the recent research studies. Very few patients have a pure type I or type II syndrome; admixtures are far more common.

DIFFERENTIAL DIAGNOSIS

The first step in the differential diagnosis is to exclude psychoses with known organic causes, e.g. complex partial seizures, drug-induced psychoses (like amphetamine-induced psychoses), metabolic disturbances, or cerebral neoplasm.

The second step is to rule out a possibility of mood disorder (mania, depression, or mixed affective disorder) or schizo-affective disorder.

The third step is exclude the possibility of other non-organic psychoses like delusional disorders, or acute and transient psychotic disorders (ATPD).

PROGNOSIS

The prognostic factors in schizophrenia are summarized in Table 5.5.

COURSE AND OUTCOME

Since the time of Kraepelin, when the disorder was conceptualized as dementia precox, schizophrenia has been associated with a progressive downhill course, with a large number of patients hospitalized in mental asylums.

However, the longitudinal studies suggest that this pattern occurs in only a minority of patients. According to a major study (Luc Ciompi 1980), where 5661 cases were followed up for an average of 36.9 years, the outcome was as follows:

- Complete remission (27%)
- Remission with minor residual deficit (22%)
- Intermediate outcome (24%)
- Severe disability (18%)
- Unstable or uncertain outcome (9%)

So, almost 50% patients showed complete or near complete recovery, and only 18% showed severe disability with only 9% needing institutionalization.

A Study of Factors Associated with Course and Outcome of Schizophrenia (SOFACOS) was conducted by ICMR (Indian Council of

TABLE 5.6. IPSS OUTCOME

Outcome Average	Nine countries	India	Nigeria	Denmark
Extremely good and good outcome	51%	66%	86%	35%

Medical Research) at 3 centres (Vellore, Madras and Lucknow) in India. A total of 386 patients were followed up for a period of 5 years (1981 to 1986), at the end of which the outcome was as follows:

- Very favorable outcome (27%)
- Favorable outcome (40%)
- Intermediate outcome (31%)
- Unfavorable outcome (2%)

So, about 2/3rd (67%) of the patients had a favorable outcome as compared to 50% in Luc Ciompi's study.

IPSS (International Pilot Study on Schizophrenia), conducted on 811 schizophrenic patients selected in 1968-1969 [patients selected from 9 countries, namely USA, Columbia, UK, Czechoslovakia, USSR (now CIS), India, Nigeria, Denmark and China], found similar outcome results.

The course and prognosis of schizophrenia is better in the developing countries like India, than in developed countries (Table 5.6).

In ICD-10, the course of schizophrenia is specified under *continuous; episodic with progressive deficit; episodic with stable deficit; episodic remittent; incomplete remission;* or *complete remission*. If the period of observation is less than one year, the course is not specified.

Some studies have suggested that longer the DUP (duration of untreated psychosis), worse is the outcome, undelining the importance of early diagnosis and treatment of schizophrenia.

There is an increased mortality in patients with schizophrenia by almost one and a half times. The most important cause of death is suicide, the life-time risk of which is 5-10 times higher in schizophrenia as compared to normal population.

ETIOLOGY

The etiology of schizophrenia is currently unknown. However, several theories have been propounded; these include the following:

I. Biological Theories

1. Genetic Hypothesis

About 10% of first degree relatives (and 3% of second degree relatives and 2% of third degree relatives) of schizophrenic patients have schizophrenia, as compared with the 0.5-1% prevalence rate in the general population.

The concordance rate for monozygotic twins is 46% and for dizygotic twins is 14%. If one parent has schizophrenia, the chances of the child developing schizophrenia are 10-14%. However, if both parents have schizophrenia, chances of the child developing schizophrenia increase to about 46%.

Therefore, genetic factors are very important in making an individual vulnerable to schizophrenia. However, the environmental factors are probably important in precipitating an episode in some individuals.

2. Biochemical Theories

Schizophrenia is presently thought to be probably due to a functional increase of dopamine at the post-synaptic receptor, though other neurotransmitters like serotonin (especially 5-HT_2 receptors), GABA and acetylcholine are also presumably involved.

3. Brain imaging

Cranial CT Scan, MRI Scan, and post-mortem studies show *enlarged ventricles* (not amounting to hydrocephalus) and *mild cortical atrophy* (with an overall reduction in brain volume and cortical grey matter by 5-10%) in some patients of schizophrenia.

PET (positron emission tomography) scan shows hypofrontality and decreased glucose utilization in the dominant temporal lobe. Attempts are being made to localize symptoms of schizophrenia (like auditory

TABLE 5.7. ANTIPSYCHOTIC DOSAGE IN SCHIZOPHRENIA

Drug	Oral Dose Range (mg/day)	Parenteral Dose (mg/day)	Equivalent Oral Dose (Equal To 100 mg. CPZ)
A. TYPICAL OR TRADITIONAL ANTIPSYCHOTICS			
1. Chlorpromazine (CPZ)	300-1500	50-100 IM	100
2. Thioridazine	300-800	—	90-100
3. Trifluoperazine	15-60	1-5 IM	5
4. Haloperidol	5-100	5-20 IM/IV	2
5. Pimozide	4-12	—	2
6. Triflupromazine	100-400	30-60 IM	25
7. Prochlorperazine	45-150	40-80 IM	15
8. Flupenthixol	3-10	—	—
9. Loxapine	25-150	—	10
10. Zuclopenthixol	50-150	50-100 IM	—
B. ATYPICAL OR NEWER ANTIPSYCHOTICS			
11. Clozapine	25-450	—	50
12. Risperidone	2-8	—	1-2
13. Olanzapine	5-20	—	2-3
14. Ziprasidone	40-160	—	20

hallucina-tions, negative symptoms) to the various brain regions by PET studies.

4. Other Theories

The following findings also point towards a biological basis of schizophrenia.

Antipsychotics, which act by blocking the dopamine (D_2) receptor, cause significant improvement in schizophrenia and relapse occurs on stopping antipsychotic medication. The newer, atypical antipsychotics (like risperi-done) are D_2-5-HT_2 antagonists.

Drugs, like LSD, amphetamines and mescaline, can cause schizophrenia-like symptoms in normal subjects. Organic mental disorders with schizophrenia-like symptoms may be seen in Huntington's chorea (early stages), homocystinuria, acute intermittent porphyria, Wilson's disease and hemachromatosis.

Soft neurological signs (SNS), minor physical anomalies, and impaired eye tracking (smooth pursuit eye movements) are more often seen in patients with schizophrenia than in normal persons.

Viral and auto-immune factors have been implicated by some, while others (Weinberger) have suggested a neurodevelopmental hypothesis.for schizophrenia.

II. Psychological Theories

1. Stress

Increased number of stressful life events before the onset or relapse probably has a triggering effect on the onset of schizophrenia, in a vulnerable (e.g. genetic vulnerability) person (*Stress-vulnerability hypothesis*).

Increased EE or *expressed emotions* (e.g. hostility, critical comments, emotional over-involvement) of 'significant others' in the family can lead to early relapse.

2. Family Theories

Several theories have been propounded in the past but are currently of doubtful value. These include 'schizophrenogenic mothers', lack of 'real' parents, dependency on mother, anxious mother, parental marital schism or skew, double-bind theory, communication deviance, and pseudo-mutuality.

Several other theories have also been propounded but are currently of doubtful value as theories of causation.

3. Information Processing Hypothesis

Disturbances in attention, inability to maintain a set, and inability to assimilate and integrate percepts are common findings in schizophrenia. Schizophrenics may at first be overly attentive to stimuli but later may reduce or exclude attention to stimuli. There is possibly a breakdown in the *internal representation* of mental events.

4. Psychoanalytical Theories

According to Freud, there is regression to the pre-oral (and oral) stage of psycho-sexual development, with the use of defense mechanisms of denial, projection, and reaction formation (see Table 17.1). There is a loss of ego-boundaries (described by Federn), with a loss of touch with reality.

III. Socio-Cultural Theories

Although the prevalence of schizophrenia is quite uniform across cultures, it was found to be more common in lower socio-economic status in some studies. This has now been explained due to a *'downward social drift'* which is a result of schizophrenia rather than its cause.

Slightly higher rates of schizophrenia have been found among some migrants, not only among the "first generation" migrants but also among the "second generation.

MANAGEMENT

The management of schizophrenia can be discussed under the following headings:

1. Somatic treatment
   a) Pharmacological treatment
   b) Electro-convulsive therapy (ECT)
   c) Others.
2. Psychosocial treatment and rehabilitation.

1. Pharmacological Treatment

The first drug to be used with beneficial effect in schizophrenia was reserpine (*Rauwolfia serpentina* extract), in India by Sen and Bose (1931). Reserpine is no longer used for treatment of schizophrenia.

Antipsychotics were formally discovered by Delay and Deniker in 1952. Since their introduction, they have changed the outcome of schizophrenia significantly. These are discussed in detail in Chapter 15. Only some relevant points are mentioned here.

The commonly used antipsychotics are listed in Table 5.7 with their routinely used dosage.

Risperidone, olanzapine, trifluoperazine, haloperidol, ziprasidone, and chlorpromazine are commonly used in acute stages. Atypical antipsychotics, like risperidone, olanzapine and ziprasidone are also useful when negative symptoms (e.g. social withdrawal, emotional blunting and apathy) are prominent, in chronic schizophrenia.

Clozapine, another atypical antipsychotic, is available in the Indian market. Clinical trials have shown that clozapine is effective in about 30% of patients who had no beneficial response to traditional antipsychotics. However, as it can cause agranulocytosis and seizures as side-effects, it should be used with caution.

Drug treatment is usually given in the *outpatient setting* as:

1. There are very few number of psychiatric beds in our country,
2. Majorities of families are willing to care for the patients at home, and
3. Majority of patients do not require hospi talization.

However, *hospitalization* is indicated if there is:

1. Neglect of food and water intake,
2. Danger to self or others,
3. Poor drug compliance,
4. Significant neglect of self care, or
5. Lack of social support.

In presence of *acute excitement*, haloperidol 10-20 mg IV or IM, with/without 10 mg diazepam or 50 mg of promethazine can be given. Chlorpromazine 50-100 mg IM can also be given but painful injection abscess at the injection site may develop. Chlorpromazine should never be given IV, as severe hypotension can occur.

A majority of patients require *maintenance treatment* with antipsychotics to prevent relapse. Although there are no clear-cut rules, generally treatment is continued for 6 months to 1 year for the first episode, for 1 to 2 years for the subsequent episodes, and for indefinite period for repeated episodes or persistent symptoms. However, the decision regarding the duration of treatment in a particular case has to be assessed individually by the treating psychiatrist.

To ensure drug compliance, depot preparations with long duration of action can be used. The following preparations are presently available in India:

1. Fluphenazine decanoate, 25-50 mg IM is given every 2-3 weeks.
2. Penfluridol, 20-60 mg oral is given every week.
3. Flupenthixol decanoate, 20-40 mg IM, given every 2 weeks.
4. Haloperidol decanoate, 100-250 mg IM, given every 4 weeks.
5. Zuclopenthixol decanoate, 200-400 mg IM, given every 2-4 weeks.

Many patients require adjuvant antiparkinsonian medication to prevent extrapyramidal side-effects, e.g. trihexiphenidyl 6 mg/day, biperidin 6 mg/day, orphenadrin 150 mg/day, procyclidine 7.5 mg/day. This is particularly true if the patient is receiving traditional antipsychotics (like haloperidol), though one of the atypical antipsychotics, namely risperidone, also causes extrapyramidal symptoms.

Ideally during the hospitalization, no patient should receive anticholinergic antiparkinsonian medication till the extrapyramidal side-effects appear. Anticholinergics can worsen cognitive function, have an abuse potential, can cause delirium (especially in elderly), can worsen or contribute to negative symptoms in schizophrenia, and may increase the risk of TD (tardive dyskinesia). But, often a majority of patients do receive anticholinergics in addition to traditional antipsychotics.

Antipsychotics probably act by blocking postsynaptic dopamine (D_2) receptors probably in the meso-limbic system. Other receptors like 5-HT, muscarinic receptors and GABA are also probably important. Atypical antipsychotics are also called as SDAs (Serotonin-Dopamine Antagonists) beacuse of their action on both dopamine and 5-HT.

2. Electroconvulsive Therapy (ECT)

Schizophrenia is not a primary indication for ECT. Indications for ECT in schizophrenia include:

1. Catatonic stupor.
2. Uncontrolled catatonic excitement.

3. Acute exacerbation not controlled with drugs.
4. Severe side-effect with drugs, in presence of untreated schizophrenia.

Usually 8-12 ECTs are needed (although up to 18 have been given in poor responders), given three times a week.

3. Miscellaneous Treatments

Psychosurgery is usually not indicated in schizophrenia. When used, the treatment of choice is *limbic leucotomy* (a small subcaudate lesion with a cingulate lesion) in some cases with severe and very prominent depression, anxiety or obsessional symptoms.

Severely deteriorated patients are unlikely to benefit. The maximum benefit would be in acute episodes, but antipsychotics are far better obviously both in efficacy and safety.

Many other methods like megavitamin therapy, dialysis, malaria therapy, high dose propranolol, and insulin coma therapy have been used in past but are no longer popularly used.

5. Psychosocial Treatment

Psychosocial treatment can be divided in following steps:

i. *Psychoeducation* of the patient and especially the family regarding the nature of illness, its course and treatment. Psychoeducation helps in establishing a good therapeutic relationship with the patient (and family), an important ingredient of successful management of schizophrenia.

ii. *Group psychotherapy* is particularly aimed at
   a) teaching problem solving, and
   b) teaching communication skills.

   It is usually conducted in a form which is known as '*social skills training package*'.

iii. *Family therapy*: Apart from education, family members are also provided social skills training to enhance communication and decrease family tensions.

   Attempts are made to decrease '*expressed emotions*' (EE) of the 'significant others' in the family. The family is taught to decrease expectations and to avoid critical remarks, emotional over-involvement, and hostility.

iv. *Millieu therapy* (or therapeutic community) includes treatment in a living, learning or working environment ranging from inpatient psychiatric unit to day-care hospitals and half-way homes.

v. *Individual psychotherapy* is usually supportive in nature. Rarely, psychoanalytically oriented psychotherapy is used. However, the current consensus does not recommend the use of psychoanalytic psychotherapy in treatment of schizophrenia.

vi. *Psychosocial rehabilitation* is used, usually along with millieu therapy.

   This includes *activity therapy*, to develop the work habit, *training* in a new vocation or *retraining* in a previous skill, *vocational guidance*, independent job placement, *sheltered employment* or self-employment, and *occupational therapy*.

However, antipsychotic drug treatment in the acute stages, as well as for maintenance treatment, is the mainstay of management of schizophrenia.

Psychosocial treatment is an important adjunct to drug treatment which enhances its efficacy and leads to a more complete recovery and rehabilitation. However, it is unlikely that psychosocial treatment, in the absence of drug treatment, will be of substantial help.

6 Mood Disorders

The *emotions* can be described as two main types:

1. *Affect*, which is a *short-lived* emotional response to an idea or an event, and
2. *Mood*, which is a *sustained and pervasive* emotional response which colors the whole psychic life.

So according to these definitions, depression and mania are *'mood disorders'* and not 'affective disorders' as they have been called so frequently. Throughout this chapter (and this book), the more correct word *'mood disorder'* will be used (as in DSM-IV-TR and ICD-10).

Mood disorders have been known to man since antiquity. The Old Testament describes King Saul as suffering from severe depressive episodes responding slightly to David's soothing music. While Hippocrates coined the words mania and melancholia, it was Aretaeus who first described mania and depression occurring in the same individual.

Emil Kraepelin, borrowing from the work of Kahlbaum, Falret and Baillarger, described the manic-depressive illness as separate from dementia precox on the basis of course, clinical symptoms and outcome.

Recently, the World Health Report 2001 (WHO) has identified *unipolar depression* as the 4th cause of DALY (Disability-Adjusted Life Years) in all ages, and the 2nd Cause in 15-44 years. Unipolar depression is also the 1st Cause of YLD (Years of Life Lived with Disability) in all ages. The comparison was with all medical disorders, and not only psychiatric disorders.

The WHR-2001 estmates that there are 121 million people worldwide suffering from depression.

CLASSIFICATION

The classification of mood disorders is an area which is fraught with multiple controversies. According to the ICD-10 (CDDG), the mood disorders are classified as follows:

1. Manic episode
2. Depressive episode
3. Bipolar mood (affective) disorder
4. Recurrent depressive disorder
5. Persistent mood disorder (including cyclothymia and dysthymia)
6. Other mood disorders (including mixed affective episode and recurrent brief depressive disorder).

CLINICAL FEATURES AND DIAGNOSIS

I. Manic Episode

The life-time risk of manic episode is about 0.8-1%. This disorder tends to occur in episodes lasting usually 3-4 months, followed by complete recovery. Further episodes can be either manic or depressive.

A manic episode is characterized by following features (which should last for at least one week and cause disruption in occupational and social activities):

1. Elevated, Expansive or Irritable Mood

The elevated mood can pass through following four stages depending on the severity of manic episode:

a. *Euphoria* (mild elevation of mood): Increased sense of psychological well-being and happiness not in keeping with ongoing events. This is seen in hypomania (Stage I).
b. *Elation* (moderate elevation of mood): Feeling of confidence and enjoyment along with increased psychomotor activity. This is classical of mania (Stage II).
c. *Exaltation* (severe elevation of mood): Intense elation with delusions of grandeur; seen in severe mania (Stage III).
d. *Ecstasy* (very severe elevation of mood): Intense sense of rapture or blissfulness; seen in delirious or stuporous mania (Stage IV).

Along with these variations in elevation of mood, expansive mood may be present, which is unceasing and unselective enthusiasm for interacting with people and surrounding environment.

At times elevated mood may not be apparent; instead irritable mood may be predominant, especially when the person is stopped from doing what he wants.

There may be rapid, short lasting shifts from euphoria to depression or anger.

2. Psychomotor Activity

There is an increased psychomotor activity ranging from overactiveness and restlessness to manic excitement where the person is 'on-the-toe-on-the-go', (i.e. involved in ceaseless activity). The activity is usually goal-oriented and based on external environmental cues.

Rarely, a manic patient can go in to a stuporous state (*manic stupor*).

3. Speech and Thought

The person is more talkative than usual; describes thoughts racing in mind; develops pressure of speech; uses playful language with punning, rhyming, joking and teasing; and speaks loudly. Later, there is *'flight of ideas'* (rapidly produced speech with abrupt shifts from topic to topic, using environmental cues. Usually the connections between the shifts are apparent). When 'flight' becomes severe, incoherence may occur. On the other hand, a less severe and a more ordered 'flight', in the absence of pressure of speech, is called as *'prolixity'*.

There can be delusions (or ideas) of grandeur (grandiosity) with markedly inflated self-esteem. Delusions of persecution may some-times develop secondary to the delusions of grandeur (e.g. "I am so great that people are against me"). Hallucinations (both auditory and visual) with religious content can occur (e.g. "God appeared before me and spoke to me"). Since these psychotic symptoms are in keeping with the mood state, these are called as *'mood-congruent psychotic features'*.

Distractibility is common and results in rapid changes in speech and activity, in response to even irrelevant stimuli.

4. Goal-directed Activity

The person is unusually alert, trying to do many things at one time.

In hypomania, ability to function becomes much better and there is a marked increase in productivity and creativity. Many artists and writers have contributed significantly in such periods. As hypomania and mild forms of mania are difficult to detect if not looked for, it is really important to elicit additional historical information from reliable informants (e.g. family members).

In mania, there is marked increase in activity with excessive planning and at times execution of multiple activities. Due to being involved in so many activities and distractibility, there is decrease in functioning ability in later stages. There is marked increase in sociability even with previously unknown people. Gradually this sociability leads to an interfering behavior though the person does not recognize it as abnormal at that time.

The person becomes impulsive, shows disinhibition, sexual indiscretion and usually becomes hypersexual and promiscuous.

Due to grandiose ideation, increased sociability, overactivity and poor judgement, the manic person is involved in high-risk activities like buying sprees, reckless driving, foolish business investments, distributing money and/or personal articles to unknown persons. He is usually dressed up in gaudy and flamboyant clothes, although in severe mania there may be poor self-care.

5. Other Features

Sleep is usually reduced with a decreased need for sleep. Appetite may be increased but later there is usually decreased food intake, due to marked overactivity.

Insight into the illness is absent, especially in severe mania.

Psychotic features like delusions, hallucinations which are not understandable in the context of mood disorder (called *mood incongruent psychotic features*), e.g. delusions of persecution, may be present in some cases.

6. Absence of an Underlying Organic Cause

If manic episode is secondary to an organic cause, a diagnosis of organic mood disorder should be made.

II. Depressive Episode

The life-time risk of depression in males is 8-12% and in females is 20-26%, though the life-time risk of major depression or depressive episode is about 8%. The typical depressive episode is characterized by following features (which should last for at least two weeks):

TABLE 6.1. SOMATIC SYNDROME IN DEPRESSION (ICD-10)

The *somatic syndrome* is characterized by:

a. Significant decrease in appetite or weight
b. Early morning awakening, atleast 2 (or more) hours before the usual time of awaking
c. Diurnal variation, with depression being worst in the morning
d. Pervasive loss of interest and loss of reactivity to pleasurable stimuli
e. Psychomotor agitation or retardation.

1. Depressed Mood

The most important feature is the sadness of mood or loss of interest and/or pleasure in almost all activities (*pervasive sadness*), present throughout the day (*persistent sadness*). This sadness of mood is quantitatively as well as qualitatively different from sadness encountered in normal depression or grief. The depressed mood varies little from day to day and is often not responsive to environmental stimuli.

The loss of interest in daily activities results in social withdrawal, decreased ability to function in occupational and interpersonal areas and decreased involvement in previously pleasurable activities. In severe depression, there may be complete *anhedonia* (inability to experience pleasure).

2. Depressive Ideation/cognitions

Sadness of mood usually is associated with pessimism. This results in 3 common types of depressive ideas, i.e.

a. Hopelessness ('there is no hope in future due to pessimism').
b. Helplessness ('no help is possible').
c. Worthlessness ('feeling of inadequacy and inferiority').

The ideas of worthlessness can lead to self-reproach and guilt-feelings. Other features are difficulty in thinking, difficulty in concentra-

TABLE 6.2. SUICIDAL RISK: IMPORTANT FACTORS

Suicidal risk is much more in the presence of following factors:

a. Presence of marked hopelessness
b. Males; age > 40; unmarried, divorced or widowed
c. Written or verbal communication of suicidal intent and/or plan
d. Early stages of depression
e. Recovering from depression (At peak of depression, patient is usually either too depressed or too retarded to commit suicide)
f. Period of 3 months from recovery.

tion, indecisiveness, slowed thinking, subjective poor memory, lack of initiative and energy. Often there are ruminations (repetitive, intrusive thoughts) of pessimistic ideas. Thoughts of death and preoccupation with death are not uncommon.

Suicidal ideas may be present. In severe cases, Delusions of nihilism (e.g. 'world is coming to an end', 'there is no brain in the skull', 'intestines have rotted away') may occur.

3. Psychomotor Activity

In younger patients (< 40 year old), retardation is more common which is characterized by slowed thinking and activity, decreased energy and monotonous voice. In severe form, patient becomes stuporous (depressive stupor).

In older patients (e.g. post-menopausal women), agitation is commoner with marked anxiety, restlessness (inability to sit still, hand-wriggling, picking at body parts or other objects) and subjective feeling of unease.

Anxiety is a frequent accompaniment of depression. Irritability may present as easy annoyance and frustration in day-to-day activities, e.g. unusual anger at the noise made by children in the house.

4. Physical Symptoms

Multiple physical symptoms (like heaviness of head, vague body aches) are common in elderly depressives and depressive patients from developing countries (e.g. India). Hypochondriacal features may be present in up to a quarter of depressives presenting for treatment. These physical symptoms are almost always present in severe depressive episode.

Another common symptom is complaints of reduced energy and easy fatiguability. Patients, therefore, not surprisingly attribute their symptoms to physical cause(s).

5. Biological Functions

Disturbance of biological functions is common with insomnia (sometimes hypersomnia), loss of appetite and weight (sometimes hyperphagia and weight gain) and loss of sexual drive.

When the disturbance is severe, it is called as melancholia (*somatic syndrome* in ICD-10, Diagnostic Criteria for Research). The somatic syndrome of depression is described in Table 6.1.

The presence of somatic syndrome in depressive disorder signifies more severe and more biological nature of the disturbance. It often also implies a good response to somatic methods of treatment (e.g. pharmacotherapy, ECT).

6. Psychotic Features

15-20% of depressed patients have delusions, hallucinations, grossly inappropriate behavior or stupor. Psychotic features can be mood-congruent (e.g. nihilistic delusions, delusions of guilt, delusions of poverty, stupor) which are understandable in the light of depressed mood, or can be mood-incongruent (e.g. delusions of control) which are not directly related to depressive mood.

TABLE 6.3. SUBTYPES OF BIPOLAR DISORDER

1. **Bipolar I**
   Characterized by episodes of severe mania and severe depression.
2. **Bipolar II**
   Characterized by episodes of hypomania (not requiring hospitalization) and severe depression.

7. Suicide

Suicidal ideas in depression, if expressed, should be taken seriously. Although there is a risk of suicide in every depressed patient with suicidal ideation, presence of certain factors increases the risk of suicide (Table 6.2).

8. Absence of an Underlying Organic Cause

If depressive episode is secondary to an organic cause, a diagnosis of organic mood disorder should be made.

In ICD-10, the severity of depressive episode is defined as mild, moderate or severe, depend-ing primarily on the number of the symptoms, but also on the severity of symptoms and the the degree of impairment.

III. Bipolar Mood (Affective) Disorder

This disorder, earlier known as manic depressive psychosis (MDP), is characterized by recurrent episodes of mania episode and depression in the same patient at different times. These episodes can occur in any sequence. Patients with recurrent episodes of mania (unipolar mania) are also classified here as they are rare and often resemble the bipolar patients in their clinical features.

The current episode in bipolar mood disorder is specified as: hypomanic, manic without psychotic symptoms, manic with psychotic symptoms, mild or moderate depression, severe depression without psychotic symptoms, severe depression with psychotic symptoms, mixed, or in remission.

Bipolar mood disorder is further classified in to bipolar I and bipolar II disorders (Table 6.3).

IV. Recurrent Depressive Disorder

This disorder is characterized by recurrent (at least two) depressive episodes (unipolar depression). The current episode in recurrent depressive disorder is specified as: mild, moderate, severe without psychotic symptoms, severe with psychotic symptoms, or in remission.

V. Persistent Mood Disorder

These disorders are characterized by persistent mood symptoms which last for more than 2 years (1 year in children and adolescents) but are not severe enough to be labeled as even hypomanic or mild depressive episode. If the symptoms consist of persistent mild depression, the disorder is called as *dysthymia*; and if symptoms consist of persistent instability of mood between mild depression and mild elation, the disorder is called as *cyclothymia*.

VI. Other Mood Disorders

This category includes the diagnosis of mixed affective episode. This is a frequently missed diagnosis. In this type, full clinical picture of depression and mania is present either at the same time intermixed, or alternates rapidly with each other (*rapid cycling*), without a normal intervening period of euthymia.

COURSE AND PROGNOSIS

Bipolar mood disorder has an earlier age of onset (third decade) than recurrent depressive (unipolar) disorder. Unipolar depression is common in two age groups: late third decade and fifth to sixth decades.

An average manic episode lasts for 3-4 months while a depressive episode lasts from

TABLE 6.4. PROGNOSTIC FACTORS IN MOOD DISORDERS

Good Prognostic Factors
1. Acute or abrupt onset
2. Typical clinical features
3. Severe depression
4. Well adjusted premorbid personality
5. Good response to treatment.

Poor Prognostic Factors
1. Co-morbid medical disorder(s), personality disorder(s) or alcohol dependence
2. Double depression (acute depressive episode superimposed on chronic depression or dysthymia)
3. Catastrophic stress or chronic ongoing stress
4. Unfavorable early environment
5. Marked hypochondriacal features, or mood-incongruent psychotic features
6. Poor drug compliance.

4-6 months. Unipolar depression lasts usually longer than bipolar depression.

With rapid institution of treatment, the major symptoms of mania are controlled within 2 weeks and of depression within 6-8 weeks.

Nearly 40% of depressives with episodic course improve in 3 months, 60% in 6 months and 80% improve with in a period of one year. 15-20% of patients develop a chronic course of illness, which may last for two or more years. Chronic depression is usually characterized by less intense depression, hypochondriacal symptoms, presence of co-morbid disorders (like dysthymic disorder, alcohol dependence, personality disorders and medical disorders), presence of ongoing stressors and unfavorable early environment.

As the age advances, the normal intervals between two episodes shorten and, the duration of the episodes and their frequency increase. Although not all patients have relapses, it has been estimated that up to 75% of patients have a second episode within 5 years.

Some patients of bipolar mood disorder have more than 4 episodes per year; they are called *rapid cyclers*. 70-80% of rapid cyclers are women. When the phases of mania and depression alternate very rapidly (in matter of hours or days), the condition is called as *ultra-rapid cycling*.

Some of the factors associated with rapid cycling include the use of tricyclic anti-depressants, low thyroxin levels, being a female patient, bipolar II pattern of illness, and the presence of neurological disease.

There is an increased mortality in patients with mood disorders by almost two times the general population. The most important cause of death is suicide, the life-time risk of which is 10-15 times higher in depression. Patients with depression also have higher mortality rates from cardiovascular diseases and co-morbid alcohol and drug dependence. Patients with depression also exhibit a variety of disturbances in immune function.

PROGNOSIS

Classically, the prognosis in mood disorders is described as better than in schizophrenia. The good and poor prognostic factors in mood disorders are described in Table 6.4.

ETIOLOGY

Over the years, a vast amount of data has emerged probing the etiology of mood disorders. The etiology of mood disorders is currently unknown. However, several theories have been propounded; these include:

I. Biological Theories

The following findings and theories point towards a biological basis of mood disorders.

1. Genetic Hypothesis

The life-time risk for the first degree relatives of bipolar mood disorder patients is 25%, and

TABLE 6.5. SOME COMMONLY USED ANTIDEPRESSANTS

Generic Name	Equivalent Dose (To 25 mg of IMI)	Usual Therapeutic Range (mg/day)
1. Imipramine (IMI)	25	150-300
2. Amitriptyline	25	150-300
3. Doxepine	25	150-300
4. Mianserin	10	30-120
5. Trazodone	50	300-600
6. Dotheipin	25	150-300
7. Clomipramine	25	75-250
8. Nortriptyline	25	150-300
9. Citalopram	—	10-40
10. Mirtazapine	—	15-45
11. Fluoxetine	—	10-60
12. Paroxetine	—	10-40
13. Amoxapine	50	150-300
14. Tianeptin	—	37.5
15. Bupropion	—	150-450
16. Venlafaxine	—	75-375
17. Sertraline	—	50-200
18. Fluvoxamine	—	50-200
19. Moclobemide	—	300-600

of recurrent depressive disorder patients is 20%. The life-time risk for the children of one parent with mood disorder is 27% and of both parents with mood disorder is 74%. The concordance rate in *bipolar disorders* for monozygotic twins is 65% and for dizygotic twins is 20% and the concordance rate in *unipolar depression* for monozygotic twins is 46% and for dizygotic twins is 20%.

Therefore, genetic factors are very important in making an individual vulnerable to mood disorders, particularly so in bipolar mood disorders. However, environmental factors are also probably important.

2. Biochemical Theories

There are several biochemical hypotheses for the the causation of mood disorders. The mmonoamine hypothesis suggests abnormality in monoamine [catecholamine (norepinephrine and dopamine) and serotonin] system in the central nervous system at one or more sites. Acetylcholine and GABA are also presumably involved.

The earlier models of a functional increase (in mania) or decrease (in depression) of amines at the synaptic cleft now appear simplistic, though urinary and CSF levels of amine metabolites indicate decreased norepinephrine and/or 5-HT function in depression, and increased norepinephrine and/or 5-HT function in mania.

Postsynaptic events involving the second messenger system, and alterations in receptor number and function, are also important in addition to the synaptic and presynaptic events. The effects of antidepressants and mood stabilizers in mood disorders also provide additional evidence to the biochemical hypothesis of mood disorders.

Patients suffering from severe depression with suicidal intent/attempt have a marked decrease in the serotonergic function, evidenced by decreased urinary and plasma 5-HIAA levels and post-mortem studies.

3. Neuroendocrine Theories

Mood symptoms are prominently present in many endocrine disorders, like hypothyroidism, Cushing's disease, Addison's disease.

Endocrine function is often disturbed in depression with cortisol hypersecretion, non-suppression with dexamethasone challenge (DST or Dexamethasone suppression test), blunted TSH response to TRH, and blunted GH (growth hormone) production during sleep.

The neuroendocrine and biochemical mechanisms are closely inter-related.

4. Sleep Studies

Sleep abnormalities are common in mood disorders (e.g. decreased need for sleep in mania; insomnia and frequent awakenings in depression). In depression, commonly observed abnormalities are decreased REM latency (i.e. the time between falling asleep and the first REM period is decreased), increased duration of the first REM period, and delayed sleep onset.

5. Brain Imaging

In mood disorders, brain imaging studies (CT scan/MRI scan of brain, PET scan, and SPECT) have yielded inconsistent, yet suggestive findings (e.g. ventricular dilatation, changes in blood flow and metabolism in several parts of brain, like prefrontal cortex, anterior cingulate cortex, and caudate).

II. Psychosocial Theories

1. Psychoanalytic Theories

In depression, loss of a libidinal object, introjection of the lost object, fixation in the oral sadistic phase of development, and intense craving for narcissism or self-love have been postulated as theories.

Mania represents a *reaction formation* (see Table 17.1) to depression according to psychodynamic theory.

2. Stress

Increased stressful life events before the onset or relapse probably have a *formative* rather than a precipitating effect. Increased stressors in the early development are probably more important in depression.

3. Cognitive and Behavioral Theories

The mechanisms of causation of depression according to these approaches is depressive negative cognition (cognitive theory), learned helplessness (animal model), and anger directed inwards. These concepts are useful in the treatment of mild depression.

Several other theories have also been propounded but are currently of doubtful value as theories of causation of depression.

DIFFERENTIAL DIAGNOSIS

The first step in the differential diagnosis is to exclude psychoses with known organic causes, e.g. *organic* (especially drug-induced) *mood disorders* and *dementia* (differential diagnosis from depressive pseudodementia).

The second step is to rule out a possibility of *acute and transient psychotic disorders, schizo-affective disorder*, and rarely *schizophrenia*.

The third step is exclude the possibility of other non-organic psychoses like *delusional disorders*.

The fourth step is exclude the possibility of *adjustment disorder with depressed mood*, *generalized anxiety disorder* (with a few symptoms of depression), *grief reaction*, and *obsessive compulsive disorder* (with or without secondary depression).

MANAGEMENT

I. Somatic Treatment

1. Antidepressants

Antidepressants are the treatment of choice for a vast majority of depressive episodes. The commonly used antidepressants with their usual range of therapeutic dosage are listed in Table 6.5. (Antidepressants are discussed in detail in Chapter 15).

The usual starting dose is about 75-150 mg of imipramine equivalent. The clinical improvement is assessed after about two weeks. In case of non-improvement, the dose can usually be increased up to 300 mg of imipramine equivalent.

It should be remembered that it may take up to 3 weeks before any appreciable response may be noticed. Before stopping or changing a drug, the particular drug should be given in a dose of 300 mg imipramine equivalent for at least 6 weeks.

A variety of antidepressants are available in the market. Since almost all antidepressants are equal in antidepressant efficacy and there is no single antidepressant effective for all depressed patients, the choice of antidepressant is often dictated by other factors. These factors include cost and ease of availability of drug, the side-effect profile of the drug, past history of response and (any) co-morbid medical or psychiatric disorders. An individualized choice has to be made in each patient keeping these various factors in mind.

Imipramine, amitriptyline and other related drugs are called *tricyclic antidepressants—TCAs*. The newer antidepressants like *selective serotonin reuptake inhibitors - SSRIs* (fluoxetine, sertraline, citalopram), mirtazapine, and venlafaxine have very little anticholinergic side-effects and, hence, are safer drugs to use in elderly patients with cardiac disease or benign hypertrophy of prostate.

The antidepressant dosage are monitored on the basis of clinical improvement. Routine monitoring of blood levels is not usually indicated.

For the first, uncomplicated, episode of depression, the patient should receive full therapeutic dose of the chosen antidepressant for a period of 6-12 months, after achieving full remission. It is wise to taper the antidepressant medication when treatment is to be stopped after the continuation phase.

There are three phases of treatment: *acute treatment* (till remission occurs), *continuation treatment* (from remission till end of treatment), and *maintenance treatment* (to prevent further recurrences). Maintenance treatment may be indicated in the following patients:

i. Partial response to acute treatment.
ii. Poor symptom control during the continuation treatment.
iii. More than 3 episodes (90% chances of recurrence).
iv. More than 2 episodes with early age of onset, or recurrence within 2 years of stopping antidepressants, or severe and/or life-threatening depression, or family history of mood disorder.
v. Chronic depression (> 2 years) or double depression.

About 20-35% of depressed patients are *refractory* to antidepressant medication. The management of a treatment refractory depressed patient is best done by a psychiatrist, often at a tertiary care centre. These patients may require one of the following alternatives:

i. A change of antidepressant (*Switch*),
ii. Combination of two types of antidepressants (e.g. TCA with SSRI),

iii. Augmentation with lithium,
iv. Augmentation with T_3 or T_4,
v. Augmentation with antipsychotics,
vi. Electroconvulsive therapy, or
vii. Use of newer and experimental techniques.

One type of depression, namely delusional depression (depression with *psychotic* features), is usually refractory to antidepressants alone. The treatments of choice are:

i. Antidepressants with ECT, or
ii. Antidepressants with antipsychotics, or
iii. Antidepressants with lithium.

2. ECT (Electroconvulsive therapy)

The indications for ECT in depression are:

i. Severe depression with suicidal risk.
ii. Severe depression with stupor, severe psychomotor retardation, or somatic syndrome.
iii. Severe treatment refractory depression.
iv. Delusional depression (psychotic features).
v. Presence of significant antidepressant side-effects or intolerance to drugs.

Severe depression with suicidal risk is the first indication for use of ECT. The prompt use of ECT can be life-saving.

The response is rapid, resulting in marked improvement. Usually 6-8 ECTs are needed, given three times a week. (When 6 ECTs are given, the usual pattern is 3 in the 1st week, 2 in the 2nd week and 1 in the 3rd week). However, the improvement is not sustained after stopping the ECTs. So, antidepressants have to be given along with ECTs to maintain the improvement achieved. The safety of this procedure has been well established.

ECT can also be used for acute manic excitement, if it is not adequately responding to antipsychotics and lithium.

3. Lithium

Lithium (Li) is currently the drug of choice for treatment of manic episode (acute phase) as well as for prevention of further episodes in bipolar mood disorder. It has also been used in treatment of depression with less success. (Lithium is discussed in detail in Chapter 15).

There is a 1-2 week lag period before any appreciable response is observed. So, for the treatment of acute manic episode, antipsychotics are usually administered along with lithium, to provide cover for the first few weeks.

The usual therapeutic dose range is 900-1500 mg of lithium carbonate ($LiCO_3$) per day. The treatment is closely monitored by repeated blood levels, as the difference between therapeutic and lethal blood levels is not very wide.

Therapeutic blood lithium = 0.8-1.2 mEq/L

Prophylactic blood lithium = 0.6-1.2 mEq/L

A blood lithium level of more than 2.0 mEq/L may be associated with toxicity, while a level of more than 2.5-3.0 mEq/L may be lethal.

Although lithium is indicated for therapeutic use in all manic episodes, the preventive use is best in usually those bipolar patients where the frequency of episodes is 1-3 per year or 2-5 per two years.

The common acute toxic symptoms are neurological while the common chronic side-effects are nephrological and endocrinal (usually hypothyroidism).

The important investigations before starting lithium therapy are complete general physical examination, CBC, EKG, urine routine examination, 24 hour urine volume, renal function tests, and thyroid function tests.

4. Antipsychotics

Antipsychotics are an important adjunct in the treatment of mood disorder. The commonly used drugs are risperidone, haloperidol, olanzapine, and chlorpromazine. The indications are:

i. Acute manic episode

- Along with mood stabilizers for the first few weeks before their effect appears.
- Where mood stabilizers are not effective, not indicated, or have significant side-effects.
- Given parenterally (IM or IV) for emergency treatment of mania.

ii. Delusional depression

The commonly used drugs are olanzapine, risperidone, ziprasidone, haloperidol, and chlorpromazine, although any antipsychotic can be used.

5. Other Mood Stabilizers

These include:

i. Sodium valproate

- For acute treatment of mania and prevention of bipolar mood disorder.
- Particulary useful in those patients who are refractory to lithium..
- The dose range is 1000-3000 mg/day (The therapeutic blood levels are 50-100 mg/ml).
- It has a faster onset of action than lithium or carbamazepine, so can be used in acute treatment of mania effectively.

ii. Carbamazepine and Oxcarbazepine

- For acute treatment of mania and prevention of bipolar mood disorder.
- Particulary useful in those patients who are refractory to lithium and valproate.
- Particulary effective when EEG is abnormal (although this is not necessary for the use of carbamazepine).
- The dose range is 600-1600 mg/day (The therapeutic blood levels are 6-12 mg/ml).

iii. Benzodiazepines

Clonazepam is used for the treatment of manic episode rarely alone but more often as an adjuvant to antipsychotics. The other benzodiazepines, like lorazepam (IV as well as oral), are useful adjuncts in the management of acute mania.

iv. *Topiramate*

v. *Lamotrigine,* for bipolar depression.

vi. T_3 *and* T_4 for the treatment of rapid cyclers and resistant depression, as adjunct.

6. Other Treatments

Psychosurgery is resorted to only in exceptional circumstances. In depressive episode, which is either chronic or persistently recurrent with a limited or absent response to other modes of treatment, one of the following procedures may be performed:

i. Stereotactic subcaudate tractotomy, or
ii. Stereotactic limbic leucotomy.

In carefully selected patients, the results are reported to be satisfactory. However, in the present scenario, psychosurgery is very rarely used in routine clinical practice.

II. Psychosocial Treatment

Although somatic treatment is the primary mode of management in major mood disorders, psychosocial treatment may be indicated in certain cases. These include:

i. As an adjunct to somatic treatment.
ii. In mild cases of depression.
iii. Certain selected cases.

These methods are (see Chapter 18 for details):

1. Cognitive Behavior Therapy

Cognitive therapy (CT) or cognitive behavior therapy (CBT) aims at correcting the depressive negative cognitions (ideations) e.g. hopelessness, worthlessness, helplessness and pessimistic ideas, and replacing them by new cognitive and behavioral responses.

It is useful in mild to moderate, non-bipolar depression and can be used along with somatic treatment.

2. Interpersonal Therapy

Interpersonal therapy (IPT) attempts to recognize and explore interpersonal stressors, role disputes and transitions, social isolation, or social skills deficits, which act as precipitants for depression. It is useful in the treatment of mild to moderate unipolar depression, with or without antidepressants.

3. Psychoanalytic Psychotherapy

The short-term psychoanalytic psychotherapies aim at changing the personality itself rather than just ameliorating the symptoms. Their usefulness is uncertain, particularly in a florid depressive or manic episode.

4. Behavior Therapy

This includes the various short-term modalities like social skills training; problem solving techniques, assertiveness training, self-control therapy, activity scheduling and decision-making techniques.

It is useful in mild cases of depression.

5. Group Therapy

Group psychotherapy can be useful in mild cases of depression.

6. Family and Marital Therapy

Apart from educating the family about the nature of illness and usefulness of somatic treatment, family therapy has not been found very useful in mood disorders. Another use is to decrease the intrafamilial and interpersonal difficulties, and to reduce or modify stressors, which may help in a faster and more complete recovery. The main purpose is to ensure on continuity of treatment (e.g. lithium prevention in bipolar patients) to ensure adequate drug compliance.

OTHER SYNDROMES OF DEPRESSION AND MANIA

Involutional Melancholia

Described by Kraepelin, this is a form of severe depression which occurs in the involutional period (i.e. 40-65 years of age). It is characterized by marked agitation, psychotic features like delusions of persecution, tactile and auditory hallucinations, and multiple somatic symptoms (or hypochondriacal delusions). Presently, it is no longer thought of as an independent entity but is included as a part of depressive episode.

Mixed Anxiety-Depressive Disorder

This disorder is characterized by the presence of depressive and anxiety symptoms which result in significant distress or disability in the person. The symptoms should not meet the criteria of either an anxiety disorder or a mood disorder.

This disorder is apparently seen more frequently in medical outpatient departments and primary care centres. Several cases probably exist in general population, but rarely come to medical attention.

In clinical practice, it is useful to consider a diagnosis of either a mood disorder or an anxiety disorder, before attempting a diagnosis of mixed anxiety-depressive disorder.

Masked Depression

In masked depression, the depressive mood is not easily apparent and is hidden by somatic symptoms. It is especially common in elderly, where somatic symptoms range from chronic pain, insomnia, atypical facial pain, paresthesias, to even drug and alcohol abuse. Sometimes, a more detailed examination will bring out the tell-tale symptomatology of depression.

The treatment is with antidepressants.

Depressive Equivalents

These are certain conditions which although are not a part of the depressive syndrome but are still thought be comparable to depression. Some of these show a clinical response with the antidepressant treatment while others are related due to multiple and complex reasons. These disorders include agoraphobia, chronic pain, paresthesias, panic attacks, alcoholism, drug abuse, hysteria, obsessive compulsive disorder and eating disorders (anorexia nervosa and bulimia nervosa).

This term presently has an uncertain nosological status.

Atypical Depressions

These are depressive syndromes which do not present with classical or typical features of depression. They include:

1. *Depression with predominant anxiety*: This anxiety is subjective in contrast to the objective restlessness in agitated depression. The treatment is by antidepressants.
2. *Phobic-anxiety-depersonalization syndrome (PAD syndrome)*: Described by Roth, this syndrome is commoner in women aged 20-40 years. It is characterized by diffuse anxiety, multiple phobias (like agoraphobia and claustrophobia), panic attacks, depersonalization, derealization and depressive features. The treatment is by antidepressants. ECTs may make the condition worse.
3. *Non-endogenous depression*: Atypical depression of the non-endogenous type is characterized by absence of neurotic traits and significant stressful life events. This differentiates it from neurotic or reactive depression.
4. *Hysteroid-dysphoric depression*: In this type, there are marked fluctuations of mood from near normal to severe depression. Any stress leads to an abrupt onset of depression with marked anxiety, pallor and changes in physical appearance. The person usually has histrionic (hysterical) personality traits.

Atypical depression usually has an onset in the teens and runs a chronic course. Hypersomnia, hyperphagia, reactive nature of symptoms, 'rejection sensitivity' and lethargy ('leaden paralysis') are some of the characteristic features.

The importance of diagnosing atypical depression lies in the fact that many of these patients respond better to MAOIs (monoamine oxidase inhibitors), although SSRIs and TCAs should be tried first.

Double Depression

This is a major depressive episode (usually acute) superimposed on an underlying dysthymia or neurotic depression (usually chronic). The response to treatment is usually poor.

Agitated Depression

This is a type of severe depression with marked motor restlessness or agitation. It is either seen alone or along with involutional melancholia. It is common after the age of 40 years.

The treatment usually requires addition of antipsychotics to the antidepressant therapy.

Seasonal Mood Disorder

This is either a bipolar mood disorder or recurrent depressive episode which tends to occur in the same season on each occasion. It is usually more commonly seen in women.

For example, in a bipolar seasonal mood disorder, depression would tend to occur in the same months every time (usually winter months), while mania would occur in the months of some other season every episode. (usually summer months). This is thought to be due to changes in the length of the day (and light) and its effect on hypothalamus. The characteristic symptoms of winter depression are dysphoria, decreased activity and atypical depressive symptoms (increased fatigue, increased sleep, increased appetite and weight, and carbohydrate craving). The prevalence of winter seasonal mood disorder increases with increasing latitude.

The treatment, in addition to the usual modes of management, also includes *phototherapy,* which consists of increasing the number of hours of daylight (using artificial, full-spectrum, white light of 2,500-10,000 lux intensity, in the early morning, with eyes open) for the treatment of depression.

Secondary Depression and Secondary Mania

Depressive episode and manic episode can occur secondary to certain physical diseases and drugs. These have been discussed under organic mood disorders (Chapter 3).

Neurotic Depression

Neurotic depression is usually characterized by the following clinical features:

1. Presence of mild to moderate depression.
2. Depression usually occurs in response to a stress but is often disproportionate to the severity of stress.
3. Other neurotic symptoms like, anxiety, obsessive symptoms, phobic symptoms, multiple somatic symptoms, are often present.
4. Preoccupation with the stress is common.

The course of neurotic depression is usually chronic, with fluctuations. Delusions, hallucinations and other psychotic features are characteristically absent. The other common features include:

1. Reactivity of mood is preserved, i.e. the patient is able to emotionally react to the events occurring in his surroundings.
2. There may be insomnia or hypersomnia. There is usually difficulty in initiating sleep and sometimes difficulty in awakening in the morning.
3. The mood may be worse in the evening, after the whole day has been spent. The mood may also become better in social gatherings and in some recreational activities.
4. Suicidal threats and gestures are more common than completed suicide. However, as suicide may be completed accidentally, all such threats should be taken seriously.

An episode of major depression may become superimposed on an underlying neurotic depression. This is known as *double depression.*

Neurotic depression has been renamed as *dysthymia* or *dysthymic disorder* in DSM-IV-TR and ICD-10. This category does not require the presence of stress as a precipitating factor, and does not put emphasis on the presence of other neurotic symptoms or traits. It is defined as any mild depression which is not severe enough to be called depressive episode, and lasts for two years or more. This is more common in females, with an average age of onset in late third decade.

A large number of psychotherapies have been advocated for neurotic depression. The choice of therapy mainly rests on the therapist's expertise in a particular mode of therapy. Two important issues which need to be addressed in the therapeutic relationship are:

i. Dependency needs of the patient, and
ii. Manipulative behavior.

Supportive psychotherapy is an important adjunct to the treatment.

When depression is significant and/or is not responding to psychotherapy, *tricyclic antidepressants* should be used. As mixed depression and anxiety are very common, addition of benzodiazepines to antidepressants may be needed for the first one or two weeks.

For non-responders to TCAs and SSRIs, and/or when other neurotic symptoms (e.g. hysterical or hypochondriacal symptoms, or depersonalization) are prominent, MAOIs are drugs of choice. Occasionally, amphetamines (e.g. methylphenidate) may be useful in mild depression; however, there is a significant risk of dependence.

7
Other Psychotic Disorders

The major non-organic psychotic disorders are schizophrenia and mood disorders. In addition to these two, there are other non-organic psychoses some of which have been sometimes labeled as *third psychoses* or *other psychotic disorders* (Psychosis is defined in Table 7.1). These conditions are discussed in this chapter.

TABLE 7.1. DEFINITION OF PSYCHOSIS

The term *psychosis* is defined as:

1. Gross impairment in reality-testing (contact with reality).
2. Marked disturbance in personality, with impairment in social, interpersonal and occupational functioning.
3. Marked impairment in judgement and absent understanding of the current symptoms and behavior (loss of insight).
4. Presence of the characteristic symptoms like delusions and hallucinations.

PERSISTENT DELUSIONAL DISORDERS

This category in ICD-10 includes all disorders in which persistent delusions are the prominent and most important clinical features.

1. Delusional Disorder

This disorder, also previously called *paranoid disorder*, is characterized by the following clinical features:

1. Persistent (delusions must be present for at least 3 months)
   i. Delusions of persecution (being persecuted against),
   ii. Delusions of grandeur (inflated self-esteem and self image),
   iii. Delusions of jealousy (infidelity),
   iv. Somatic (hypochondriacal) delusions,
   v. Erotomanic delusions (delusions of love), or
   vi. Other non-bizarre delusions.
2. Absence of significant or persistent hallucinations.
3. Absence of organic mental disorders, schizophrenia and mood disorders.

The common etiology appears to be an abrupt change in the environment, e.g. in prison inmates, and in immigrants (to a different culture), though stressors are not evident in several other cases. Probably the etiology of delusional disorders is multifactorial.

It is a disorder with usually a relatively stable and chronic course. It is characterized by well-systematized delusions of non-bizarre type. The emotional response and behavior is understandable in the light of delusions. The behavior outside the limits of delusions is almost normal. Very often, these individuals carry on a near normal social and occupational life without arousing suspicion regarding the delusional disorder. It is only when the area of delusions is probed or confronted that the personality disorganization is evident.

When the content of delusions is predominantly persecutory (as is most often the case), it is important to differentiate delusional disorder from paranoid schizophrenia and paranoid personality disorder (Table 7.2).

TABLE 7.2. DIFFERENTIAL DIAGNOSIS OF DELUSIONAL DISORDERS

Parameters	Paranoid Schizophrenia	Delusional Disorder (Paranoid disorder)	Paranoid Personality Disorder
1. General behavior	Eccentricities, mannerisms, stereotypies, decreased self care, social withdrawal, guarded and evasive	Eccentricities, suspiciousness, decreased social interaction	Restrained social interaction
2. Personality	Disorganized (Although deterioration is much less than in other types of schizophrenia	Disturbed in delusional area, Near normal in other areas	No deterioration
3. Thought disorder	Delusions, Schneiderian FRS, loosening of associations, formal thought disorder; delusions may be bizarre	Non-bizarre delusions which are well-systematized, No other thought disorder	No thought disorder
4. Hallucinations	Auditory hallucinations common	Uncommon. If present, are not persistent	Absent
5. Contact with reality	Markedly disturbed	Disturbed in delusional area	Intact
6. Insight	Absent	Absent	Present
7. Affect/mood in relation to thought	Often inappropriate	Appropriate	Appropriate

When the content of delusions is predominantly jealousy (infidelity) involving the spouse, it is called as *Othello syndrome* or *conjugal paranoia*.

A syndrome of late paraphrenia has been described in the elderly. Although it was earlier considered a subtype of delusional disorders, it is presently diagnosed under paranoid schizophrenia.

When the content of delusions is predominantly the presence of hypochondriacal delusions, it is called as *monosymptomatic hypochondriacal psychosis* (MHP), *delusional parasitosis*, or *hypochondriacal paranoia*. The common delusions include infestations by worms or foreign bodies, emitting a foul odor (*delusional halitosis*), body (or its parts) being ugly or misshapen (*delusional dysmorphophobia*).

When the content of delusions is erotic (erotomanic), it is called as *Clerambault's syndrome* or *erotomania*. Occurring most often in women, there is an erotic conviction that a person with higher status is in love with the patient.

When the content of delusions is predominantly grandiose, then the patient usually has delusions with religious or political content and may believe self to be a leader with 'higher' aims of spreading peace, making war or spreading a message in the world.

2. Other Persistent Delusional Disorders

This is a residual category in ICD-10 for other persistent delusional disorders which do not fulfill the criteria for delusional disorders. The examples of disorders included here are:

1. Delusions associated with persistent hallucinatory voices (but a diagnosis of schizophrenia can not be made).
2. Delusional disorders with a duration of less than 3 months.

Differential Diagnosis

The conditions from which delusional disorders should be differentiated include paranoid schizophrenia, mania, depression, paranoid personality disorder and organic delusional disorder (Table 7.2).

Treatment

1. Antipsychotics are used to control agitation and psychotic features. For MHP (monosymptomatic hypochondriacal psychosis) or delusional disorder with somatic (hypochondriacal) delusions, pimozide is the drug of choice.
2. Supportive psychotherapy.
3. Antidepressants and/or ECT may be needed for secondary depression.

INDUCED DELUSIONAL DISORDER

This is a rare delusional disorder characterized by a sharing of delusions between usually two (folie å deux) or occasionally more persons (folie å trios, folie å quatre, folie å famille) who usually have closely knit emotional bond. Only one person has 'genuine' delusions due to an underlying psychiatric disorder, most often schizophrenia or delusional disorder.

On separation of the two, the dependent individual may give up his/her delusions and the patient with the 'genuine' delusions should be treated appropriately.

ACUTE AND TRANSIENT PSYCHOTIC DISORDERS

A large number of psychiatrists, especially from the developing countries like India, reported that many patients developed an acute psychotic disorder that neither followed the course of schizophrenia nor resembled mood disorders in clinical picture, and that usually had a better prognosis than schizophrenia.

In a study conducted by the Indian Council of Medical Research (ICMR) on acute psychoses (1989), the following findings were apparent:

1. 85% of patients exhibited full recovery.
2. The recovery occurred in several cases in the absence of treatment.
3. 50% of patients had a psychological stressor and 20% of patients had a somatic stressor before the onset.
4. The onset occurred in less than 48 hours in 50% of cases.

ICD-10 has included a new category of 'acute and transient psychotic disorders' in the section on 'schizophrenia, schizotypal and delusional disorders'.

According to ICD-10 (CDDG), these disorders have an abrupt (less than 48 hours) or acute (less than 2 weeks) onset. The onset is often associated with an easily identifiable acute stress, though not necessarily always so, that would be regarded as stressful to most people in similar circumstances, within the culture of the person concerned. The typical events would be bereavement, unexpected loss of partner or job, marriage, or the psychological trauma of combat, terrorism, and torture. Long-standing difficulties or problems are not included here as stressful.

Acute onset is probably associated with a good outcome, and it seems that more abrupt the onset, the better is the outcome. A complete recovery usually occurs within 2-3 months, often even much earlier.

These disorders should not satisfy the criteria for organic mental disorders, psychoactive substance use disorders, schizophrenia, or mood disorders.

The subtypes of acute and transient psychotic disorders include the following:

1. Acute polymorphic psychotic disorder without symptoms of schizophrenia.

2. Acute polymorphic psychotic disorder with symptoms of schizophrenia.
3. Acute schizophrenia-like psychotic disorder.
4. Other acute predominantly delusional psychotic disorders.

The various subtypes of acute and transient psychotic disorders are further classified as:

i. without associated acute stress, and
ii. with associated acute stress.

1. Acute Polymorphic Psychotic Disorder Without Symptoms of Schizophrenia

According to ICD-10 (CDDG), this disorder is characterized by an acute onset (from a non-psychotic state to a clearly psychotic state within 2 weeks) and polymorphic picture (unstable and markedly variable clinical picture that changes from day to day or even from hour to hour).

There are several types of hallucinations and/or delusions, changing in both type and intensity from day to day or within the same day. Marked emotional turmoil which ranges from intense feelings of happiness and ecstasy to anxiety and irritability, is also frequently present.

This disorder is particularly likely to have an abrupt onset (within 48 hours) and a rapid resolution of symptoms; in a large proportion of cases there is no obvious precipitating stress. If the symptoms persist for more than 3 months, the diagnosis should be changed. In spite of the variety of symptoms, none should be present with sufficient consistency to fulfill the criteria for schizophrenia or mood disorder.

2. Acute Polymorphic Psychotic Disorder Without Symptoms of Schizophrenia

According to ICD-10 (CDDG), this disorder meets the descriptive criteria for acute polymorphic psychotic disorder but in which typically schizophrenic symptoms are also consistently present.

If the schizophrenic symptoms persist for more than 1 month, the diagnosis should be changed to schizophrenia.

3. Acute Schizophrenia-like Psychotic Disorder

According to ICD-10 (CDDG), this disorder is characterized by an acute onset of a psychotic disorder in which the psychotic symptoms are comparatively stable and fulfill the criteria for schizophrenia but have lasted for less than 1 month.

Some degree of emotional variability or instability may be present, but not to the extent described in acute polymorphic psychotic disorder. The criteria for acute polymorphic psychotic disorder should not fulfilled.

If the schizophrenic symptoms persist for more than 1 month, the diagnosis should be changed to schizophrenia.

4. Other Acute Predominantly Delusional Psychotic Disorders

According to ICD-10 (CDDG), this disorder is characterized by an acute onset of a psychotic disorder in which comparatively stable delusions or hallucinations are the main clinical features, but do not fulfill the criteria for schizophrenia. Delusions of persecution or reference are common, and hallucinations are usually auditory (voices talking directly to the patient). The criteria for neither schizophrenia nor acute polymorphic psychotic disorder are fulfilled.

If delusions persist for more than 3 months, the diagnosis should be changed to persistent delusional disorder. If only hallucinations persist for more than 3 months, the diagnosis should be changed to other non-organic psychotic disorder.

Differential Diagnosis

The conditions from which acute and transient psychotic disorders should be differentiated are organic mental disorders, psychoactive substance use disorders, schizophrenia, mood disorders, and delusional disorders.

Prognosis

The good prognostic factors in acute and transient psychotic disorders are as follows:

1. Well adjusted premorbid personality.
2. Absence of family history of schizophrenia.
3. Presence of severe precipitating stressor before onset.
4. Sudden onset of symptoms.
5. Presence of affective symptoms, confusion, perplexity and disorientation in the clinical picture.
6. Short duration of symptoms.
7. First episode.

Treatment

1. Antipsychotics are the mainstay of treatment, and are used to control agitation and psychotic features. Usually lower doses of antipsychotics are needed. However, in the initial stages the patient may not take oral medication. In such cases, parenteral administration of antipsychotics (with or without benzodiazepines, e.g. lorazepam or diazepam) is needed. Long term use of antipsychotics should be avoided in these patients.
2. ECT may be needed in case with marked agitation and emotional turmoil, and in cases where there is a danger to self and/or others.
3. Antidepressants may be rarely needed as adjuvants in some cases with associated depression.
4. Psychotherapy and other psychological interventions may be needed in cases with associated stress. Such management is usually done after the acute episode is under control and the patient can communicate his/her fears and anxieties.

SCHIZOAFFECTIVE DISORDER

This is a disorder which lies on the borderland between schizophrenia and mood disorders. In this disorder, the symptoms of schizophrenia and mood disorders are prominently present within the same episode. The symptoms of both disorders may be present simultaneously or may follow within few days of each other.

It is of 3 types:

1. Schizoaffective disorder, manic type.
2. Schizoaffective disorder, depressed type.
3. Schizoaffective disorder, mixed type.

The course is usually episodic (particularly in manic subtype), although a chronic course in some patients has been described (particularly in depressed subtype). The prognosis is better than that in schizophrenia but is worse than that in mood disorders.

The treatment is with lithium, antipsychotics, antidepressants and/or electroconvulsive therapy (ECT), depending on the symptomatology.

CAPGRAS' SYNDROME (THE DELUSION OF DOUBLES)

A syndrome that is closely related to delusional disorders, it is characterized by a delusional conviction that other persons in the environment are not their real selves but are their own doubles.

There are 4 types:

1. Typical Capgras' syndrome (*Illusion des sosies*): Here the person sees a familiar person as a stranger who is imposing as the familiar person.
2. *Illusion de Fregoli*: The person falsely identifies strangers as familiar persons.

3. *Syndrome of subjective doubles*: The person's own self is perceived as being replaced by a double.
4. *Intermetamorphosis*: Here the patient's misidentification is complete (including not only the 'external appearance' as in the previous three types, but also the personality).

The syndrome is commonly seen in psychotic conditions with delusional sympto-matology like, paranoid schizophrenia (most frequently), delusional disorders and organic delusional disorder.

The treatment is of the underlying disorder.

REACTIVE PSYCHOSIS

Reactive psychosis is characterized by following features:

1. A sudden onset of symptoms.
2. Presence of a major stress before the onset (The quantum of stress should be severe enough to be stressful to a majority of people).
3. A clear temporal relation between stress and the onset of psychotic symptoms.
4. No organic cause underlying the psychosis.

The usual duration of illness is less than one month and recovery is usually complete.

Currently a majority of cases of reactive psychosis would be classified under acute and transient psychotic disorder with associated stress (in ICD-10) or brief reactive psychosis (DSM-IV-TR).

8

Neurotic, Stress-Related and Somatoform Disorders

The terms *neurosis* (Table 8.1) and *psychosis* are currently not widely used, partly as their definitions and descriptions are far from perfect (i.e. there are exceptions to the rules), partly because they have psychodyna-mic connotations, and partly because DSM-IV does not use them. Although the ICD-10 still uses the term *neurotic* in the classification, it discourages the use of the terms neurosis and psychosis.

In ICD-10 (CDDG), *'neurotic, stress-related and somatoform disorders'* have been classified into the following types:

1. Phobic anxiety disorder,
2. Other anxiety disorders (called simply *anxiety disorder* in this book),
3. Obsessive compulsive disorder,
4. Reaction to severe stress, and adjustment disorders,
5. Dissociative (conversion) disorders,
6. Somatoform disorders, and
7. Other neurotic disorders.

TABLE 8.1. DEFINITION OF NEUROSIS

The term *neurosis* is defined as:

1. The presence of a symptom or group of symptoms which cause subjective distress to the patient.
2. The symptom is recognized as undesirable (i.e. insight is present).
3. The personality and behavior are relatively preserved and not usually grossly disturbed.
4. The contact with reality is preserved.
5. There is an absence of organic causative factors.

ANXIETY DISORDER

Anxiety is the commonest psychiatric symptom in clinical practice and anxiety disorders are one of the commonest psychiatric disorders.

Anxiety is a normal phenomenon which is characterized by a state of apprehension or unease arising out of anticipation of danger. Anxiety is differentiated from fear, as fear is an apprehension in response to an external danger while in anxiety the danger is largely unknown.

Normal anxiety becomes pathological when it causes significant subjective distress and/or impairment in functioning of the individual.

Some authors separate anxiety into 2 types:

1. *Trait anxiety:* This is a habitual tendency to be anxious in general and is exemplified by 'I often feel anxious'.
2. *State anxiety*: This is the anxiety felt at the present moment exemplified by 'I feel anxious now'. Persons with trait anxiety often have episodes of state anxiety.

The symptoms of anxiety can be broadly classified in two groups: physical and psychic (Table 8.2).

TABLE 8.2. SYMPTOMS OF ANXIETY

1. Physical Symptoms

A. Motoric Symptoms

Tremors, Restlessness, Muscle twitches, Fearful facial expression

B. Autonomic and Visceral Symptoms

Palpitations, Tachycardia, Sweating, Flushes, Dyspnea, Hyperventilation, Dry mouth, Frequency and hesitancy of micturition, Dizziness, Diarrhea, Mydriasis

2. Psychic Symptoms

A. Cognitive Symptoms

Poor concentration, Distractibility, Hyperarousal, Vigilance or scanning

B. Perceptual Symptoms

Derealization, Depersonalization

C. Affective Symptoms

Diffuse, unpleasant, vague sense of apprehension, Fearfulness, Inability to relax, Irritability, Feeling of impending doom (when severe)

D. Other Symptoms

Insomnia (initial), Exaggerated startle response.

1. Generalized Anxiety Disorder

This is characterized by an insidious onset in the third decade and a stable, usually chronic course which may or may not be punctuated by repeated panic attacks (episodes of acute anxiety). The symptoms of anxiety should last for at least a period of 6 months for a diagnosis of generalized anxiety disorder to be made.

The one year prevalence of generalized anxiety disorder is 2.5-8%. It is the commonest psychiatric disorder in the general population.

As anxiety is a cardinal feature of almost all psychiatric disorders, it is important to exclude other diagnoses. The most important differential diagnosis is from depressive disorders and from organic anxiety disorder.

2. Panic Disorder

This is characterized by discrete episodes of acute anxiety. The onset is usually in early third decade with often a chronic course. The panic attacks occur recurrently every few days. There may or may not be an underlying generalized anxiety disorder.

The episode is usually sudden in onset, lasts for a few minutes and is characterized by very severe anxiety. Classically the symptoms begin unexpectedly or 'out-of-the-blue'. Usually there is no apparent precipitating factor.

The differential diagnosis is from organic anxiety disorder (Chapter 3) (e.g. secondary to hypoglycemia, hyperthyroidism, pheochromo-cytoma) and cardiac disorders (e.g. MVPS - mitral valve prolapse syndrome).

The life time prevalence of panic disorder is 1.5-2%, with 3-4% reporting sub-syndromal panic symptoms (i.e. panic symptoms not severe enough to qualify for panic disorder). Panic disorder is seen 2-3 times more often in females. Panic disorder can present either alone or with agoraphobia.

Etiology

The cause of anxiety disorders is not clearly known. There are many theories of which more than one may be correct.

1. Psychodynamic Theory

According to this theory, anxiety is a signal that something is disturbing the internal psychological equilibrium. This is called as *signal anxiety*. This signal anxiety arouses the ego to take defensive action which is usually in the form of *repression*, a primary defense mechanism. Ordinarily when repression fails, other secondary defense mechanisms, like conversion, isolation, are called into action.

In anxiety, repression fails to function adequately and the secondary defense mechanisms are *not* activated. Hence, anxiety comes to the forefront.

Developmentally, primitive anxiety is manifested as somatic symptomatology while developmentally advanced anxiety is signal anxiety.

Panic anxiety, according to this theory, is closely related to the separation anxiety of childhood.

2. Behavioral Theory

According to this theory, anxiety is viewed as an unconditioned inherent response of the organism to painful or dangerous stimuli. In anxiety and phobias, this becomes attached to relatively neutral stimuli by conditioning.

Behavioral approach is more helpful in treatment rather than in explaining the cause of anxiety.

3. Cognitive Behavioral Theory (CBT)

According to cognitive behavior theory, in anxiety disorders, there is evidence of selective information processing (with more attention paid to threat-related information), cognitive distortions, negative automatic thoughts (NATs) and perception of decreased control over internal and external stimuli.

4. Biological Theory

i. Genetic evidence

15-20% of the first degree relatives of patients with anxiety disorder exhibit anxiety disorders themselves. The concordance rate in the monozygotic twins of patients with panic disorders is as high as 80% (4 times more than dizygotic twins).

ii. Chemically induced anxiety states

Infusion of sodium lactate, isoproterenol and caffeine; ingestion of yohimbine and inhalation of 5% CO_2 can produce panic episodes in predisposed individuals. Administration (oral) of MAOIs before lactate infusion protects the individual from panic attack, thus providing a probable clue to the biological model of anxiety.

iii. GABA-benzodiazepine receptors

This is one of the most recent advances in the search for etiology of anxiety disorders. Benzodiazepine receptors are distributed widely in the central nervous system. Presently, two types have been identified. The type I (ω_1) is GABA and chloride independent, while type II (ω_2) is GABA and chloride dependent.

GABA (Gamma amino butyric acid) is the most prevalent inhibitory neurotransmitter in the central nervous system. It has been suggested that an alteration in GABA levels may lead to production of clinical anxiety. The fact that the benzodiazepines (which facilitate GABA transmission, thereby causing a generalized inhibitory effect on the CNS) relieve anxiety and benzodiazepine-antagonists (e.g. flumazenil) and inverse agonists (e.g. β-carbolines) cause anxiety, lends heavy support to this hypothesis.

iv. Other neurotransmitters

Norepinephrine, 5-HT, dopamine, opioid receptors and neuroendocrine dysfunction have also been implicated in the causation of anxiety disorders.

v. Neuroanatomical basis

Locus ceruleus, limbic system, and prefrontal cortex are some of the areas implicated in the etiology of anxiety disorders. Regional cerebral blood flow (rCBF) is increased in anxiety, though vasoconstriction occurs in severe anxiety.

vi. Organic anxiety disorder

This disorder is characterized by the presence of anxiety which is secondary to the various medical disorders (e.g. hyperthyroidism, pheochromocytoma, coronary artery disease). If anxiety can occur secondary to medical disorders, it is possible that anxiety has a biological basis.

Treatment

The treatment is usually multi-modal.

1. Psychotherapy

Psychoanalytic psychotherapy is not usually indicated, unless characterological (personality) problems coexist. Usually supportive psychotherapy is used either alone, when anxiety is mild, or in combination with drug therapy. The establishment of a good therapist-patient relationship is often the first step in psychotherapy.

2. Relaxation Techniques

In patients with mild to moderate anxiety, relaxation techniques are very useful. These techniques are used by the patient himself or herself as a routine exercise every day and also whenever anxiety-provoking situation is at hand.

The techniques include Jacobson's progressive relaxation technique, yoga, pranayama, self-hypnosis, and meditation (including TM-transcendental meditation).

3. Other Behavior Therapies

These include cognitive behavioral therapy (CBT), biofeedback and hyperventilation control. These methods are important adjuncts to treatment.

4. Drug Treatment

The differential response of generalized anxiety and panic to drug treatment has lead to what is called as the *pharmacological dissection of anxiety disorders*.

The drugs of choice for generalized anxiety are benzodiazepines, and for panic, antidepressants. Both benzodiazepines and antidepressants are discussed in detail in Chapter 15. It is useful to begin treatment of panic disorders with small doses of antidepressants (e.g. imipramine and fluoxetine).

Alprazolam, a benzodiazepine drug, which has antianxiety as well as antidepressant properties, is useful in the treatment of both generalized anxiety and panic disorders. Clonazepam is also useful in the treatment of panic disorders.

β-blockers like propranolol and atenolol are particularly useful in the management of anticipatory anxiety (e.g. anxiety occurring before going on stage, before examinations). Care must be exercised in the use of propranolol in the patients with history of asthma, bradycardia or heart block. Atenolol does not cross the blood brain barrier and takes care of only peripheral symptoms of anxiety. It also has less likelihood of causing bronchial constriction than propranolol.

Buspirone is a new antianxiety drug (discussed in Chapter 15) which does not have any dependence potential, unlike benzodiazepines. It takes 2-3 weeks before its action is apparent. It may be preferable to benzodiazepines for the long term management of anxiety disorder. It, however, has no role in the management of panic disorder.

PHOBIC DISORDER

Phobia is defined as an irrational fear of a specific object, situation or activity, often leading to persistent avoidance of the feared object, situation or activity.

The characteristic features of phobia are described in Table 8.3.

The common types of phobias are:

1. Agoraphobia,
2. Social phobia, and
3. Specific (Simple) phobia.

1. Agoraphobia

This is an example of irrational fear of situations. It is the commonest type of phobia encountered in clinical practice. Women out-

TABLE 8.3. PHOBIA: CHARACTERISTIC FEATURES

1. Presence of the fear of an object, situation or activity.
2. The fear is out of proportion to the dangerousness perceived.
3. Patient recognizes the fear as irrational and unjustified (Insight is present).
4. Patient is unable to control the fear and is very distressed by it.
5. This leads to persistent avoidance of the particular object, situation or activity.
6. Gradually, the phobia and the phobic object become a preoccupation with the patient, resulting in marked distress and restriction of the freedom of mobility (afraid to encounter the phobic object; *phobic avoidance*).

number men in suffering from agoraphobia in the Western countries.

It is characterized by an irrational fear of being in places away from the familiar setting of home. Although it was earlier thought to be a fear of open spaces only, now it includes fear of open spaces, public places, crowded places, any other place from *where there is no easy escape to a safe place*.

In fact, the patient is afraid of all the places or situations from where escape may be difficult or help may not be available, if he suddenly develops embarrassing or incapacitating symptoms. These embarrassing or incapacitating symptoms are the classical symptoms of panic.

A full-blown panic attack may occur (*agoraphobia with panic disorder*) or only a few symptoms like dizziness or tachycardia may occur (*agoraphobia without panic disorder*).

As the agoraphobia increases in severity, there is a gradual restriction in normal day-to-day activities. The activity may become so severely restricted that the person becomes self-imprisoned at home. One or two persons (usually close relations) may be relied upon, with whom the patient can leave home. Hence, the patient becomes severely dependent on these *phobic companion(s)*.

2. Social Phobia

This is an example of irrational fear of activities or social interaction, characterized by an irrational fear of performing activities in the presence of other people or interacting with others. The patient is afraid of his own actions being viewed by others critically, resulting in embarrassment or humiliation.

There is marked distress and disturbance in daily functioning. Examples are fear of blushing (*erythrophobia*), eating, public speaking, public performance (e.g. on stage), participating in groups, writing in public (e.g. signing a check), speaking to strangers (e.g. for asking for directions), dating, speaking to authority figures, and urinating in a public lavatory (*shy bladder*). Sometimes, alcohol (and rarely other drugs) is used to overcome the anxiety occurring in social situations.

3. Specific (Simple) Phobia

In contrast to agoraphobia and social phobia where the stimuli are generalized, in specific phobia the stimulus is usually circumscribed. This is an example of irrational fear of objects situations.

It is characterized by an irrational fear of a specified object or situation. Anticipatory anxiety leads to persistent avoidant behavior, while confrontation with the avoided object or situation leads to panic attack. Gradually, the phobia spreads to other objects and situations (commonly).

The disorder is diagnosed only if there is marked distress and/or disturbance in daily functioning, in addition to fear and avoidance of the specified object or situation. Examples of simple phobia are *acrophobia* (fear of high places), *zoophobia* (fear of animals), *xenophobia* (fear of strangers), *algophobia* (fear of pain), and *claustrophobia* (fear of closed places).

The list of specific phobias is virtually endless.

Course

The phobias are more common in women with an onset in late second decade or early third decade. Typically, the onset is sudden without any apparent cause. The course is usually chronic with gradually increasing restriction of daily activities. Sometimes, phobias are spontaneously remitting.

Etiology

1. Psychodynamic Theory

As discussed in the etiology of anxiety disorders, anxiety is usually dealt with *repression*. When repression fails to function adequately, other secondary defense mechanisms of ego come into action. In phobia, this secondary defense mechanism is *displacement*. By displacement, anxiety is transferred from a really dangerous or frightening object to a neutral object. These two objects are connected by symbolic associations. The neutral object chosen unconsciously is the one which can be easily *avoided* in day-to-day activity, in contrast to the frightening object (frightening to the patient only, due to oedipal genital drives).

In agoraphobia, loss of parents in childhood and separation anxiety have been theorized to contribute to causation.

From a psychobiological perspective, the traumatic experiences of childhood may affect the child's developing brain in such a manner that the child becomes susceptible to anxiety and fear in childhood.

2. Behavioral Theories

Here, phobia is explained as a conditioned reflex. Initially, the anxiety provoked by a naturally frightening or dangerous object occurs in contiguity with a second neutral object. If this happens often enough, the neutral object becomes a conditioned stimulus for causing anxiety.

This theory does not explain all the features of phobic disorders adequately but is very helpful in planning treatment.

3. Biological Theories

All phobias, especially agoraphobia, are closely linked to panic disorders. It has been suggested that probably the biological models of panic apply to phobias too. But the evidence for this view is not strong at present, except for the importance of genetic factors in specific phobias of blood-injury type. There is also some evidence for the presence of familial factors in social phobias.

Differential Diagnosis

The differential diagnoses include anxiety disorder, panic disorder, major depression, avoidant personality disorder, obsessive compulsive disorder, delusional disorder, hypochondriasis, and schizophrenia.

Treatment

Most patients with phobic disorder rely on avoidance to manage their fears and anxieties. As long as they find ways to limit their lives within the limitations imposed by phobias, they experience little, if any, anxiety. When they are forced to face the phobic situation, anxiety mounts and they seek treatment. Patients with more than one phobias and presence of panic symptoms often seek treatment earlier.

The treatment approach is usually multimodal.

1. Psychotherapy

Psychodynamically oriented psychotherapy is not usually helpful in treatment of phobias. This approach is indicated when there are characterological or personality difficulties as well.

Supportive psychotherapy is helpful adjunct to behavior therapy and drug treatment. *Cognitive behavior therapy* can be used to break the anxiety patterns in phobic disorder.

2. Behavior Therapy

If properly planned, this mode of treatment is usually successful. As the behavioral therapies are discussed in Chapter 18, only the names of important techniques are mentioned here.

i. Flooding.
ii. Systematic desensitization.
iii. Exposure and response prevention.
iv. Relaxation techniques.

3. Drug Treatment

The drugs used in the treatment of phobia are:

i. Benzodiazepines (Chapter 15) are given to reduce the anticipatory anxiety. *Alprazolam* is believed to have anti-phobic, anti-panic and anti-anxiety properties. So, it is the drug of choice when benzodiazepines are used. Long-term follow-up of double-blind trials are needed before it is firmly established as an anti-phobic. The other drugs used include clonazepam, lorazepam and diazepam.
ii. Among the antidepressants (discussed in Chapter 15), SSRIs are currently drugs of choice, with *paroxetine* being the most widely used and effective drug. Other SSRIs, like *fluoxetine* and *sertraline* are also very effective.
   Other antidepressants e.g. *imipramine* (TCA) and *phenelzine* (MAOI), are also helpful in controlling the panic attacks associated with phobias, thereby decreasing the distress.

As mentioned earslier, multiple approaches are usually combined together in treatment of a particular patient.

OBSESSIVE-COMPULSIVE DISORDER

An *obsession* is defined as:

1. An idea, impulse or image which intrudes into conscious awareness repeatedly.
2. It is recognized as one's own idea, impulse or image but is ego-alien (foreign to one's personality).
3. It is recognized as irrational and absurd (insight is present).
4. Patient tries to resist against it but is unable to.
5. Failure to resist leads to marked distress.

Differentiation has to be made from delusion and thought insertion.

A *delusion* is recognized as one's own idea but is not recognized as ego-alien. It is strongly believed, hence it is never thought to be irrational and is never resisted.

Thought insertion is not thought of as one's own idea, but somebody else's thought being forcibly inserted into one's mind.

An obsession is usually associated with a compulsion.

A *compulsion* is defined as:

1. A form of behavior which usually follows obsessions.
2. It is aimed at either preventing or neutralizing the distress or fear arising out of obsession
3. The behavior is not realistic and is either irrational or excessive.
4. Insight is present, so the patient realizes the irrationality of compulsion.
5. The behavior is performed with a sense of subjective compulsion (urge or impulse to act).

Compulsions may diminish the anxiety associated with obsessions.

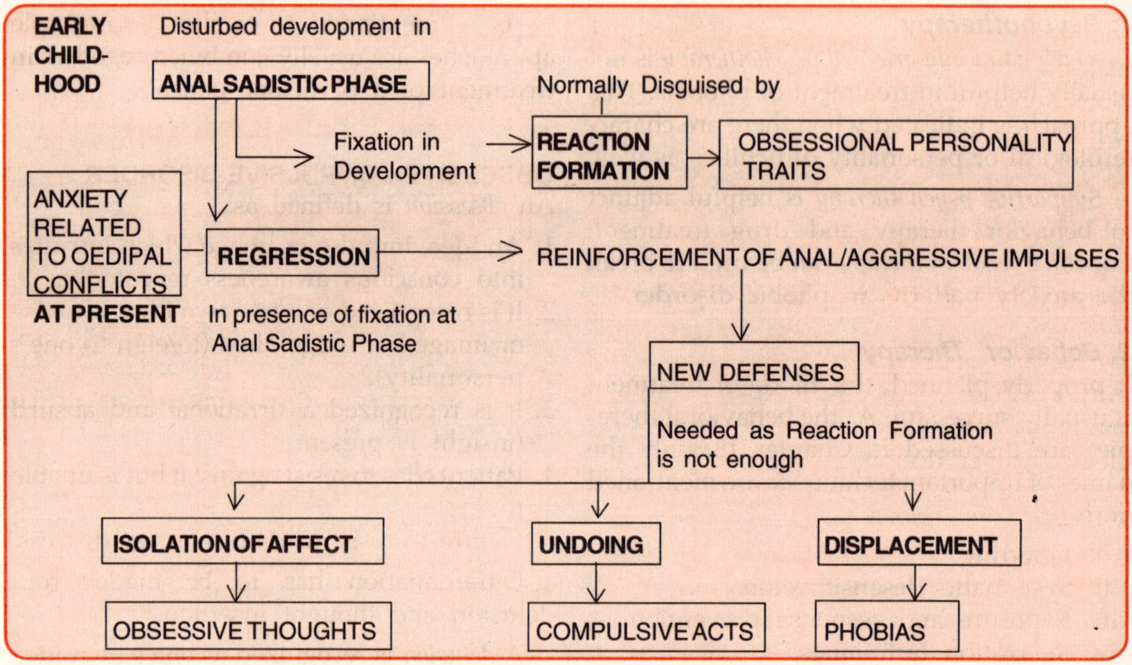

FIG. 8.1. PSYCHODYNAMIC THEORY OF OBSESSIVE COMPULSIVE DISORDER

Epidemiology, Course and Outcome

In India, obsessive compulsive disorder (OCD) is more common in unmarried males, while in other countries no sex differences are reported. This disorder is commoner in persons from upper social strata and with high intelligence. Average age of onset is late third decade (i.e. late 20s) in India, while in Western countries the onset is earlier in life.

Recent studies show the life-time prevalence of OCD to be as high as 2-3%, though the Indian data shows a lower prevalence rate. Although classically thought to have a steady *chronic* course, the longitudinal profile of this disorder can also be *episodic*.

A summary of long-term follow-up studies shows that about 25% remained unimproved over time, 50% had moderate to marked improvement while 25% had recovered completely.

Clinical Syndromes

ICD-10 classifies OCD in to three clinical subtypes:

1. Predominantly obsessive thoughts or ruminations,
2. Predominantly compulsive acts (compulsive rituals), and
3. Mixed obsessional thoughts and acts.

Depression is very commonly associated with obsessive compulsive disorder. It is estimated that at least half the patients of OCD have major depressive episodes while many other have mild depression. *Premorbidly* obsessional or anankastic personality disorder or 'traits' may be commoner than in rest of the population.

Four clinical syndromes have been described in literature, although admixtures are commoner than pure syndromes.

1. Washers

This is the commonest type. Here the *obsession* is of *contamination* with dirt, germs, body excretions and the like. The *compulsion* is *washing* of hands or the whole body, repeatedly many times a day. It usually spreads on to washing of clothes, washing of bathroom, bedroom, door knobs and personal articles gradually.

The person tries to avoid contamination but is unable to, so washing becomes a ritual.

2. Checkers

In this type, the person has multiple *doubts*, e.g. the door has not been locked, kitchen gas has been left open, counting of money was not exact, etc. The *compulsion* of course is *checking* repeatedly to remove the doubt. Any attempt to stop the checking leads to mounting anxiety. Before one doubt has been cleared, other doubts may creep in.

3. Pure Obsessions

This syndrome is characterized by repetitive intrusive thoughts, impulses or images which are *not* associated with compulsive acts. The content is usually sexual or aggressive in nature. The distress associated with these obsessions is dealt with by *counter-thoughts* (e.g. counting) and not by behavioral rituals.

A variant is *obsessive rumination*, which is a preoccupation with thoughts. Here the person ruminates in his mind about pros and cons of the thought concerned, repetitively.

4. Primary Obsessive Slowness

A relatively rare syndrome, it is characterized by severe obsessive ideas and/or extensive compulsive rituals, in the relative absence of manifested anxiety. This leads to marked slowness in daily activities.

Etiology

Multiple causative factors have been explored but no clear etiology is known. The important theories are:

1. Psychodynamic Theory

Freud found obsessions and phobias to be psychogenetically related. This theory can be explained in a flow diagram (Fig. 8.1).

Isolation of Affect

By this defense mechanism, ego removes the affect (*isolates the affect*) from the anxiety-causing idea. The idea is thus weakened, but remains still in consciousness. The affect however becomes free and attaches itself to other *neutral ideas* by symbolic associations. Thus, these neutral ideas are made anxiety-provoking and turned into *obsessions*. This happens only when *isolation of affect* is not fully successful. When it is fully successful, both the idea and affect are repressed and there are *no* obsessions.

Undoing

This defense mechanism leads to compulsions, which prevent or *undo* the feared consequences of obsessions.

Reaction formation results in formation of obsessive compulsive personality traits rather than contributing to obsessive compulsive symptoms, while *displacement* leads to formation of phobic symptoms. These defense mechanisms are discussed in Table 17.1.

This mechanism has been explained in slight detail as this theory attempts to describe the probable causation of OCD in a remarkably systematic manner. Whether it is true or not, however, is a matter of conjecture.

Thus, the psychodynamic theory explains OCD by a defensive regression to anal-sadistic phase of development with the use of isolation, undoing and displacement to produce obsessive-compulsive symptoms.

2. Behavioral Theory

This theory explains *obsessions* as conditioned stimuli to anxiety (similar to *phobias*). *Compulsions* have been described as learned behavior which decrease the anxiety associated with obsessions. This decrease in anxiety positively reinforces the compulsive acts and they become stable learned behaviors.

Behavioral or learning theory is *not* able to explain the causation of OCD adequately but is very useful in its treatment.

3. Biological Theories

i. Obsessive compulsive symptoms can occur secondary to many illnesses like von Economo's encephalitis, basal ganglia lesions, Gilles de la Tourette syndrome, and hypothalamic and third ventricle lesions.

ii. Obsessive compulsive disorder is found in 5-7% of first degree relatives of patients with OCD.

iii. Psychosurgery is successfully used for treatment of OCD.

iv. Biochemically, the central 5-HT system seems to be involved in OCD, as specific serotonin reuptake inhibitors (SSRIs) are useful in treatment of OCD.

Some authors pointed at cingulum (gyrus) as the probable site of lesion, while others have found EEG abnormalities most marked over the temporal lobes.

However, at the present moment, there is no conclusive evidence for OCD having a clearly proven organic etiology.

Treatment

1. Psychotherapy

i. Psychoanalytic psychotherapy is used in certain selected patients, who are psychologically oriented.

ii. Supportive psychotherapy is an important adjunct to other modes of treatment. Supportive psychotherapy is also needed by the family members.

2. Behavior Therapy

Behavior modification is an effective mode of therapy, with a success rate as high as 80%, especially for the compulsive acts.

The techniques used are listed below (They are described in Chapter 18):

i. Thought-stopping (and its modifications).
ii. Response prevention.
iii. Systematic desensitization.
iv. Modeling.

3. Drug Treatment

i. Benzodiazepines (e.g. alprazolam, clonazepam) have a limited role in controlling anxiety as adjuncts.

ii. *Antidepressants*: Some patients may improve dramatically with specific serotonin reuptake inhibitors (SSRIs). *Clomipramine* (75-300 mg/day), a non-specific serotonin reuptake inhibitor (SRI), is the first drug used effectively in the treatment of OCD. The response is better in presence of depression, but many patients with pure OCD also improve substantially.
Fluoxetine (20-80 mg/day) is a good alternative to clomipramine. *Fluvoxamine* (50-200 mg/day) is marketed as a specific anti-obsessional drug, while paroxetine (20-40 mg/day), and sertraline (50-200 mg/day) are also effective in some patients.

iii. *Antipsychotics*: These are occasionally used in low doses (e.g. haloperidol, risperidone, olanzapine, pimozide) in the treatment of severe, disabling anxiety.

iv. Buspirone has also been used beneficially as an adjunct for augmentation in some patients.

4. Electroconvulsive Therapy

In the presence of severe depression with obsessive compulsive disorder, ECT may be needed. ECT is particularly indicated when there is a risk of suicide and/or when there is a poor response to other modes of treatment. However, ECT is not the treatment of first choice in OCD.

5. Psychosurgery

Psychosurgery can be used in treatment of OCD that has become intractable, and is not responding to other methods of treatment.

The best responders are those who have significant associated depression although pure obsessives do also respond. The main benefit is the marked reduction in associated distress and severe anxiety.

The procedures which can be employed are:

i. Stereotactic limbic leucotomy.
ii. Stereotactic subcaudate tractotomy.

Psychosurgery is usually followed by intensive behavior therapy aimed at rehabilitation. However, with the easy availabilty of SSRIs, and good response of OCD to SSRIs and other pharmacological measures, psychosurgery is very rarely used for the treatment of OCD.

Very often, a comprehensive treatment of obsessive-compulsive disorder requires that multiple treatment modalities (e.g. drug treatment and behavior therapy) be combined in a specific manner suitable to the particular patient being treated at the time.

DISSOCIATIVE AND CONVERSION DISORDERS

The word *hysteria* has been used in so many contexts by psychiatrists, physicians and non-professionals that it no longer has any one meaning. These various contexts are:

1. Impulsive, uncontrolled behavior (impulse dyscontrol).
2. Manipulative, dramatic, exhibitionistic, emotional and/or seductive behavior (histrionic personality traits).
3. Absence of objective signs of an organic illness.
4. Presence of multiple vague somatic symptoms, especially in a female patient (masked depression, somatization disorder or Briquet's hysteria).
5. Hypochondriasis.
6. Any mental illness.
7. Presence of certain symptoms which are not explainable in the context of present organic illness (functional overlay, conversion symptoms).
8. Difficult patient; poor doctor-patient communication.
9. 'Sick' role or 'abnormal illness behavior'.
10. Psychosomatic disorders.
11. Malingering.
12. Psychosexual dysfunctions.

This list is not exhaustive. Therefore, it is not surprising that the word *hysteria* has been removed from DSM-IV as well as ICD-10. The term hysteria has been replaced in ICD-10 by 'dissociative (conversion) disorders' and in DSM-IV-TR, by conversion and dissociative disorders.

Epidemiology

Hysteria (comprising of conversion, dissociation and somatization disorder) constitutes 6-15% of all OPD diagnoses and 14-20% of all neurotic disorders. Females usually outnumber males, but in children the percentage is similar in boys and girls.

1. Conversion Disorder

Conversion disorder is characterized by the following clinical features:

1. Presence of symptoms or deficits affecting motor or sensory function, suggesting a medical or neurological disorder.
2. Sudden onset.
3. Development of symptoms usually in the presence of a significant psychosocial stressor(s).
4. A clear temporal relationship between stressor and development or exacerbation of symptoms.
5. Patient does not intentionally produce symptoms.
6. There is usually a 'secondary gain' (though not required by ICD-10 for diagnosis).

TABLE 8.4. DISSOCIATIVE CONVULSIONS AND EPILEPTIC SEIZURES

Clinical Points	Epileptic Seizures	Dissociatve Convulsions (Hysterical Fits)
1. Attack pattern	Stereotyped, known clinical patterns	Absence of any established clinical pattern. Purposive body movements occur
2. Place of occurrence	Anywhere	Usually indoors or at safe places
3. Warning	Both prodrome and aura are stereotyped	Variable
4. Time of day	Anytime. Can occur during sleep	Never occur during sleep
5. Tongue bite	Usually present	Usually absent. cheek and lip bite may be present
6. Incontinence of urine and feces	Can occur	Very rare
7. Injury	Can occur	Very rare. If occurs, it is minor or may be accidental
8. Speech	No verbalization during the seizure	Verbalization may occur during the fit
9. Duration	Usually about 30-70 sec. (Short)	20 - 800 sec. (Prolonged)
10. Head turning	Unilateral	Side to Side turning
11. Eye gaze	Staring, if eyes are open	Avoidant gaze
12. Amnesia	Complete	Partial
13. Neurological signs	Present, e.g. upgoing plantars	Absent
14. Post-ictal confusion	Present	Absent
15. Stress	Present in 25%	Present much more often
16. EEG - Iner-ictal	Usually abnormal	Usually normal
- Ictal	Abnormal	Normal
17. Serum prolactin	Increased in post-ictal period (15-20 minutes after seizure; returns back to normal in 1 hour)	Usually normal

7. Detailed physical examination and investigations do not reveal any abnormality that can explain the symptoms adequately.
8. The symptom may have a 'symbolic' relationship with the stressor/conflict.

There are usually *two* types of disturbances in conversion disorder; motor and sensory. Autonomic nervous system is typically not involved, except when voluntary musculature is involved, e.g. vomiting, globus hystericus.

In ICD-10 (CDDG), conversion disorder is subsumed under 'dissociative disorders of movement and sensation', a subtype under 'dissociative (conversion) disorders'. It is further classified in to dissociative motor disorders, dissociative anesthesia and sensory loss, and dissociative convulsions.

1. Dissociative Motor Disorders

The *motor disturbance* usually involves either

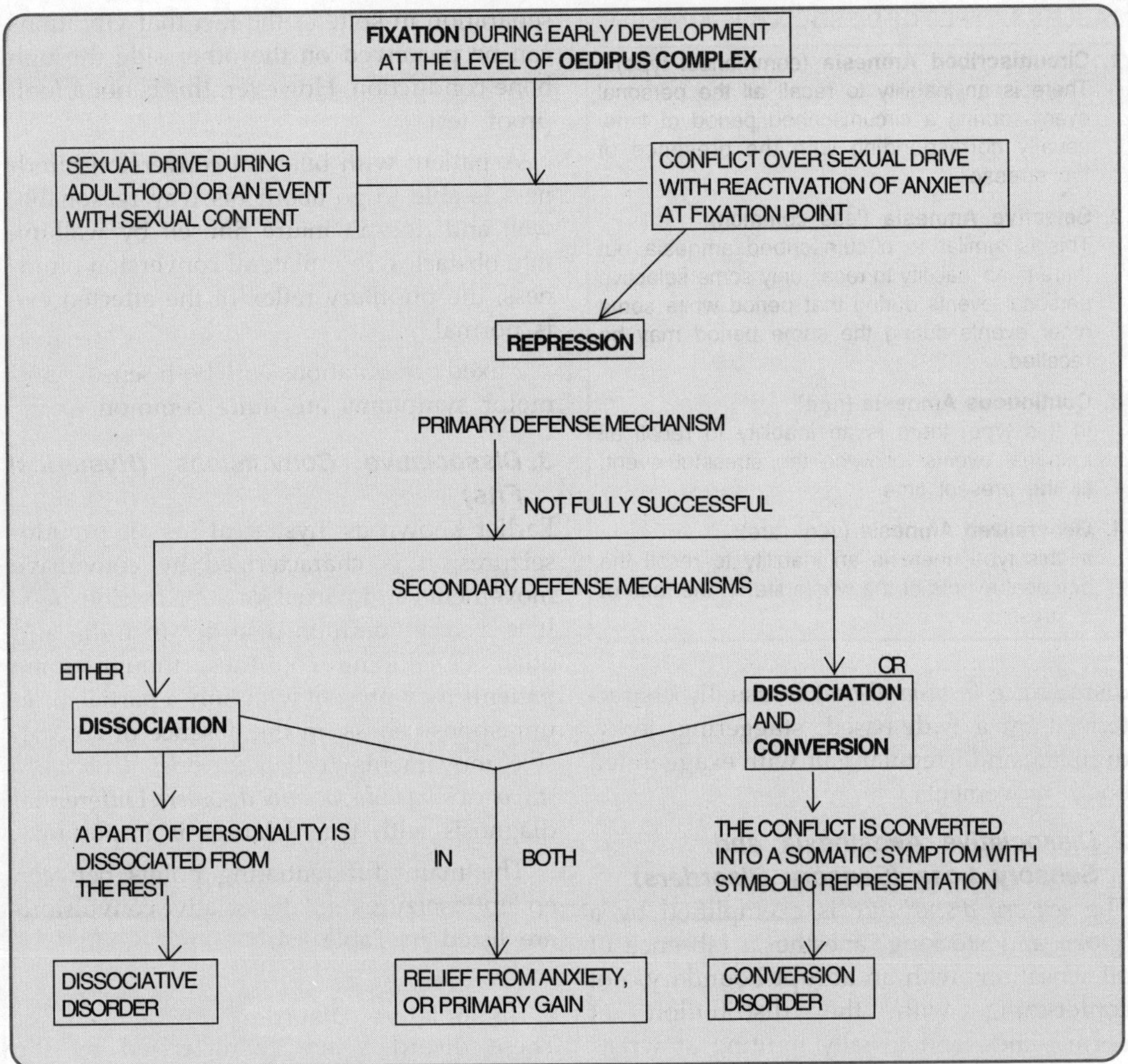

FIG. 8.2. PSYCHODYNAMIC THEORY OF DISSOCIATIVE (CONVERSION) DISORDER

paralysis or abnormal movements. The *'paralysis'* may be a monoplegia, paraplegia or quadriplegia. Classically, the symptom distribution is according to the patient's knowledge of nervous system. Examination shows normal or voluntarily increased tone and normal reflexes. However, a prolonged 'paralysis' may lead to the development of contractures.

The *'abnormal movements'* range from tremors, choreiform movements, gait disturbances to convulsive movements. These movements either occur or increase when attention is directed towards them, and may disappear when patient is watched unobserved. These movements do not fit the 'typical' clinical picture of the abnormal involuntary movement disorders. The gait

TABLE 8.5. TYPES OF DISSOCIATIVE AMNESIA

1. **Circumscribed Amnesia** (commonest type):
   There is an inability to recall all the personal events during a circumscribed period of time, usually corresponding with the presence of the stressor.
2. **Selective Amnesia** (less common):
   This is similar to circumscribed amnesia but there is an inability to recall only some selective personal events during that period while some other events during the same period may be recalled.
3. **Continuous Amnesia** (rare):
   In this type, there is an inability to recall all personal events following the stressful event, till the present time.
4. **Generalized Amnesia** (very rare):
   In this type, there is an inability to recall the personal events of the whole life, in the face of a stressful life event.

disturbance (*astasia abasia*) is usually characterized by a wide-based, staggering, jerky, dramatic and irregular gait with exaggerated body movements.

2. Dissociative Anesthesia and Sensory Loss (Sensory Disorders)

The *sensory disturbance* is exemplified by a 'glove and stocking' anesthesia (absence of all sensations with an abrupt boundary, not confor-ming with the distribution of dermatomes, and usually limiting at wrists and ankles), hemianesthesias, blindness or contracted visual fields ('tubular vision') and deafness. The detailed examination usually shows absence of objective signs of the particular illness and the disturbance is usually based on patient's knowledge of that illness.

Sensory disturbances are inconsistent with the anatomic patterns expected. Often all sensory modalities (like touch, pain, temperature and position sense) are affected at the same level. In conversion disorder, the loss of vibration sense maintains a strict midline separation in spite of the fact that vibrations can be perceived on the other side through bone conduction. However, this is not a fool-proof test.

A patient with bilateral conversion blindness is able to go about his way reasonably well and doesn't injure himself by walking into obstacles. In unilateral conversion blindness, the pupillary reflex of the affected eye is normal.

Mixed presentations with both sensory and motor symptoms are quite common.

3. Dissociative Convulsions (Hysterical Fits)

Earlier known as 'hysterical fits' or pseudoseizures, it is characterized by convulsive movements and partial loss of consciousness. It is a very common disorder in India and other developing countries, though some patients may present with only a partial, brief unresponsiveness, in the absence of convulsive movements (called as *brief dissociative stupor* or *simple dissociative disorder*). Differential diagnosis with true seizures is important.

The main differentiating points between epileptic seizures and dissociative convulsions are listed in Table 8.4.

2. Dissociative Disorder

These disorders are characterized by the following clinical features:

1. Disturbance in the normally integrated functions of consciousness, identity and/ or memory.
2. Onset is usually sudden and the disturbance is usually temporary. Recovery is often abrupt.
3. Often, there is a precipitating stress before the onset. There is a clear temporal relationship between the stressor and the onset of the illness. A frequent stressful situation is an ongoing war.

4. A 'secondary gain' resulting from the development of symptoms may be found.
5. Detailed physical examination and investigations do not reveal any abnormality that can explain the symptoms adequately.

The common clinical types are described below:

1. Dissociative Amnesia

This is the commonest clinical type of dissociative disorder. Occurring mostly in adolescent and young adults (females more than males, except in war), it is characterized by a sudden inability to recall important personal information (amnesia), particularly concerning stressful or traumatic life events. The amnesia can not be explained by everyday forgetfulness and there is no evidence of an underlying medical illness.

Most often, dissociative amnesia follows a traumatic or stressful life situation. Sometimes, imagined stressors or expression of 'forbidden' impulses may also precipitate the onset of amnesia.

This amnesia is of four types (Table 8.5). During the amnesic period, there may be slight clouding of consciousness. In the post-amnesic period, the awareness of disturbance of memory is present.

2. Dissociative Fugue

Dissociative fugue is characterized by episodes of wandering away (usually from home). During the episode, the person usually adopts a new identity with complete amnesia for the earlier life. The onset is usually sudden, often in the presence of severe stress. The termination too is abrupt and is followed by amnesia for the episode, but with recovery of memories of earlier life. The characteristic feature is the assumption of a purposeful new identity with absence of awareness of amnesia.

Important differential diagnosis is from fugue states seen in complex partial seizures or temporal lobe epilepsy, where there is no assumption of a new identity; confusion or disorientation is present during the episode and usually there is no precipitating stress.

3. Multiple Personality (Dissociative Identity) Disorder

In this dissociative disorder, the person is dominated by two or more personalities of which only one is being manifest at a time. These personalities are usually different, at times even opposing. Each personality has a full range of higher mental functions, and performs complex behavior patterns.

Usually one personality is not aware of the existence of the other(s), i.e. there are amnesic barriers between the personalities. Both the onset and termination of control of the each personality is sudden.

4. Trance and Possession Disorders

Trance and possession disorders (*possession hysteria*) are characterized by the control of person's personality by a 'spirit', during the episodes. Usually the person is aware of the existence of the other (i.e. 'possessor'), unlike in multiple personality. This disorder is very commonly seen in India and certain African countries.

5. Other Dissociative Disorders

Ganser's syndrome (*hysterical pseudodementia*) is commonly found in prison inmates. The characteristic feature is *vorbeireden* which is also called as 'approximate answers'. The answers are wrong but show that the person understands the nature of question asked. For example; when shown a red pen, the patient calls it blue.

Etiology

The etiological theories of dissociative (and

conversion) disorders are predominantly of three types:

1. Psychodynamic Theory

The explanation given by this theory can be summarized in a flow diagram (Fig 8.2). For further details regarding defense mechanisms and Freudian theory, see Tables 17.1 and 17.2.

2. Behavioral Theory

According to this theory, dissociative (and conversion) symptoms are learned responses in the face of stress. For the first time, the symptom may be learned from surrounding environment (e.g. seeing a paralyzed patient).

Development of the symptom brings about psychological relief by avoidance of stress and is thus secondarily reinforced.

3. Biological Theory

The biological basis of dissociative (conversion) disorders is far from proven. Some long-term studies (e.g. Slater) have found that up to 80% of patients, diagnosed as 'hysteria', were later found to have physical illnesses. However, replications of such studies have not found such high figures.

Conversion symptoms are frequently seen in patients of epilepsy and it may at times be difficult to differentiate between true and pseudoseizures. Similarly, 'conversion-release' symptoms are seen in some cerebral cortex lesions. However, these are only conversion *symptoms* and are not dissociative (and conversion) *disorders* [other points for diagnosis of dissociative (conversion) disorders are not present]. Hence, these are of doubtful help in elucidating the etiology of dissociative (and conversion) disorders.

Diagnosis

Diagnosis is *not* merely based on the absence of objective signs of physical illness, although it is very important to exclude an underlying or associated physical illness. The presence of positive points in history and examination should be present, before a diagnosis of dissociative (and conversion) disorders can be made.

These positive points are the characteristic clinical features listed previously. As dissociative (and conversion) disorders and physical illness can be co-existing, a detailed examination is a must. Dissociative (conversion) symptoms appearing for the first time in an elderly male, especially in a male more than 40 years old, a strong suspicion of underlying physical or major psychiatric illness should be kept in mind.

Other clinical features of dissociative (conversion) disorders include *la-belle-indifférence*, which is a lack of concern towards the symptoms, despite the apparent severity of disability produced. Although earlier thought to be a hallmark of dissociative (conversion) disorders, it is now known to be present even in physical illnesses. Also, it is not always present in dissociative (conversion) disorders.

Premorbid histrionic personality traits are often present, although a personality disorder is less common.

Treatment

1. Behavior Therapy

Since hysterical patients are *attention seeking* and their symptoms increase with focus of attention, the symptoms should be ignored; the patients treated as normals, and *not* given a *sick-role;* and any improvement should be encouraged.

Since these patients are also very *suggestible,* they respond quickly to the above mentioned methods, and a consistently firm attitude.

When there is a *sudden, acute symptom,* its prompt removal may prevent habituation and future disability. This may be achieved by one of the following methods:

i. Strong suggestion for a return to normalcy.
ii. *Aversion therapy* (liquor ammonia; aversive electric stimulus; pressure just above eyeballs or tragus of ear; closing the nose and mouth) may occasionally be employed in resistant cases.
But, its use has been decried as it tends to get over-used; may harm the patient; violates the basic human rights of the patient; and lends a wrong mental picture of the patient in the physician's mind, of a 'manipulator' needing punishment.
iii. Amplification of suggestion with hypnosis, free-association, intravenous amytal or thiopentone, or intravenous diazepam.

2. Psychotherapy with Abreaction

Abreaction is bringing to conscious awareness, thoughts, affects and memories for the first time. This may be achieved by:
i. Hypnosis.
ii. Free association.
iii. Intravenous barbiturates (thiopentone) or diazepam.

The aim of abreaction with IV thiopentone is, both, to make the conflicts conscious and to make the patient more suggestible to therapist's advice. Once the conflicts have become conscious and their affects (emotions) have been released, the conversion/dissociative symptom disappears.

3. Supportive Psychotherapy

This is especially needed when the conflict and current problems have become conscious and have to be faced in routine life. It is an important adjunct to treatment.

4. Psychoanalysis

This mode of treatment is chosen not on the basis of conversion/dissociative symptoms but on the total personality structure of the patient. Many patients respond remarkably well. The total length of therapy is usually five years or more.

5. Drug Therapy

Drug treatment has a very limited role in dissociative (and conversion) disorders (apart from the use of IV thiopentone, amytal or diazepam in abreaction and suggestion). Few patients have disabling anxiety (although anxiety as a rule is rather uncommon in hysteria) and may need short-term benzodiazepines.

SOMATOFORM DISORDERS

The somatoform disorders are characterized by repeated presentation with physical symptoms which do not have any adequate physical basis (and are not explained by the presence of other psychiatric disorders), and a persistent request for investigations and treatment despite repeated assurances by the treating doctors.

In ICD-10, somatoform disorders are divided into the following categories.

1. Somatization Disorder

Somatization disorder is characterized by the following clinical features:

1. Multiple somatic symptoms in the absence of any physical disorder.
2. The symptoms are recurrent and chronic (of many years duration); at least 2 year duration is needed for diagnosis.
3. The symptoms are vague, presented in a dramatic manner, and involve multiple organ systems. The common symptoms are *gastrointestinal* (abdominal pain, beltching, nausea, vomiting, regurgitation), *abnormal skin sensations* (numbness, soreness, itching, tingling, burning), and *sexual and menstrual complaints* (menorrhagia, dysmenorrhea, dyspareunia).
4. There is frequent change of treating physicians.

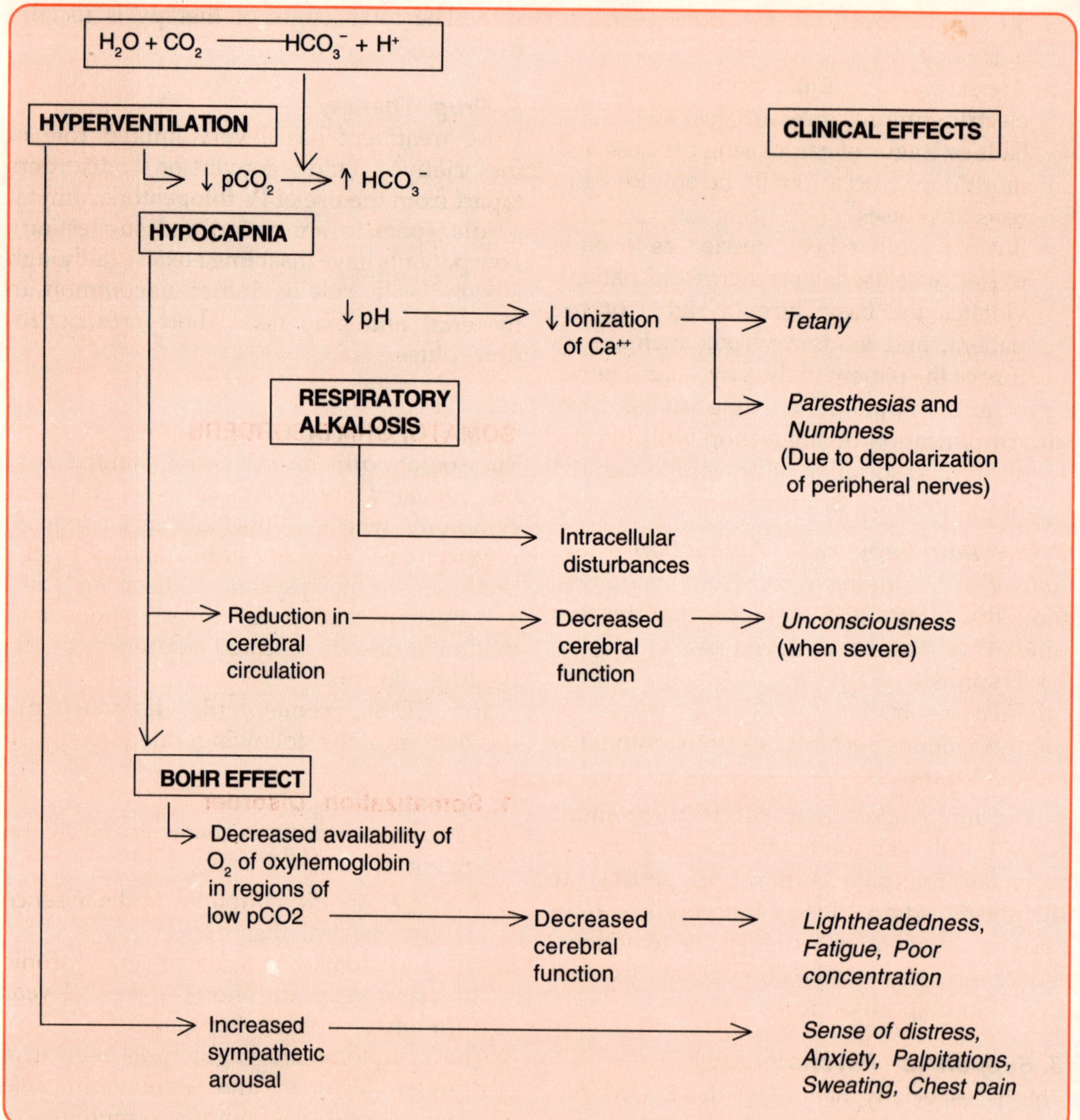

FIG. 8.3. PHYSIOLOGY OF HYPERVENTILATION SYNDROME

5. Persistent refusal to accept the advice or reassurance of several doctors that there is no physical explanation for the symptoms.
6. Some degree of impairment of social and family functioning attributable to the nature of the symptoms and resulting behavior.
7. Presence of conversion symptoms is common.

This disorder usually begins in second or third decade of life and is much more common in females. In the first degree relatives of somatization disorder patients, somatization disorder (in females), and alcoholism and psychopathy (in males) are common.

Histrionic personality traits or disorder may also be present.

Differential Diagnosis

It is important to rule out physical disorders before making a diagnosis of somatization disorder. Particularly those physical disorders, which often present with apparently vague and multiple somatic symptoms, must be kept in mind. This is especially so if the onset of symptoms is in the later part of life (> 30 years of age; more so if > 40 years of age) and in male patients.

These physical disorders include:

1. Multiple sclerosis.
2. Hypothyroidism.
3. Acute intermittent porphyria.
4. Systemic lupus erythematosis (SLE).
5. Hyperparathyroidism.
6. Carcinoma pancreas.

Somatization is sometimes an 'idiom of distress' in the absence of a diagnosable psychiatric disorder. However, certain psychiatric disorders also must be ruled out.

1. *Schizophrenia*: In the initial stages, multiple somatic symptoms may be present but later typical features of schizophrenia are manifested.

2. *Major depression*: Particularly in India, multiple somatic symptoms are common in major depression. The presence of depressed mood, depressive ideation and disturbances of biological functions in major depression help in differentiation. Occasionally differential diagnosis with *masked depression* may be difficult.

3. *Hypochondriasis*: In *somatization disorder*, there are multiple, vague somatic symptoms, while in *hypochondriasis*, normal body functions or minor somatic symptoms are interpreted as the presence of a serious body disease.

4. *Conversion disorder*: Although conversion symptoms are common in somatization disorder, they are classified separately. The number of symptoms in conversion disorder is far less (one or two) than in somatization disorder (usually more than ten).

5. *Delusional disorders*: Somatic delusions may be present in delusional disorders (e.g. monosymptomatic hypochondriacal psychosis). In delusional disorders, there is a delusional conviction of somatic symptoms with far fewer number of symptoms..

Treatment

The treatment is often difficult. It mainly consists of:

1. Supportive psychotherapy: The treatment of choice is supportive psychotherapy. The first step is to enlist the patient in the therapeutic alliance by establishing a rapport. It is useful to demonstrate the link between psychosocial conflict(s) and somatic symptoms, if it is apparent.
   In chronic cases, 'symptom reduction' rather than 'complete cure' might be a reasonable goal.
2. Behavior modification: After rapport is established, attempts at modifying behavior are made, for example ignoring symptoms, and positively reinforcing 'good' beahvior.
3. Relaxation therapy, with graded physical exercises.
4. Drug therapy: Antidepressants and/or benzodiazepines can be given on a short term basis for associated depression and/or anxiety. Benzodiazepines should be used with caution, as the risk of drug abuse is high in these patients.

2. Hypochondriasis (Hypochondriacal Disorder)

Hypochondriasis is defined as a persistent preoccupation with a fear or belief of having one or more serious disease(s), based on person's own interpretation of normal body function or a minor physical abnormality.

The other important features are:

1. Complete physical examination and investigations do not show presence of any significant abnormality.
2. The fear or belief persists despite assurance to the contrary by showing normal reports to the patient.
3. The fear or belief is *not* a delusion. Patient may agree, regarding the possibility of his exaggerating the graveness of situation, at that time.
4. Preoccupation with medical terms and syndromes is common. Repeated change of physicians is common.

The usual age of onset is in late third decade. The course is usually chronic with remissions and relapses. Obsessive personality traits and narcissistic personality features are frequently seen, in addition to associated anxiety and depression.

Etiology

The cause of hypochondriasis is not known. The important theories are mentioned below:

1. Psychodynamic Theory

Hypochondriasis is believed to be based on a narcissistic personality, caused by a narcissistic libido. Here other parts of body become erotogenic zones, which act as substitutes for genitals. Hypochondriac organs symbolize the genitals.

This is only a theoretical construct.

2. As a Symptom of Depression

Hypochondriacal symptoms are commonly present in major depression. In fact according to some, hypochondriasis is almost always a part of another psychiatric syndrome, most commonly a mood disorder. Thus, hypochondriasis has been visualized as a *masked depression* or *depressive equivalent*. However, this has not been proven till now.

Treatment

The treatment is often difficult. It consists of:

1. Supportive psychotherapy.
2. Treatment of associated or underlying depression and/or anxiety, if present.

3. Somatoform Autonomic Dysfunction

According to ICD-10 (CDDG), in this disorder, symptoms are presented by the patient as if they were due to a physical disorder of an organ system that is predominantly under autonomic control, e.g. heart and cardiovascular system (e.g. palpitations), upper gastrointestinal tract (aerophagy, hiccough), lower gastro-intestinal tract (flatulence, irritable bowel), respiratory system (hyperventilation), genitourinary system (dysuria), or other organ systems.

There is preoccupation with and distress with the possibility of a serious (but often unspecified) disorder of the particular organ system. Physical examination and investigations do not show presence of any significant abnormality. The preoccupation persists despite repeated assurances and explanations.

Treatment

The treatment consists of:

1. Supportive psychotherapy.
2. Drug treatment: The symptoms of anxiety and/or depression usually respond to benzodiazepines (e.g. alprazolam) and antidepressants (e.g. imipramine).

Some common disorders are described in some detail below:

A. Hyperventilation Syndrome (HVS)

This is a very common clinical syndrome which is often missed, particularly when not present in its full blown form. The syndrome is characterized by a habit of hyperventilation which becomes particularly marked in presence of a psychosocial stress, or any emotional upheaval.

In its *mild form*, it is characterized by excessive fatigue, chest pain, headache, palpitations, sweating and a feeling of 'lightheadedness'. In *severe* hyperventilation syndrome, carpopedal spasm (tetany), paresthesias and loss of consciousness may occur.

These symptoms are produced by hypocapnia (or a decrease in arterial pCO_2). The sequence of events in hyperventilation syndrome is explained in the diagram below (Fig. 8.3).

The diagnosis is easy. Apart from clinical history and presence of frequent 'sighing' during the interview, a simple test would demonstrate the symptomatology. The patient is asked to breathe rapidly and deeply for 2-3 minutes. This produces the classical physical symptoms. If carried on longer, tetany and unconsciousness would result.

Treatment

1. Relaxation techniques: Jacobson's progressive muscular relaxation, autohypnosis or hypnosis, *yoga*, transcendental meditation, or biofeedback.
2. Teaching relaxed breathing techniques, which include,
   i. Breathing more from the abdomen, thus avoiding the use of accessory muscles of expiration.
   ii. Slow respiration with passive expiration, without muscular effort.
   iii. Short rest cycle to be voluntarily introduced after each respiratory cycle.
3. Treatment of underlying anxiety or depression, if present, with benzodiazepines or tricyclic antidepressants.
4. *Breathing-in-bag technique*: The aim of this technique is to have the patient rebreathe expired air. This prevents the decrease in pCO_2 which causes physical symptoms, or causes an increase in pCO_2 where physical symptoms have already developed. Rebreathing in a plastic bag, which is carried by the patient, quickly reverts the symptoms.

B. Irritable Bowel Syndrome (IBS)

This is a common syndrome often called by a large variety of names, like spastic colitis, irritable colon syndrome, nervous diarrhea, mucus colitis, colon neurosis. The principal abnormality is a disturbance of bowel mobility which is modified by psychosocial factors. The patients usually present with one or more of the following symptoms:

1. Abdominal pain, discomfort or cramps.
2. Alteration of bowel habits (diarrhea or constipation).
3. Sensation of incomplete evacuation.

Very often all three (abdominal pain, and diarrhea alternating with constipation) are present together; also associated is flatulence. The patients often describe their stools in a dramatic manner.

It is a fairly common disorder occurring in nearly 40% of all patients attending a gastroenterology (GE) clinic. Although females more frequently have IBS in America, in India males are more often affected. It is more or less a stable disorder with frequent exacerbations.

The typical mode of onset or exacerbation is with occurrence of a psychosocial stressor or emotional upheaval. Physiologically, there are two changes possible in the bowel motility.

1. Hypomotility, which is often associated with painless diarrhea.
2. Hypermotility, which presents clinically as painful constipation or rarely painful diarrhea.

Treatment

1. A stable and trustful doctor-patient relationship.
2. Supportive psychotherapy is best carried out in medical or GE clinic by the treating physician. These patients often resent psychiatric referrals.
3. Identification of current life stressors and environmental manipulation and/or coping skills aimed at dealing with stressors are very helpful.
4. Antianxiety and antidepressant medication may be helpful at times. At other times, they just act like placebos.
5. Symptomatic management is often unsuccessful. However, prokinetic agents (e.g. cisapride) may sometimes be useful. A trial of fibre (wheat bran, psyllium, methylcellulose) is reasonable in some patients of irritable bowel syndrome.

C. Premenstrual Syndrome

Premenstrual syndrome or premenstrual tension (as it is commonly called) is characterized by a variety of physical, psychological and behavioral symptoms occurring in the second half of menstrual cycle. Typically, the symptoms start after a few days of ovulation, reach a peak about 4-5 days before menstruation and disappear usually around menstruation. The period between menstruation and next ovulation is normal.

The syndrome is characterized by feelings of irritability, depression, crying spells, restlessness and anxiety. These are associated with changes in appetite; signs and symptoms of water retention (like pedal edema, weight gain, swelling of breasts, sense of bloating of abdomen); gastroenterological changes; headache and fatigue.

The etiology is probably multifactorial. The biological factors include faulty luteinization, excess of esterogens, progesterone deficiency. The psychosocial factors encompass education, expectations and attitudes towards menstruation and femininity ('tension' about menstruation).

TABLE 8.6. DEPERSONALIZATION: CAUSES

1. Psychiatric Disorders
- i. Depersonalization disorder
- ii. Phobic-anxiety-depersonalization (PAD) syndrome
- iii. Anxiety disorder
- iv. Panic disorder
- v. Agoraphobia
- vi. Schizophrenia
- vii. Depression

2. Neurological Disorders
- i. Complex partial seizures
- ii. Migraine
- iii. Cerebral tumors (especially affecting the non-dominant parietal lobe)
- iv. Encephalitis

3. Other Causes
- i. Hyperventilation
- ii. Alcohol and drug dependence
- iii. Hypoglycemia
- iv. Fatigue (in normals)
- v. Grief
- vi. Sensory deprivation

Treatment

1. The treatment of water retention by giving diuretics, and restricting fluid and electrolyte intake. Thiazide diuretics are often prescribed but spironolactone is superior.
2. Psychotherapy may be helpful in some cases where conflicts regarding menstruation and/or femininity are present.
3. Hormonal treatment with oral or parenteral progesterone has been recommended by some, with good results.
4. In resistant cases, other drugs like lithium, bromocriptine, antidepressants and antianxiety agents have been used.

4. Persistent Somatoform Pain Disorder

It was previously called as psychogenic pain disorder. In this disorder, persistent, severe and distressing pain is the main feature which is, either grossly in excess of what is expected from physical findings, or inconsistent with the anatomical distribution of nervous system. Preoccupation with pain is common.

There is often a precipitating stressful event and secondary gain may be present. Repeated change of physicians *(doctor-shopping)* is common. The affected person often assumes a 'sick-role' or an 'invalid-role'. Abuse and dependence of analgesics and minor tranquilizers is common, particularly when the course is chronic.

This disorder is more common in females, with an onset in third or fourth decade of life.

Treatment

1. The patients usually refuse psychiatric intervention.
2. Drug therapy should be avoided as the risk of iatrogenic drug abuse is high.
3. In the absence of other modes of successful treatment, a supportive relationship with a physician will prevent doctor-shopping and provide relief.

5. Other Somatoform Disorders

In ICD-10, this category includes other somatoform disorders not classified in the previous four categories, e.g. 'globus hystericus', psychogenic torticollis, psychogenic pruritus, psychogenic dysmenorrhea, teeth-grinding.

OTHER NEUROTIC DISORDERS

In ICD-10, the other neurotic disorders are divided into the following categories:

1. Neurasthenia

According to ICD-10 (CDDG), this disorder is characterized by:

1. Either persisting and distressing complaints of increased fatigue after mental effort, or persistent and distressing complaints of bodily weakness and exhaustion after minimal effort.
2. At least two of the following: feelings of muscular aches and pains, dizziness, tension headaches, sleep disturbances, inability to relax, irritability, and dyspepsia.
3. Any autonomic or depressive symptoms present are not sufficiently persistent and severe to fulfill the criteria for any of the more specific mental disorders.

This is a poorly defined syndrome and its independence as a diagnosis is doubtful.

A differential diagnosis with *CFS (chronic fatigue syndrome)* and other medical and psychiatric disorders presenting with fatigue is important before diagnosing neurasthenia.

CFS is characterized by profound fatigue (present at rest, and made worse by physical and mental effort), muscle pains, headache, sore throat, functional impairment and non-specific 'soft' physical signs, e.g. mild fever, mild lymphadenopathy. CFS is diagnosed in absence of medical or other psychiatric disorder, though neuropsychiatric symptoms may be present.

2. Depersonalization Disorder

(Depersonalization-Derealization Syndrome)

Depersonalization is characterized by alteration in the perception or experience of self, so that the feeling of one's own reality is temporarily changed or lost. It is an *'as if'* phenomenon. The person affected is not delusionally convinced about the change, but instead describes it to have occurred, as-if.

This is often accompanied by *derealization*, which is an alteration in the perception or experience of external world, so that the feeling of reality of external world is temporarily changed or lost. This too is an 'as if' phenomenon. Derealization is a larger concept which encompasses depersonalization also.

As both depersonalization and derealization occur in many other disorders (Table 8.6), the term depersonalization disorder should be used only when other disorders have been ruled out.

The other associated clinical features include:

1. The episodes of depersonalization and/or derealization causing significant social, interpersonal or occupational impairment. The episodes recur frequently.
2. The onset and termination of episodes is sudden.
3. Marked distress and anxiety results, as the experience is highly unpleasant. Insight into the illness is present.
4. Feeling of loss of control on one's action and speech may occur.
5. The episodes occur in the presence of a clear sensorium.

The age of onset is usually late second or early third decade. The course is usually chronic.

Treatment

The treatment is usually not successful. The various methods which can be tried are:

1. Supportive psychotherapy.
2. Drug therapy with antidepressants, amphetamines or antipsychotics.

3. Other Specified Neurotic Disorders (Culture Bound Syndromes)

In ICD-10, this category includes miscellaneous disorders which are of uncertain etiology and nosological status, and which occur in certain cultures, e.g. *dhat syndrome, koro, latah, wihtigo, piblokto* and *amok*. These are called as *culture-bound syndromes*, as they are localized to certain geographical areas only, and are not seen in the Western, developed countries.

A. Dhat Syndrome

Dhat syndrome is a culture-bound syndrome, which is prevalent in the Indian subcontinent. This is characterized by:

1. Complaint of passage of *'dhat'* in urine.
2. Multiple somatic symptoms.
3. Asthenia (physical or mental exhaustion).
4. Anxiety or depression may be present.
5. Sexual dysfunction may occur.

'Dhat' is a whitish discharge passed in urine and believed to be semen by the patient. According to a socio-cultural belief prevalent in the Indian society, semen is an extremely precious body element which is produced from many drops of blood. Hence, it follows that loss of semen will lead to weakness and sexual dysfunction. Often, masturbatory anxiety and overconcern with nocturnal emissions are associated with other clinical symptoms.

Treatment

1. *Counseling*: This is the most important method directed towards removing the misconceptions regarding apprehension of semen loss. This is combined with sex education in general. Specifically, fears regarding masturbation and nocturnal emissions are allayed.
2. *Symptomatic treatment*: The treatment of underlying anxiety, depression, hypochondriasis and/or sexual dysfunction may also be required.

B. Amok

Amok is characterized by a sudden, unprovoked episode of rage, in which the affected person runs about (runs *'amok'*) and indiscriminately injures or kills any person who is encountered on the way. It is usually seen in south-east Asia (e.g. Malaysia).

C. Koro

Koro is a culture-bound syndrome seen in Asia (including India). The affected male person has the belief that his penis is shrinking and may disappear in to his abdominal wall and he may die. Females are affected infrequently, with a corresponding belief that their breasts (and vulva) are shrinking.

Koro often spreads rapidly to other members of the community in an epidemic form. It is usually based on culturally elaborated fears regarding nocturnal emission and masturbation.

D. Wihtigo (Windigo)

This syndrome is seen in native American-Indians. The affected person has the belief that he has been transformed in to a *wihtigo*, a cannibal monster, occurring especially during times of starvation.

E. Piblokto (Arctic Hysteria)

This culture-bound syndrome occurs in Iskimos. The affected person is often a female, who screams and tears off her clothes, and throws herself on ice in extemely cold conditions. She may imitate the cry of a bird or an animal. The episode usually lasts for 1-2 hours, followed by amnesia for the events. It is probably a type of dissociative disorder.

F. Latah (Startle Reaction)

This syndrome is reported form south-east Asia and Japan. Occurring more often in women, *latah* is characterized by presence of automatic obedience, echolalia, and echopraxia. It is often precipitated by a sudden stimulus.

G. Some Indian Culture-bound Syndromes

In addition to Dhat syndrome, amok and koro (described above), the other culture-bound syndromes seen in India include *Suchi-bai* (*purity mania*), *ascetic syndrome*, *nupital psychosis*, and *Jhin-jhinia*.

REACTION TO STRESS AND ADJUSTMENT DISORDERS

This category in ICD-10 consists of those disorders which are temporally related to an exceptionally stressful life event (acute stress reaction and post-traumatic stress disorder) or a significant life change (adjustment disorders) immediately before the onset.

1. Acute Stress Reaction

According to ICD-10 (CDDG), in this disorder there is an immediate and clear temporal relationship between an exceptional stressor (e.g. death of a loved one, natural catastrophe, accident, rape) and the onset of symptoms. The symptoms show a mixed and changing picture. This disorder is more likely to develop in presence of physical exhaustion and in extremes of age. It is more commonly seen in females and people with poor coping skills.

The symptoms range from a 'dazed' condition, anxiety, depression, anger, despair, overactivity or withdrawal, and constriction of the field of consciousness. The symptoms resolve rapidly (with in few hours usually) if removal from stressful environment is possible. If the stress continues or can not be reversed, resolution of symptoms begins after 1-2 days and is usually minimal after about 3 days.

Treatment

The treatment consists of removal of the patient from the stressful environment and helping the patient to 'pass through' the stressful experience. IV benzodiazepines (e.g. diazepam) may be needed in case with marked agitation.

2. Post-Traumatic Stress Disorder (PTSD)

According to ICD-10 (CDDG), this disorder arises as a delayed and/protracted response to an exceptionally stressful or catastrophic life event or situation which is likely to cause pervasive distress in almost any person (e.g. disasters, war, rape or torture, serious accident). The symptoms of PTSD may develop, after a period of latency, with in 6 months after the stress or may be delayed beyond this period.

PTSD is characterized by recurrent and intrusive recollections of the stressful event either in *flashbacks* (images, thoughts, or perceptions) and/or in dreams. There is an associated sense of re-experiencing of the stressful event. There is marked *avoidance* of the events or situations that arouse recollections of the stressful event, along with marked symptoms of anxiety and increased arousal.

The other important clinical features include partial amnesia for some aspects of the stressful event, feeling of numbness, and anhedonia (inability to experience pleasure).

Treatment

The treatment consists of the following measures:

1. *Prevention*: Anticipation of disasters in the high risk areas, with the training of personnel in disaster management.
2. *Disaster management*: Here the speed of providing help is of paramount importance. This is also a preventive measure.
3. *Supportive psychotherapy*.
4. *Drug treatment*: Antidepressants and benzodiazepines are useful in treatment if anxiety and/or depression are important components of the clinical picture.

3. Adjustment Disorders

Adjustment disorders are one of the most common psychiatric disorders seen in clinical practice. They are most frequently seen in adolescents and women. Although adjustment disorder is often precipitated by one or more stressors, it often represents a maladaptive response to the stressful life event(s).

In ICD-10, this disorder is characterized by those disorders which occur within 1 month of a significant life change (stressor). This disorder usually occurs in those individuals who are vulnerable due to poor coping skills or personality factors. It is assumed that the disorder would not have arisen in the absence of the stressor(s). The duration of the disorder is usually less than 6 months, except in the case of prolonged depressive reaction.

The various subtypes include brief depressive reaction, prolonged depressive reaction, mixed anxiety and depressive reaction, with predominant disturbance of other emotions, with predominant disturbance of conduct, and with mixed disturbance of emotions and conduct. Most patients recover within a period of three months.

Treatment

1. *Supportive psychotherapy* remains the treatment of choice.
2. *Crisis intervention* is useful in some patients, by helping to quickly resolve the stressful life situation which has led to the adjustment disorder.
3. Stress management training.
3. Coping skills training.
4. *Drug treatment* may be needed in some patients for the management of anxiety (benzodiazepines) and/or depressive symptoms (antidepressants).

9

Disorders of Adult Personality and Behavior

SPECIFIC PERSONALITY DISORDERS

Personality is defined as a deeply ingrained pattern of behavior that include modes of perception, relating to and thinking about oneself and the surrounding environment.

Personality traits are normal, prominent-aspects of personality. *Personality disorders* result when these personality traits become abnormal, i.e. become inflexible and maladaptive, and cause significant social or occupational impairment, or significant subjective distress.

Although personal distress may occur in some personality disorders, classically the abnormal personality traits are 'ego-syntonic'. This is in sharp contrast to the symptoms in neurotic disorders, which are ego-dystonic and hence cause significant distress to the patient. So, unlike the patients with neurotic disorders, personality disorder patients do not usually seek psychiatric help unless other psychiatric symptoms co-exist.

Although personality disorders are usually recognizable by early adolescence, they are not typically diagnosed before early adult life. The symptoms continue unchanged through the adult life and usually become less obvious in the later years of life (after 40 years of age).

The prevalence of personality disorders in the general population is 5-10%. Often symptoms of more than one personality disorder are present in one person. In fact, it is now believed that the occurrence of mixed personality disorders (i.e. co-morbidity) is commoner than single (pure) personality disorders.

In DSM-IV-TR, the personality disorders are coded on Axis II and have been divided into three clusters (Table 9.1).

In addition to these three clusters, passive-aggressive personality disorder and depressive personality disorder have been

TABLE 9.1. PERSONALITY DISORDERS CLUSTERS (DSM-IV-TR)

1. Cluster-A (Odd and eccentric)

Personality disorders (PDs), thought to be on a 'schizophrenic-continuum'. These are:

i. Paranoid PD
ii. Schizoid PD
iii. Schizotypal PD

2. Cluster-B (Dramatic, emotional and erratic)

Personality disorders (PDs), thought to be on a 'psychopathic continuum'. These are:

i. Antisocial PD
ii. Histrionic PD
iii. Narcissistic PD
iv. Borderline PD

3. Cluster-C (Anxious and fearful)

Personality disorders (PDs), characterized by 'introversion'. These are:

i. Avoidant PD
ii. Dependent PD
iii. Obsessive-compulsive PD

included in the section on 'Criteria provided for further study' in DSM-IV-TR.

In ICD-10, the personality disorders are listed under section on 'Disorders of adult personality and behavior'.

Diagnosis

According to the ICD-10 (CDDG), the diagnostic guidelines for *specific personality disorder* include conditions not directly attributable to gross brain damage or disease, or to another psychiatric disorder, meeting the following criteria:

1. Markedly dysharmonious attitudes and behavior, involving usually several areas of functioning, e.g. affectivity, arousal, impulse control, ways of perceiving and thinking, and style of relating to others;
2. The abnormal behavior pattern is enduring, of long standing, and not limited to episodes of mental illness;
3. The abnormal behavior pattern is pervasive and clearly maladaptive to a broad range of personal and social situations;
4. The above manifestations always appear during childhood or adolescence and continue into adulthood;
5. The disorder leads to considerable personal distress but this may only become apparent late in its course;
6. The disorder is usually, but not invariably, associated with significant problems in occupational and social performance.

Clinical Subtypes

1. Paranoid Personality Disorder

According to the ICD-10 (CDDG), the diagnostic guidelines for paranoid personality disorder include the following features (in addition to features of personality disorders in general, described above). Clear evidence is usually required of the presence of *at least three* of the traits or behaviors given in the clinical description.

1. Excessive sensitiveness to setbacks and rebuffs.
2. Tendency to bear grudges persistently, i.e. refusal to forgive insults and injuries or slights.
3. Suspiciousness and a pervasive tendency to distort experience by misconstruing the neutral or friendly actions of others as hostile or contemptuous.
4. A combative and tenacious sense of personal rights, out of keeping with the actual situation.
5. Recurrent suspicions, without justification, regarding sexual fidelity of spouse or sexual partner.
6. Tendency to experience excessive self-importance, manifest in a persistent self-referential attitude.
7. Preoccupation with unsubstantiated 'conspiratorial' explanations of events, both immediate to the patient and in the world at large.

The patients may become involved in litigation on small issues. The disorder is commoner in men. It is more common in minority groups and immigrants.

Psychodynamically, the underlying defense mechanism is *projection.*

The paranoid personality disorder is found premorbidly in some patients of paranoid schizophrenia. But whether it predisposes to the development of paranoid schizophrenia, is not known. Differential diagnosis is from delusional (paranoid) disorders and paranoid schizophrenia.

Treatment

1. Individual psychotherapy.
2. Supportive psychotherapy.

The response to treatment is usually poor. The patients often do not seek treatment on their own and may resent treatment. Drug treatment has a very limited role.

2. Schizoid Personality Disorder

According to the ICD-10 (CDDG), the diagnostic guidelines for schizoid personality disorder include the following features (in addition to the general features of personality disorders). Clear evidence is usually required of the presence of at least three of the traits or behaviors given in the clinical description.

1. Few, if any, activities, provide pleasure.
2. Emotional coldness, detachment or flattened affectivity.
3. Limited capacity to express either warm, tender feelings or anger towards others.
4. Apparent indifference to either praise or criticism.
5. Little interest in having sexual experiences with another person (taking into account age).
6. Almost invariable preference for solitary activities.
7. Excessive preoccupation with fantasy and introspection.
8. Lack of close friends or confiding relationships (or having only one) and of desire for such relationships.
9. Marked insensitivity to prevailing social norms and conventions.

The features of this disorder may overlap with paranoid and schizotypal personality disorders, which too belong to the Cluster-A. Psychotic features are absent. It is more common in men.

Psychodynamically, it is supposed to result from 'cold and aloof' parenting in a child with introverted temperament. However, this hypothesis is far from proven in the research conducted so far.

Like all personality disorders, schizoid personality disorder has an onset in early childhood with stable course over the years. Earlier it was believed to predispose to development of schizophrenia, but later studies have failed to replicate the findings.

Treatment

1. Individual psychotherapy.
2. Psychoanalysis.
3. Gradual involvement in group psychotherapy.

The patients often do not seek treatment on their own. The response to treatment is usually not good. Drug treatment has a very limited role.

3. Schizotypal Disorder (Schizotypal Personality Disorder)

According to the ICD-10 (CDDG), this disorder is not classified under specific personality disorders but instead along with schizo-phrenia. The diagnostic guidelines for specific personality disorder include the following features.

A disorder characterized by eccentric behavior and anomalies of thinking and affect which resemble those seen in schizophrenia, though no definite and characteristic schizophrenic anomalies have occurred at any stage. At least three or four of the following should be present continuously or episodically for a period of at least 2 years:

1. Inappropriate or constricted affect (the individual appears cold and aloof).
2. Behavior or appearance that is odd, eccentric, or peculiar.
3. Poor rapport with others and a tendency to social withdrawal.
4. Odd beliefs or magical thinking, influencing behavior and inconsistent with subcultural norms.
5. Suspiciousness or paranoid ideas.
6. Obsessive ruminations without inner resistance, often with dysmorphophobic, sexual or aggressive contents.
7. Unusual perceptual experiences including somatosensory (bodily) or other illusions, depersonalization or derealization.
8. Vague, circumstantial, metaphorical, overelaborate, or stereotyped thinking, mani-

fested by odd speech or in other ways, without gross incoherence.
9. Occasional transient quasi-psychotic episodes with intense illusions, auditory or other hallucinations, and delusion-like ideas, usually occurring without external provocation.

This disorder lies between schizoid personality disorder and schizophrenia on a schizophrenic continuum. Differentiation from simple schizophrenia, schizoid personality disorder, and paranoid personality disorder is not clearly demarcated. It is more common in individuals related to schizophrenics and is believed to be part of the genetic 'spectrum' of schizophrenia. Its onset, evolution and course are usually those of a personality disorder. It usually runs a chronic course.

Treatment

The response to treatment is usually poor, except for brief psychotic episodes.

1. Psychoanalysis.
2. Individual psychotherapy.
3. Drug therapy: Antipsychotics have been used without much benefit. The role of antipsy-chotics in treatment is limited to brief psychotic episodes.

4. Antisocial/Dissocial Personality Disorder

According to the ICD-10 (CDDG), the diagnostic guidelines for dissocial (antisocial) personality disorder include the following clinical features. Clear evidence is usually required of the presence of at least three of the traits or behaviors given in the clinical description. This disorder is synonymous with psychopathy and sociopathy, but does not always mean criminal behavior.

1. Callous unconcern for the feelings of others.
2. Gross and persistent attitude of irresponsibility and disregard for social norms, rules and obligations.
3. Incapacity to maintain enduring relationships, though having no difficulty in establishing them.
4. Very low tolerance to frustration and a low threshold for discharge of aggression, including violence.
5. Incapacity to experience guilt and to profit from experience, particularly punishment.
6. Marked proneness to blame others, or to offer plausible rationalizations, for the behavior that has brought the patient in to conflict with society.

There may also be persistent irritability as an associated feature. Conduct disorder during childhood and adolescence, though no invariably present, may further support the diagnosis.

There are no psychotic features in this disorder. Earlier antisocial personality disorder was divided into four clinical types namely:

1. Aggressive psychopath,
2. Inadequate psychopath,
3. Creative psychopath, and
4. Sexual psychopath.

As these are not discrete groups and their characteristic symptoms merge with one another, they are no longer classified in this manner. Although no clear etiology is known, several genetic, environmental and biological factors are associated with this disorder. These factors include more than normal prevalence of antisocial personality disorder in father; presence of impulsive and inconsistent parents; presence of soft neurological signs, non-specific EEG abnormalities; and presence of conduct and/or attention deficit disorder in childhood.

This disorder is diagnosed more commonly in males. The course is usually chronic; however, there is some decrease in the symptoms after the fifth decade of life in some patients.

Treatment

Patients often do not seek psychiatric help and if they do, under pressure from legal authorities, the therapeutic alliance is not often sustained.

1. Individual psychotherapy.
2. Psychoanalysis.
3. Group psychotherapy and self-help groups.
4. Drug therapy: Pharmacotherapy is of little help. Earlier claims, of beneficial effect of *pericyazine* (an antipsychotic drug) in certain behavior patterns of antisocial personality disorder, have not been substantiated.

5. Histrionic Personality Disorder

According to the ICD-10 (CDDG), the diagnostic guidelines for histrionic personality disorder include the following clinical features. Clear evidence is usually required of the presence of at least three of the traits or behaviors given in the clinical description.

1. Self-dramatization, theatricality, exaggerated expression of emotions (*dramatic emotion-ality*).
2. Suggestibility, easily influenced by others or by circumstances.
3. Shallow and labile affectivity.
4. Continual seeking for excitement, appreciation by others, and activities in which the person is the center of attention (*Attention-seeking attitude*).
5. Inappropriate seductiveness in appearance or behavior.
6. Over-concern with physical attractiveness.

Associated features may include egocentricity, self-indulgence, continuous longing for appreciation, feelings that are easily hurt, and persistent manipulative behavior to achieve own needs.

Tantrums or anger outbursts are common. The actions are not planned for long-term goals, instead they seek instant satisfaction and approval. Exhibitionistic traits like dressing flamboyantly, mannerisms of speech and motor behavior are present. There is an attempt to look charming, beautiful and seductive. Suicidal gestures may be made. Interpersonal relationships are often stormy and ungratifying.

This disorder is more common in females. Hysteria (conversion and dissociation disorder) was previously thought to be more common in the presence of histrionic personality disorder, but recent studies have failed to prove this relationship.

Psychodynamically, there are intense dependency needs. The defense mechanisms used most often are *acting out* and *dissociation*.

Treatment

Psychoanalysis and psychoanalytic psychotherapy are the modes of treatment which are most successful.

The treatment is often useful in removal of a few symptoms only.

6. Narcissistic Personality Disorder

A relatively new concept, this disorder is characterized by:

1. Ideas of grandiosity and inflated sense of self-importance.
2. Preoccupation with fantasies of unlimited success.
3. Attention seeking, dramatic behavior, needs constant praise, and unable to face criticism.
4. Lack of empathy with others, with exploitative behavior.
5. Shaky self-esteem, underlying sense of inferiority, easily depressed by minor events.

Treatment

Individual psychotherapy probably helps, but data available is not sufficient for comment.

7. Emotionally Unstable Personality Disorder

According to the ICD-10 (CDDG), emotionally unstable personality disorder is described as a disorder in which there is a marked tendency to act impulsively without consideration of the consequences, together with affective instability. This disorder is further classified in to two types: impulsive type and borderline type.

The *impulsive type* is characterized by emotional instability and lack of impulse control. Outbursts of violence or threatening behavior are common, particularly in response to criticism by others.

The *borderline type* is characterized by emotional instability; in addition, patient's own self-image, aims, and internal preferences (including sexual) are often unclear or disturbed. There are usually chronic feelings of emptiness. A liability to become involved in intense and unstable relationships may cause repeated emotional crises and may be associated with excessive efforts to avoid abandonment and a series of suicidal threats or acts of self-harm, (although these may occur without obvious precipitants).

The borderline type is also known as *borderline personality disorder* (DSM-IV-TR), the characteristic features of which include the following:

1. Significant and persistent disturbance of identity of self. e.g. 'who am I'. There is marked uncertainty about major issues in life.
2. Unstable and intense interpersonal relationship patterns.
3. Impulsivity.
4. Unstable emotional responses, with rapid shifts. Anger outbursts may occur.
5. Chronic feelings of boredom or emptiness with inability to stay alone.
6. Deliberate self harm is common in the form of self-mutilation, suicidal gestures, or accident-proneness.

Borderline personality disorder includes *ambulatory schizophrenia* and *pseudoneurotic schizophrenia*, which were earlier thought to be subtypes of schizophrenia.

Psychodynamically, *splitting* is the defense mechanism employed in borderline personality disorder.

There is a considerable overlap between borderline, narcissistic and antisocial (dissocial) personality disorders. Major depressive episodes occur commonly in this disorder.

Treatment

1. Psychoanalytic psychotherapy.
2. Supportive psychotherapy.
3. Drug therapy: Antidepressants have been used with success in certain patients. Major depressive episode, if occurs, necessitates antidepressant therapy with or without ECTs. Occasionally antipsychotics, lithium, and carbamazepine have been used when aggression and impulsivity are prominent.

Drug therapy is not the treatment of choice in borderline personality disorder.

8. Anxious (Avoidant) Personality Disorder

According to the ICD-10 (CDDG), the diagnostic guidelines for anxious (avoidant) personality disorder include the following features. Clear evidence is usually required of the presence of at least three of the traits or behaviors given in the clinical description.

1. Persistent and pervasive feelings of tension and apprehension.
2. Belief that one is socially inept, personally unappealing, or inferior to others.
3. Excessive preoccupation with being criticized or rejected in social situations.
4. Unwillingness to become involved with people unless certain of being liked.
5. Restrictions in lifestyle because of need to have physical security.
6. Avoidance of social or occupational activities that involve significant interpersonal contact because of fear of criticism, disapproval, or rejection.

Associated features may include hypersensitivity to rejection and criticism.

These patients do not enter into interpersonal relationships unless they are very sure of uncritical approval. This disorder is an epitome of what is often called as *inferiority complex*. Secondary depression is very common.

Treatment

1. Individual psychotherapy.
2. Group psychotherapy.
3. Behavior therapy: In particular, social skills training and assertiveness training are useful.

The response to treatment is usually satisfactory.

9. Dependent Personality Disorder

According to the ICD-10 (CDDG), the diagnostic guidelines for dependent personality disorder include the following features. Clear evidence is usually required of the presence of at least three of the traits or behaviors given in the clinical description.

1. Encouraging or allowing others to make most of one's important life decisions.
2. Subordination of one's own needs to those of others on whom one is dependent, and undue compliance with their wishes.
3. Unwillingness to make even reasonable demands on the people one depends on.
4. Feeling uncomfortable or helpless when alone, because of exaggerated fears of inability to care for oneself.
5. Preoccupation with fears of being abandoned by a person with whom one has a close rela-tionship, and of being left to care for oneself.
6. Limited capacity to make everyday decisions without an excessive amount of advice and reassurance from others.

Associated features may include perceiving oneself as helpless, incompetent, and lacking stamina.

There may be an overlap with avoidant and passive-aggressive personality disorders. Some patients exhibit *masochistic character*. They repetitively establish close interpersonal relationships which result in punishment.

Treatment

1. Individual psychotherapy.
2. Group psychotherapy.
3. Behavior therapy in the from of assertiveness training is useful.

The response to treatment is usually good.

10. Obsessive-Compulsive (Anankastic) Personality Disorder

According to the ICD-10 (CDDG), the diagnostic guidelines for anankastic personality disorder include the following clinical features. Clear evidence is usually required of the presence of at least three of the traits or behaviors given in the clinical description.

1. Feelings of excessive doubt and caution.
2. Preoccupation with details, rules, lists, order, organization or schedule.
3. Perfectionism that interferes with task completion.
4. Excessive conscientiousness, scrupulousness, and undue preoccupation with productivity to the exclusion of pleasure and interpersonal relationships.
5. Excessive pedantry and adherence to social conventions.
6. Rigidity and stubbornness.
7. Unreasonable insistence by the patient that others submit to exactly his or her way of doing things, or unreasonable reluctance to allow others to do things.
8. Intrusion of insistent and unwelcome thoughts or impulses.

This disorder is more often diagnosed in males, and is common in premorbid personality of obsessive compulsive disorder (OCD) patients. Major depressive episodes are frequent.

Psychodynamically, this disorder is believed to result from fixation at anal sadistic phase, with the employment of *reaction formation* as a defense mechanism.

Treatment

These patients retain insight, hence seek psychiatric help on their own.

1. Psychoanalysis.
2. Group therapy.

11. Passive-Aggressive Personality Disorder

This disorder is not listed as a personality disorder in both ICD-10 and DSM-IV-TR, and is characterized by the following clinical features:

1. Significant and persistent *passive resistance* to demands for adequate social and occupational performance.
2. Stubborness, intentional inefficiency, procrastination, unjustified protests, 'forgetfulness' and/or dawdling are used to achieve the purpose.

Passive resistance is viewed as expression of 'covert anger' or 'retroflexed anger'. This behavior is often chosen in spite of the fact that a more direct and active way of showing an opinion and/or resisting was possible.

An overlap with dependent personality disorder is common. Secondary depression may develop.

Treatment

1. Supportive psychotherapy.
2. Behavior therapy: Social skills training and assertiveness training is helpful.
3. Group therapy.
4. Drug therapy: Antidepressants may be needed for secondary depression.

ENDURING PERSONALITY CHANGES, NOT ATTRIBUTABLE TO BRAIN DAMAGE AND DISEASE

This new category in ICD-10 includes disorders of adult personality and behavior which develop following catastrophic or excessive prolonged stress, or following a severe psychiatric illness, in people with no personality disorder. The presence of brain damage or disease which may cause similar clinical features should be ruled out.

HABIT AND IMPULSE DISORDERS

This category includes disorders like pathological gambling, pyromania, kleptomania, trichotillomania, and intermittent explosive disorder. The disorders in this heterogeneous group are characterized by impulsive behavior which the patient can not resist or control. There may be a feeling of release of tension by doing the act and a feeling of guilt after the act is over.

Pathological gambling is characterized by 2 or more episodes of gambling per year which have no profitable outcome, but are continued despite personal distress and interference with personal functioning in daily living. The person has an intense urge to gamble which is difficult to control and can not stop gambling by effort of will. Preoccupation with thoughts or mental images of gambling and situations surrounding gambling is often present.

Pyromania (pathological fire-setting) is characterized by 2 or more acts of fire-setting without an apparent motive. There is an intense urge to set fire to objects, with a feeling of tension before the act and a sense of relief afterwards. There is often a preoccupation with thoughts or mental images of fire-setting and situations surrounding fire-setting.

Kleptomania (pathological stealing) is characterized by 2 or more thefts, in which there is stealing without apparent motive of personal gain or gain for another person. There is an intense urge to steal, with a feeling of tension before the act and a sense of relief afterwards.

Trichotillomania (compulsive hair-pulling) is characterized by noticeable hair loss caused by person's persistent and recurrent failure to resist impulses to pullout hair. There is an intense urge to pull out hair with mounting tension before the act and a sense of relief afterwards. There is no pre-existent skin lesion or inflammation, and hair pulling is not secondary to any delusion or hallucination.

Management of impulse control disorders consists of behavior therapy (e.g. aversion therapy), cognitive behavior therapy, individual psychotherapy, and occasionally pharmacotherapy (e.g. carbamazepine for intermittent explosive disorder; fluoxetine for trichotillomania).

GENDER IDENTITY DISORDERS

These disorders of adult personality and behavior are discussed in detail in Chapter 10.

DISORDERS OF SEXUAL PREFERENCE

These disorders of adult personality and behavior are discussed in detail in Chapter 10.

PSYCHOLOGICAL AND BEHAVIORAL DISORDERS ASSOCIATED WITH SEXUAL DEVELOPMENT AND ORIENTATION

These disorders of adult personality and behavior are discussed in detail in Chapter 10.

FACTITIOUS DISORDER (MUNCHAUSEN SYNDROME)

Munchausen syndrome (also known as hospital addiction, hospital hoboes, professional patients, polysurgis other names) is used for those patients who repeatedly simulate or fake diseases for the sole purpose of obtaining medical attention. There is no other recognizable motive (hence, it is different from *malingering*).

Factitious disorders can present with predominantly physical signs and symptoms, or psychological signs and symptoms, or combined signs and symptoms.

The patients distort their clinical histories, laboratory tests' reports, and even facts about other aspects of their lives *(pseudologia fantastica)*. Sometimes, they distort physical signs by self-inflicted injuries and secondary infections. Drug abuse, especially abuse of prescription drugs, is common.

These patients have a detailed superficial knowledge of medical terms and procedures. Evidence of earlier treatment, usually surgical procedures, is available in the form of multiple scars (e.g. '*grid-iron abdomen*'). The patients are often manipulative, convincing liars, create problems in the in-patient setting and often move out LAMA (Left-Against-Medical-Advice), usually after the surgical procedure has been performed.

The cause is not clear. Probably these patients are masochistic, seek dependency from a father-figure (e.g. the physician), attempt to maneuver control over the father-figure and see the surgical procedure as partial suicide. The early childhood of these patients is characterized by deprivation and neglect.

The prognosis is usually poor and treatment often unsuccessful. Certain points must be kept in mind by the physician (or surgeon), after the diagnosis has been made.

1. Avoid the feelings of anger, hostility and ridicule which are aroused by the discovery of factitious illness.
2. Patients should not be confronted or labeled as liars. Instead, a psychiatric consultation should be sought, as these patients need help.
3. Of course, the unnecessary surgical procedure(s) should not be carried out.

10 Sexual Disorders

The sexual disorders can be classified into four main types:

1. Gender identity disorders.
2. Psychological and behavioral disorders associated with sexual development and maturation
2. Paraphilias (disorders of sexual preference).
3. Sexual dysfunctions.

In ICD-10, gender identity disorders, disorders of sexual preference, and sexual development and orientation disorders are listed under the disorders of adult personality and behavior, while sexual dysfunctions (not caused by organic disorder or disease) are listed under the behavioral syndromes associated with physiological disturbances and physical factors.

GENDER IDENTITY DISORDERS

These disorders are characterized by disturbance in *gender identity*, i.e. the sense of one's masculinity or femininity is disturbed. This group includes:

A. Transexualism: male and female; primary and secondary.
B. Gender identity disorder of childhood.
C. Dual-role transvestism.
D. Intersexuality.

A. Transexualism

Transexualism, the severest form of gender identity disorders, is characterized by the following clinical features:

1. Normal anatomic sex.
2. Persistent and significant sense of discomfort regarding one's anatomic sex and a feeling that it is inappropriate to one's perceived gender.
3. Marked preoccupation with the wish to get rid of one's genitals and secondary sex characteristics, and to adopt the sex characteristics of the other sex (perceived-gender).
4. Diagnosis is made after puberty.

It is of two types: primary and secondary.

1. Primary Transexualism

This condition has an onset in early childhood and has a stable course over time. This is a relatively homogenous category. Primary transexuals, more than secondary transexuals, are preoccupied with sex-change or sex-reassignment surgery. There are two types:

i. male (or, male-to-female) primary transexualism.
ii. female (or, female-to-male) primary transexualism.

2. Secondary Transexualism

In contrast to the primary type, secondary transexualism has an onset later in life. This is a less severe and more heterogeneous category. The only common feature is a wish to change the anatomic sex.

This category includes effeminate homosexuals, transvestites who secondarily become transexuals and the like. A majority of these patients are male (or, male-to-female) transexuals.

The prevalence of transexualism is 1:100,000 in males and 1:400,000 in females.

Differential Diagnosis

Differential diagnosis is from the following conditions:

1. Transvestism (Fetishistic Transvestism)

Transvestism (or, fetishistic cross-dressing) is wearing (cross dressing) or using clothes traditionally of the other sex, for the purpose of sexual excitement. This is almost exclusively seen in males.

In contrast, transexuals wear clothes of other sex, because they feel a part of the other sex and, *not* for sexual excitement.

2. Cross-gender Homosexuality

Effeminate male homosexuals and masculine female homosexuals sometimes cross-dress and occasionally want a sex-change (called *pseudo-transexualism*). But unlike true primary transexualism, these patients do not feel a part of the other sex and always acknowledge themselves as homosexuals (This is in contrast to transexualism. For example, a male transexual who feels like a female, even if he has a homosexual relationship with another male, justifies it as heterosexual because 'he himself feels like a female'), and seek sex-change only to rationalize or justify their primary homosexual behavior.

Treatment

The treatment can aim at two opposite ends by either making the person reconcile with the anatomic sex, or sex-change to the desired gender.

1. Reconciliation with the Anatomic Sex

There are only *occasional* reports of achieving this purpose in primary transexuals. However, in secondary transexuals, this method may be more effective and should be employed.

The methods include:

i. Psychotherapy.
ii. Behavior therapy (e.g. aversion therapy).

2. Sex-change to the Desired Gender

This procedure is known as *sex reassignment surgery (SRS)*. The first procedure was done in 1951 (Denmark) on an American soldier, George Jorgensen who become Christine Jorgensen after SRS. The first female-to-male SRS was performed in 1956.

The procedures include hormonal treatment, phalloplasty, castration, mastectomy, hysterectomy with salpingo-ophorectomy which have been used in different combinations. The procedure is performed more often in primary transexuals.

As SRS is an almost irreversible process, the following steps are taken before assigning a patient to surgery:

1. The diagnosis of primary, stable, long-standing transexualism is confirmed.
2. A possibility of stress-induced transexualism is considered and eliminated.
3. The patient has to undergo psychotherapy for at least 3-6 months preoperatively.
4. Experimental trial in the new gender role preoperatively, to assess patient's ability to adjust in the 'new' role.
5. Limitations of SRS. explained, e.g. infertility, nonfunctional testes, etc.

The success rate in carefully planned SRS can be up to 80-90%. Postoperative psychotherapy is of utmost importance in prevention of psychiatric morbidity.

B. Dual-role Transvestism

Dual-role transvestism is characterized by wearing of clothes of the opposite sex in order to enjoy the temporary experience of membership of the opposite sex, but without any desire for a more permanent sex change (unlike transexualism). No sexual excitement accompanies the cross-dressing (unlike in fetishistic transvestism).

C. Gender-Identity Disorder of Childhood

This is a disorder similar to transexualism, with a very early age of onset (2-4 years of age). This is characterized by the following clinical features:

1. Persistent and significant desire to be of the other gender, or insistence on being of the other gender.
2. Marked distress regarding the anatomic sex, with strong denial of anatomic sex (in contrast, there is no denial of anatomic sex in transexualism).
3. Involvement in traditional activities, games and clothing pattern of the perceived gender.
4. Onset before puberty.

Although a majority of primary transexuals have gender-identity disorder of childhood in past history; only a very few of the children with gender-identity disorder, in prospective studies, actually develop transexualism.

Treatment

Treatment of gender identity disorders is similar to transexualism. When the anatomic sex and gender-identity are opposing, decision on treatment should be based on gender-identity of the patient.

D. Inter-sexuality

The patients with this disorder have gross anatomical or physiological aspects of the other sex. These aspects can be in:

i. External genitals, e.g. pseudo-hermaphroditism.
ii. Gonads, e.g. ovotestes.
iii. Internal sex organs, e.g. true hermaphrodite.
iv. Hormonal disturbances, e.g. testicular feminization syndrome, congenital adrenal hypoplasia.
v. Chromosomes, e.g. Turner's syndrome, Klinefelter's syndrome.
vi. Central nervous system (rarely), e.g. temporal lobe disorders.

PSYCHOLOGICAL AND BEHAVIORAL DISORDERS ASSOCIATED WITH SEXUAL DEVELOPMENT AND MATURATION

Disorders of sexual development and maturation include disorders where sexual orientation (heterosexual, homosexual, or bisexual) causes significant distress to the individual or disturbances in the relationships. Any type of sexual orientation by itself is not a disorder unless it causes distress or disability.

A. Sexual Maturation Disorder

This disorder usually begins in adolescence and is characterized by uncertainty regarding the gender identity or sexual orientation (heterosexual, homosexual, or bisexual). This uncertainty often leads to anxiety and depression. Sometimes, this disorder arises for the time in an individual after a period of apparently stable sexual orientation.

B. Egodystonic Sexual Orientation

In this disorder, the sexual orientation is clear. However, the individual wishes to change the orientation because of associated distress and/or psychological symptoms. This disorder is seen most commonly in homosexuality.

Homosexuality

Homosexuality, in contrast to heterosexuality, is the sexual relationship between persons of the same sex. This is a disorder only when it is the predominant, significant and persistent mode of sexual relationship for that person and is ego-dystonic (causes significant distress to the individual).

It is of two types: male homosexuality, and female homosexuality.

Female homosexuals are also called as lesbians or sapphic after Sappho, a female homosexual who lived on the Isle of Lesbos in ancient Greece, while male homosexuals are called gay.

The prevalence of homosexuality (in USA) is 4-6% of males and 1-2% of females. Another 5-10% may show bisexual orientation.

Homosexual behavior can be divided into following types:

1. Obligatory homosexuality
   - Only homosexuality
   - No heterosexuality.
2. Preferred homosexuality
   - Predominant homosexuality
   - Occasional heterosexuality.
3. Bisexuality
   - Almost equal homosexuality and heterosexuality.
4. Situational homosexuality
   - Predominant heterosexuality
   - Occasional homosexuality.
5. Latent homosexuality
   - Only heterosexuality
   - Fantasies of homosexuality.

Last few decades have seen a raging controversy on whether homosexuality is a normal phenomenon or a psychiatric disorder. At first, homosexuality was divided into two types:

a. Ego-syntonic homosexuality (no distress about homosexual behavior),
b. Ego-dystonic homosexuality (associated with marked distress),

and only ego-dystonic type was called abnormal.

Later (DSM-IIIR, 1987), homosexuality was completely dropped from psychiatric nomenclature, under social and political pressure from homosexual groups. DSM-IV-TR does not list homosexuality as a disorder, while ICD-10 mentions homosexuality under *ego-dystonic sexual orientation*.

However, one fact remains. Many homosexuals who have significant distress about their homosexual orientation and themselves seek psychiatric help should be offered treatment.

Recently, it has been speculated that homosexuality may have a genetic basis in some individuals.

Treatment

At present, the treatment is offered under the following conditions only.

1. Self-referral by a homosexual person for seeking a change in the sexual orientation towards heterosexuality.
2. Self-referral by a homosexual person for removal of distress associated with homosexuality but *not* for a change in sexual orientation.
3. Referred or brought by parents, relatives or significant others.

1. For seeking a Change in Sexual Orientation

The methods employed include:

i. Psychoanalytic psychotherapy (especially when associated with neurotic symptoms or traits).
ii. Behavior therapy: aversion therapy, covert sensitization, systematic desensitization (especially if there is a phobia of heterosexual relationship).
iii. Supportive psychotherapy.
iv. Androgen therapy (occasionally).

2. For Seeking Removal of Distress Only

The following methods may be useful:

i. Psychotherapy: psychoanalytic and supportive, depending on the personality character.
ii. Drug therapy: antidepressants and/or benzodiazepines can be used for treatment of associated depression and anxiety.

3. Referred by Others

The decision regarding treatment for this group is highly debatable. The opinions range from 'no treatment at all' to 'treatment as early as possible'. The final approach depends on the sociocultural background of the patient and the viewpoint of the therapist.

The current viewpoint is that the individuals should be informed regarding normal sexuality and homosexuality in as much detail as they want and the final decision of choosing the sexual orientation should be left to the individual. Obviously, further treatment would depend on that final choice. The individual's motivation and presence of significant distress are important factors in therapy.

C. Sexual Relationship Disorder

The gender identity disorder or disorder of sexual preference leads to difficulties in establishing and/or maintaining sexual relationships. In such a case, both diagnoses should be made.

PARAPHILIAS (DISORDERS OF SEXUAL PREFERENCE)

Paraphilias (*sexual deviations; perversions)* are disorders of sexual preference in which sexual arousal occurs *persistently and significantly* in response to objects which are not a part of normal sexual arousal (e.g. non-human objects; suffering or humiliation of self and/or sexual partner; children or non-consenting person).

These disorders include: fetishism; fetishistic transvestism; sexual sadism; sexual masochism; exhibitionism; voyeurism; frotteurism; pedophilia; zoophilia (bestiality); and others.

A. Fetishism

In fetishism, the sexual arousal occurs either solely or predominantly with a non-living object, which is usually intimately associated with the human body.

The word *fetish* means magical, i.e. the non-living object magically becomes phallic for the person.

This disorder is almost exclusively seen in males. The fetish object may include shoes, gloves, bras, underpants, stockings, etc.

Fetishism is not diagnosed if the sexual object is the wearing of clothes of opposite sex (*fetishistic transvestism*), the use of a human body part (*masturbation*), or the use of a genital-stimulating object (e.g. vibrator).

Fetishism is very often associated with masturbation.

B. Fetishistic Transvestism

This disorder occurs exclusively in heterosexual males. The person actually or in fantasy wears clothes of the opposite sex (cross-dressing) for sexual arousal. This disorder should be differentiated from dual-role transvestism and transexualism.

This disorder may be associated with fantasies of other males approaching the person who is in a female dress. Masturbation or rarely coitus is associated with cross-dressing to achieve orgasm.

To be called a disorder, this should be a persistent and significant mode of sexual arousal in the person.

C. Sexual Sadism

In this disorder, the person (the 'sadist') is sexually aroused by physical and/or psychological humiliation, suffering or injury of the sexual partner (the 'victim'). Most often the person inflicting the suffering is male, although this is not essential. The methods used range from restraining by tying, beating, burning, cutting, stabbing, to rape and killing.

D. Sexual Masochism

This is just the reverse of sexual sadism. Here the person (the 'masochist') is sexually aroused by physical and/or psychological humiliation, suffering or injury inflicted on self by others (usually 'sadists'). Most often the masochist is a female. The methods used are the same as the ones used in sexual sadism. Only there is a role reversal.

To be called a disorder, this should be a persistent and significant mode of sexual arousal in the person.

Sexual sadism and sexual masochism are often seen in the same individual and are on a continuum; therefore they are classified together as *sadomasochism* in ICD-10.

E. Exhibitionism

Exhibitionism is a persistent (or recurrent) and significant method of sexual arousal by the exposure of one's genitalia to an *unsuspecting* stranger. This is followed by masturbation to achieve orgasm. The disorder is almost exclusively seen in males, and the 'unsuspecting stranger' is usually a female (child or adult).

F. Voyeurism

This is a persistent or recurrent tendency to observe *unsuspecting* persons (usually of the other sex) naked, disrobing or engaged in sexual activity. This is followed by masturbation to achieve orgasm without the observed person(s) being aware. This is almost always seen in males. Watching pornography is not included here.

G. Frotteurism

This is a persistent or recurrent involvement in the act of touching and rubbing against an unsuspecting, non-consenting person (usually of the other sex).

Frottage is often employed in crowded places. e.g. buses, where the victim does not protest because she can not suspect that frottage can be committed there. This is often seen in adolescent males.

H. Pedophilia

Pedophilia is a persistent or recurrent involvement of an adult (age >16 years and at least 5 year older than the child) in sexual activity with prepubertal children, either heterosexual or homosexual.

This may be associated with sexual sadism. The pedophilic behavior may be either limited to incest or may spread to children outside the family. It is a common disorder.

I. Zoophilia (Bestiality)

Zoophilia as a persistent and significant involvement in sexual activity with animals is rare. Occasional or situational zoophilia is much more common.

J. Other Paraphilias

These include sexual arousal with urine (urophilia); feces (coprophilia); enemas (klismaphilia); corpses (necrophilia), among many others.

Treatment

1. *Psychoanalysis*: This is of particular help if the patient is psychological minded and has good ego strength.
2. *Behavior therapy*: Aversion therapy is the treatment of choice in severe, distressing paraphilia.
3. *Drug therapy*: Antipsychotics have been used for severe or dangerous aggression associated with paraphilias. Benperidol was earlier believed to be particularly useful but the claim has not been substantiated. Antiandrogens (cyproterone acetate or medroxyprogesterone acetate) can be used in paraphilias with excessive sexual activity.

TABLE 10.1. NORMAL HUMAN SEXUAL RESPONSE CYCLE

A normal human sexual response cycle can be divided into five phases:

1. Appetitive Phase

This is the phase which occurs before the actual sexual response cycle. This consists of sexual fantasies and a desire to have sexual activity.

2. Excitement Phase

This is the first true phase of the sexual response cycle, which starts with physical stimulation and/or by appetitive phase. The major changes during this phase are listed below:

Male

- Penile erection, due to vasocongestion of corpus cavernosa.
- Elevation of testes with scrotal sac.

Female

- Lubrication of vagina by a transudate.
- Erection of nipples (in most women).
- Erection of clitoris.
- Thickening of labia minora.

The duration of this phase is highly variable and may last for several minutes (or longer).

3. Plateau Phase

This is an intermediate phase just before actual orgasm, at the height of excitement. It is often difficult to differentiate the plateau phase from the excitement phase. The following important changes occur during this phase:

Male

- Sexual flush (inconsistent).
- Autonomic hyperactivity.
- Erection and engorgement of penis to full size.
- Elevation and enlargement of testes.
- *Dew drops* on glans penis (2-3 drops of mucoid fluid with spermatozoa).

Female

- Sexual flush (inconsistent).
- Autonomic hyperactivity.
- Retraction of clitoris behind the pupuce.
- Development of *orgasmic platform* in the lower 1/3rd of vagina, with lengthening and ballooning of vagina.
- Enlargement of breasts and labia minora; increased vaginal transudate.

The duration of this phase may last from half to several minutes.

4. Orgasmic Phase

This is the phase with a peak of sexual excitement followed by a release of sexual tension, and rhythmic contractions of pelvic reproductive organs. The important changes are as follows:

Male

- 4-10 contractions of penile urethra, prostate, vas, and seminal vesicles; at about 0.8 sec. intervals.
- Autonomic excitement becomes marked in this phase. Doubling of pulse rate and respiratory rate, and 10-40 mm. increase in systolic and diastolic BP occur.
- *Ejaculatory inevitability* precedes orgasm .
- Ejaculatory spurt (30-60 cm; decreases with age).
- Contractions of external and internal sphincters.

Female

- 3-15 contractions of lower 1/3rd of vagina, cervix and uterus; at about 0.8 sec. intervals. No contractions occur in clitoris.
- Autonomic excitement becomes marked in this phase. Doubling of pulse rate and respiratory rate, and 10-40 mm. increase in systolic and diastolic BP occur.
- Contractions of external and internal sphincters.

The duration of this phase may last from 3-15 seconds.

5. Resolution Phase

This phase is characterized by the following common features in both sexes:

- A general sense of relaxation and well-being, after the slight clouding of consciousness during the orgasmic phase.
- Disappearance of sexual flush followed by fine perspiration.
- Gradual decrease in vasocongestion from sexual organs and rest of the body.
- Refractory period for further orgasm in males varies from few minutes to many hours; there is usually no refractory period in females.

4. *Other treatments*: Castration and psychosurgery (amygdalotomy) have occasionally been used in dangerous, aggressive sexual behavior which is recurrent and persistent.

SEXUAL DYSFUNCTIONS

Sexual dysfunction is a significant disturbance in the sexual response cycle, which is not due to an underlying organic cause.

To understand sexual dysfunction, a brief outline of normal human sexual response cycle is in order (Table 10.1).

In the light of the normal human sexual response cycle, it is easier to understand the sexual dysfunctions. The common dysfunctions include the following:

I. Disorders of Appetitive Phase (Sexual Desire Disorders)

1. Hypoactive sexual desire disorder

This disorder is characterized by an absence of fantasies and desire for sexual activity which is not secondary to other sexual dysfunctions like premature ejaculation or dyspareunia. Lack or diminution of sexual desire does not imply an inability to experience sexual pleasure; it makes the initiation of sexual act less likely.

This disorder is many times more common in females (previously called as *frigidity*) and its prevalence increases with age.

The contributing factors may include fear of pregnancy, unsatisfactory past sexual experiences, marital disharmony, or fatigue. If the disorder is secondary to biological factors (like drugs, chronic medical illnesses), it should be listed under 'sexual disorders due to a general medical condition'.

2. Sexual aversion disorder and Lack of sexual enjoyment disorder

In the *sexual aversion disorder*, there is an aversion to and avoidance of all sexual activity with a sexual partner. The thought of sexual interaction is associated with negative feelings and causes anxiety. The contributing factors may include history of sexual molestation (especially in childhood), unsatisfactory past sexual experiences, or culturally induced negative feelings towards sexual matters.

In the *lack of sexual enjoyment disorder* (sexual anhedonia), the sexual response is usually is normal (which may include a normal orgasm). However, there is a feeling of lack of subjective sexual pleasure. This disorder is more common in females.

3. Excessive sexual drive

Rarely, both men (*satyriasis*) and women (*nymphomania*) may complain of excessive sexual drive as a problem.

II. Disorders of Excitement and Plateau Phase (Sexual Arousal Disorders or Failure of Genital Response)

4. Male erectile disorder (Impotence; Erectile dysfunction)

This disorder is characterized by an inability to have or sustain penile erection till the completion of *satisfactory* sexual activity. It is a common disorder.

Although a large number of physical disorders have been etiologically incriminated in the causation of male erectile disorder, the important ones are mentioned below. If the disorder is secondary to biological factors (like drugs, chronic medical illnesses), it should be listed under 'sexual disorders due to a general medical condition' (see Table 10.2).

Since many drugs impair normal sexual functioning and often cause more than one sexual dysfunction, these are listed separately in Table 10.3. The secondary sexual dysfunction is usually more profound in males.

In cases of male erectile dysfunction where biological causes have been ruled out, psychological factors should be considered in causation.

Psychological impotence usually occurs acutely. The early morning erections and erections during REM sleep (nocturnal penile tumescence; NPT) are usually preserved. These psychological factors may include one of the following conditions.

1. Ignorance regarding the sexual act.
2. Fear of failure and performance anxiety (e.g. during honeymoon).
3. Interpersonal difficulties between the sexual partners (e.g. marital conflict).
4. Anxiety disorder.
5. Mood disorder.
6. Masturbatory anxiety (and 'Dhat syndrome' in India).
7. Fatigue (e.g. after the day's hard work).
8. Fear of pregnancy, or sexually transmitted disease.
9. Fear of damaging the sexual partner or oneself.
10. Certain environmental factors (e.g. lack of privacy).
11. Lack of a consistent sexual partner.
12. Fear of commitment (in premarital and extramarital sexual relationships).
13. Poor self-image or 'inferiority complex'.
14. Sexual abuse in childhood.

In many cases of erectile dysfunction, the etiology can be mixed (i.e. organic as well as psychogenic).

TABLE 10.2. PHYSICAL CAUSES OF MALE ERECTILE DISORDER/IMPOTENCE

I. Local Genital Pathology
1. Priapism
2. Congenital malformations
3. Surgical procedures on pelvic region, e.g. perineal prostatectomy
4. Mumps
5. Elephantiasis
6. Hydrocele or varicocele.

II. Endocrine Disorders
1. Diabetes mellitus
2. Dysfunction of pituitary-adrenal-testis axis
3. Testicular atrophy, e.g. secondary to dystrophia myotonica, hemachromatosis, cirrhosis
4. Thyroid dysfunction.

III. Neurological Disorders
1. Autonomic neuropathy, e.g. in diabetes mellitus
2. Spinal cord lesions e.g. transverse myelitis
3. 3rd ventricle tumors
4. Brain damage, esp. in temporal lobe
5. Multiple sclerosis.

IV. Cardiovascular Disorders
1. Leriche syndrome.

V. Any Severe or Debilitating Systemic Illness

VI. Alcohol And Drugs.

5. Female sexual arousal disorder

This disorder is characterized by subjective as well as objective lack of sexual arousal in the form of lack of lubrication or vaginal dryness. The causes can be biological (e.g. postmenopausal) or psychological (uncommon).

III. Disorders of Orgasmic Phase (Orgasmic Disorders or Dysfunctions)

6. Male orgasmic disorder (Male anorgasmia)

Failure or marked difficulty to have orgasm, despite normal sexual excitement, during coitus. An uncommon disorder, it often presents as retarded ejaculation. The causes can be biological (e.g. post-prostate surgery, drug-induced) or psychological (e.g. marital conflicts).

7. Female orgasmic disorder (Female anorgasmia)

Failure or marked difficulty to have orgasm, despite normal sexual excitement, during coitus. This is a very common disorder. Anorgasmia can be primary or secondary. Although the disorder causes marked distress, it is rarely complained of in the clinical setting particularly in India. This is probably due to cultural factors.

The causes can be biological (e.g. endocrinal disorders like hypothyroidism, drug-induced) or psychological (e.g. marital conflicts).

8. Premature ejaculation

This disorder is defined as ejaculation before the completion of *satisfactory* sexual activity for both partners. In severe cases, it is characterized by ejaculation either before penile entry into vagina or soon after penetration. It is a very common disorder in the clinical setting.

The causes can be biological (relatively uncommon) or psychological (e.g. performance anxiety).

IV. Sexual Pain Disorders

9. Non-organic vaginismus

This disorder is characterized by an involuntary spasm of lower 1/3rd of vagina, interfering with coitus. Penile entry is either painful or impossible. Before a presumption of non-organic vaginismus, it is important to rule out organic factors (e.g. local pathology causing pain).

10. Non-organic dyspareunia

This disorder is characterized by pain in the genital area of either male or female, during coitus. Before a presumption of non-organic dyspareunia, it is important to rule out organic factors (e.g. local pathology causing pain) in both males and females.

V. Sexual Disorders Due to A General Medical Condition

The disorders listed above may occur secondary to a general medical condition; they should then be coded here.

These dysfunctions are called disorders only when they occur recurrently and persistently. Also if the sexual dysfunction is due to sexual stimulation being inadequate either in focus, intensity or duration, a diagnosis of excitement and orgasmic phase disorders is not made.

Diagnosis and Differential Diagnosis

Before making a diagnosis of sexual dysfunction, it is of paramount importance to rule out an underlying physical cause, which would need treatment.

Although the diagnosis is clinical, a detailed physical examination and laboratory investigations (e.g. blood sugar, liver function tests, thyroid function tests, hormonal profile, routine examination and culture of prostatic fluid) coupled with a good history is a must in every patient to rule out an underlying physical cause.

Certain laboratory techniques, e.g. penile plethysmograph, penile tumescence monitoring during sleep, may help in differentiating organic and non-organic sexual dysfunctions. If NPT (nocturnal penile tumescence) is abnormal, then ancillary investigations like penile vascular investigations (e.g. penile pulse pressure, penile Doppler, duplex ultrasonography, diagnostic intracavernosal vasoactive substance - papaverine injection test, arteriography, DICC - dynamic infusion cavernosomatogram and cavernosogram, and cavernosography) and penile neurological investigations (e.g. penile sensory threshold test or penile biothesiometry) may be employed.

Though searching for an organic factor responsible for sexual dysfunction is very important, a large majority of dysfunctions are psychosexual in nature. A detailed sexual and personal history is important in finding out the underlying causes. The common psychological causes of sexual dysfunction have been discussed earlier.

It should be specified whether the sexual dysfunction is psychogenic alone or biogenic factors co-exist; whether the dysfunction is

TABLE 10.3. SEXUAL DYSFUNCTIONS CAUSED BY DRUGS

Drugs	Effect on Sexual Desire	Effect on Erectile Function	Effect on Ejaculation
I. Anti-Hypertensives			
1. Methyldopa	Inhibited	Impaired	Impaired
2. Clonidine	—	Impaired	Impaired
3. Propranolol	Inhibited	Impaired	—
4. Thiazide diuretics	—	Impaired	—
5. Spironolactone	Inhibited	Impaired	Impaired
6. Guanethidine	—	Impaired	Impaired; Retrograde ejaculation
7. Hexamethonium	—	Impaired	Impaired; Retrograde ejaculation
II. Hormonal Preparations			
1. Corticosteroids	Inhibited	Impaired	Impaired
2. Estrogens	Inhibited (in males)	Impaired	Impaired
3. Androgens	Increased (in both sexes)		
III. Psychotropic Medications			
1. Tricyclic antidepressants and MAO inhibitors	+/-	Impaired	Impaired
2. SSRI antidepressants (e.g. paroxetine, fluoxetine)	+/-	Impaired	Delayed ejaculation
3. Thioridazine	Inhibited	Impaired	Retrograde & Delayed ejaculation
4. Chlorpromazine	Inhibited	Impaired	—
5. Haloperidol	—	Impaired	—
6. Trazodone	—	Priapism	—
7. Barbiturates and benzodiazepines	Increased (with low dose, due to decrease in anxiety) Decreased (with high dose)	Impaired (with high dose)	Impaired (with high dose)
8. Lithium	—	Impaired	—
9. Disulfiram	—	—	Delayed ejaculation
IV. Psychoactive Substance Use			
1. Alcohol	Increased (with low dose)	Impaired	Impaired
2. Opiates and cocaine	Inhibited	Impaired (with high dose)	Impaired
V. Others			
1. Anti-inflammatory drugs (e.g. indomethacin)	Inhibited	Impaired	—
2. L-dopa	Inhibited	—	—
3. Anticholinergic drugs (e.g. trihexiphenidyl)	—	Impaired	Impaired

life-long or acquired; and whether the dysfunction is situational or generalized.

Treatment

The treatment usually consists of one or more of the following methods:

1. Treatment of the underlying physical or psychiatric disorder, if present.

2. Psychoanalysis

This is particularly indicated when the dysfunction is more pervasive and involves personality difficulties. The goal is *not* symptom removal but is resolution of the underlying unconscious conflicts.

3. Hypnosis

Hypnosis can be used either alone or in conjunction with other therapies aiming at symptom removal. However, only suggestible patients can be hypnotized.

4. Group Psychotherapy

Patients of same sex with different sexual problems or of both sexes with similar sexual problems can be treated in group therapy sessions. The focus is usually on providing education regarding normal sexuality and to remove anxiety or guilt by sharing viewpoints in a group setting. Although occasionally used alone, it is more helpful as an adjunct to other methods of treatment.

5. Behavior Therapy

The methods commonly employed are:

i. Relaxation training, e.g. Jacobson's progressive relaxation technique.
ii. Assertiveness training.
iii. Systematic desensitization, aimed at reducing the phobic anxiety related to the sexual act, e.g. in sexual aversion disorder.
iv. Biofeedback, using a penile plethysmograph.

6. Masters' and Johnson's Technique

This is one of the most popular and successful methods of treatment for psychosexual dysfunctions. The patient is *not* treated alone, but *both the partners are treated together*. This is called as *dual-sex therapy*, where both the sexual partners are treated by a team of therapists (one male and one female), although later modifications of this technique use only one therapist.

The goal of the treatment is *symptom removal*, using simple behavioral techniques. The couple is usually seen on a weekly basis; however, the sessions can be more frequent if the couple is encountering particular difficulties during treatment.

Some common steps before starting therapy include:

1. Detailed history taking (sexual history) from each partner separately.
2. Round-table discussions aiming at,
   i. education about normal sexuality.
   ii. understanding of couple's current sexual problem(s).
   iii. enhancing communication between the partners regarding the sexual matters.
3. Behavior modification steps, depending on the type of psychosexual dysfunction.

Brief examples of the techniques used are:

1. *Sensate Focus Technique*: This is used particularly for the treatment of impotence, although is also useful in management of other dysfunctions as well. The aim is to 'discover' on body (excluding genital area) 'sensate focuses' (body areas where manipulation leads to sexual arousal). This is usually a general exercise before any sex therapy.
2. *Squeeze Technique (Seman's technique)*: This is used in premature ejaculation. The female partner is asked to manually stimulate the penis causing erection. When

the male partner experiences 'ejaculatory inevitability', the female partner 'squeezes' the penis on the coronal ridge thus delaying ejaculation.

There are similar simple techniques (e.g. orgasmic conditioning, desensitization) for the treatment of other psychosexual dysfunctions. The response rate is close to 80%, with maximum success in the treatment of premature ejaculation.

7. Oral Drug Therapy

Oral drug treatment was rarely a treatment of first choice in sexual dysfunctions till very recently. The *indications* of drug treatment are:

i. Treatment of the underlying psychiatric disorder.
ii. Intense anxiety related to sexual activity may require use of low dose benzodiazepines (e.g. alprazolam).
iii. Premature ejaculation may sometimes require treatment with thioridazine, fluoxetine, trazodone, or tricyclic antidepressants (to retard ejaculation, e.g. clomipramine).
iv. Several drugs have been used in the treatment of impotence with varying degrees of efficacy, e.g. α-blockers (e.g. yohimbine, idazoxan), opiate antagonists (e.g. naltrexone), dopamine agonists (e.g. bromocriptine, apomorphine), pentoxifylline, and topical drugs (glyceryl trinitrate, minoxidyl, papaverine and PgE_1 and E_2).
v. Recently, a drug called *Sildenafil citrate* has been introduced for the treatment of erectile dysfunction. Rapidly absorbed after oral administration, the maximum plasma concentration is reached in 30-120 minutes. It is metabolized in liver (mainly by cytochrome P450 3A4) and is converted to an active metabolite. Sildenafil has a terminal half life of about 4 hours. It is highly bound to plasma proteins and is not dialyzable. Sildenafil is a competitive and selective inhibitor of cGMP (cyclic guanosine monophosphate)-specific PDE-5 (phosphodiesterase type 5). It prevents the rate of breakdown of cGMP causing enhanced relaxation of cavernosal smooth muscle, increase in arterial flow in to corpus cavernosa, compression of subtunical veins, and hence penile erection.
   The typical dose is 50 mg (25-100 mg), 1 hour before the sexual activity. The maximum recommended dosing frequency is once a day. The drug acts only in the presence of sexual stimulation. The adverse effects include transient and mild headache, flushing, dyspepsia, and nasal congestion. Caution needs to be exercised in patients with known history of hypersensitivity, with poor cardiovascular status, with anatomical deformation of penis, with conditions that predispose to priapism, and especially those on nitrates.
vi. Hormonal treatment (e.g. androgens) should not be employed unless there is an evidence of hormonal dysfunction.

It should always be remembered that prescription of non-essential drugs may worsen sexual dysfunction.

8. Intracavernosal Injection of Vasoactive Drugs (IIVD)

Papaverine, an alkaloid and a vasoactive substance, has been used as an intracavernosal injection (either alone or along with phentolamine, phenoxybenzamine, alprostadil or prostaglandin E_1, and/or atropine), in the differential diagnosis of organic and non-organic impotence and also for the treatment of impotence.

9. Physical Devices

Various suction devices (for producing artificial penile tumescence) and penile prosthetic implants are available. Their use, however, should be limited to only those patients who suffer from organic sexual disorder or in whom a sufficient and regular trial of psychological management has been done.

10. Vascular Surgery

Rarely, vascular surgery may be needed for some patients with underlying vascular insufficiency (organic sexual disorder).

11
Sleep Disorders

SLEEP

Nearly one third of our life is spent in sleep. Every day we voluntarily go to bed and transit into an easily reversible state of relative unresponsiveness and tranquillity. This state occurs almost regularly and repetitively each day.

EEG recordings show typical features of sleep. Now, it is known that sleep is divided into two different phases:

1. *D-sleep* (desynchronized or dreaming sleep), or *REM-sleep* (rapid eye movement sleep), or *active sleep*, or *paradoxical sleep*.
2. *S-sleep* (synchronized sleep), or *NREM-sleep* (non-REM sleep), or *quiet sleep*, or *orthodox sleep*. S-sleep or NREM-sleep is further divided into 4 stages, from stage 1 to stage 4. As the person falls asleep, the person first passes through these stages of NREM-sleep.

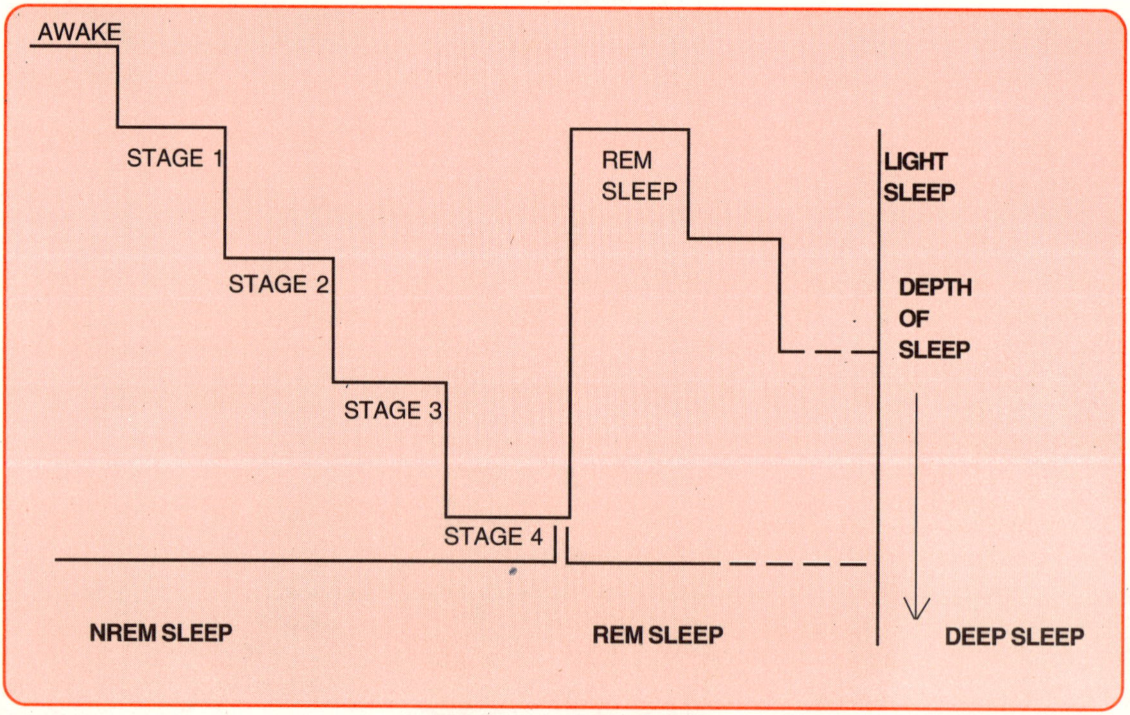

FIG. 11.1. SLEEP STAGES

EEG recording during the waking state shows α waves of 8-12 cycles/sec. frequency. The onset of sleep is characterized by a disappearance of α-activity.

Stage 1, NREM sleep is the first and the lightest stage of sleep characterized by an absence of α-waves, and low voltage, predominantly theta activity.

Stage 2, NREM sleep follows stage 1 within a few minutes and is characterized by two typical EEG changes:

i. *Sleep spindles*: regular spindle shaped waves of 13-15 cycles/sec. frequency, lasting 0.5-2.0 seconds with a characteristic waxing and waning amplitude.
ii. *K-complexes*: high voltage spikes present intermittently.

Stage 3, NREM sleep shows appearance of high voltage, 75 μV, δ-waves of 0.5-3.0 cycles/sec.

Stage 4, NREM sleep shows predominant δ-activity in EEG.

NREM sleep is followed by REM sleep which is a light phase of sleep. EEG is characterized by a return of α-waves (α-wave sleep) and other changes are similar to stage 1 NREM sleep. One of the most characteristic feature is REM or rapid (conjugate) eye movements. Also present are generalized muscular atony, penile erections, autonomic hyperactivity (increase in pulse rate, respiratory rate and blood pressure), and movements of small muscle groups, intermittently. Although it is a light stage of sleep, arousal is difficult.

These stages occur regularly throughout the whole duration of sleep. The first REM period occurs typically after 90 minutes of onset of sleep, although it can start as early as 7 minutes after going off to sleep, e.g. in narcolepsy, in major depression, and after sleep deprivation. The important time periods of various sleep stages are summarized below.

1. In an 8 hour sleep, usually 6-6½ hours are spent in NREM sleep while 1½-2 hours are in REM sleep.
2. Out of 6-6½ hour NREM sleep period, only about 70-80 minutes are spent in stage 4 sleep.
3. Maximum stage 4 sleep occurs in the first one-third of the night. In the later part, REM sleep follows stage 3 NREM sleep directly.
4. REM sleep occurs maximally in last one-third of the night. REM-sleep occurs regularly after every 90-100 minutes, with progressive lengthening of each REM period. The first REM period typically lasts for less than 10 minutes. Usually, there are 4-5 REM periods in the whole night sleep.
5. Young persons need more sleep. Sleep duration in newborn children is 16-18 hours/day with nearly 8-10 hours spent in REM sleep. As age advances, sleep duration reduces.

Certain phenomena are common just before going off to sleep (hypnagogic phenomena) and just after waking up (hypnopompic phenomena). These include a variety of illusions and simple hallucinations (both visual and auditory), jerky muscle movements involving small muscle groups, depersonal-ization and derealization.

Some of the methods of sleep study are listed in the accompanying box.

Depending on the duration of total sleep, two extremes of normal sleeping patterns have been described.

1. Long-Sleepers

These persons regularly and habitually sleep for more than 9 hours/night, and this pattern of sleep does not cause any symptoms or dysfunction.

2. Short-Sleepers

These persons regularly and habitually sleep for less than 6 hours/night, and this pattern

TABLE 11.1. METHODS OF SLEEP STUDY

To study sleep and its associated phenomena, the following techniques can be used.

1. Observation of a sleeping person for externally visible changes.
2. EEG.
3. Polysomnography (This is the preferred method in sleep research centres). It consists of:
   - i. Continuous EEG recording, particularly from occipital and parietal leads.
   - ii. EOG (electro-oculography) to record the eye movements.
   - iii. EMG (electro-myography) for muscle potential and activities.
   - iv. EKG for changes in cardiac status.
   - v. In certain cases, respiratory tracings of various kinds are used, e.g. oxymetry, expired CO_2, O_2 saturation.
   - vi. MSLT (Multiple sleep latency test): It involves repeated measures of sleep latency (i.e. time to onset of sleep).
   - vii. Penile tumescence, body temperature, GSR (galvanic skin response), and body movement are also sometimes studied.

The recordings are made throughout the night sleep.

of sleep does not cause any symptoms or dysfunction.

On comparing the long-sleepers and short-sleepers, it has been found that the time spent in stage 3 and 4 of NREM sleep is the same in both. The maximum difference is in the duration of REM sleep. The long-sleeper on an average has almost double the duration of REM sleep as compared to a short-sleeper.

SLEEP DEPRIVATION

Experimental deprivation of sleep is an important method, aimed at finding out the functions of sleep. After a few days of sleep deprivation, the EEG recording shows a gradual diminishing of a activity, with increase in lower frequency activity.

After 4-5 days of sleep deprivation, psychological symptoms become prominent. Initially there is a decrease in attention span, easy distractibility, drowsiness, decreased initiative to perform and 'micro-sleeps' lasting but a few seconds. In predisposed individuals, psychotic symptoms may appear on the fifth night characterized by break with reality, illusions and hallucinations, grossly disorganized behavior, persecutory ideation or delusions and mild disorientation and confusion. As time progresses, frank delirium may occur. Whether this type of psychosis can occur in previously normal individuals is doubtful, due to lack of sufficient research data. Ethical considerations prevent this kind of research.

Recovery after sleep deprivation is characterized by an increase in total sleep duration, lasting usually 15-16 hours. Also, there is a rebound increase in stage 3 and 4 of NREM sleep in the first few hours and an increase in REM sleep later.

FUNCTIONS OF SLEEP

Despite the accumulation of vast amount of research data regarding the physiology and biochemistry of sleep, the functions of sleep are far from clear.

It has been observed that persons sleeping for 7-9 hours per day have significantly lower rates of illness. On the other hand, certain disorders carry a higher mortality when present during sleep (especially early hours of morning), e.g. coronary artery disease, nocturnal asthma, sudden nocturnal death (in south-east Asian men), and sleep apnea.

It has been observed that there is a decrease in the metabolic rate during night sleep by 5-25%. So, conservation of energy appears to be an important function of sleep.

It also serves a restorative function for the whole body (particularly during NREM sleep) and for the brain (cognitive functions; especially during REM sleep). Further research may clarify the exact functions of the various components of the sleep cycle.

SLEEP DISORDERS

The types of sleep disorders are legion. The ASDC (Association for Sleep Disorders Centers) has done a lot of work in classifying the various sleep disorders and their classification has been adapted for use by DSM-IV and ICD-10. The sleep disorders are labeled as non-organic sleep disorders in ICD-10.

The sleep disorders are divided in 2 subtypes:

I. Dyssomnias
   1. Insomnia
   2. Hypersomnia
   3. Disorders of sleep-wake schedule.

II. Parasomnias
   1. Stage 4 disorders
   2. Other disorders.

I. Dyssomnias

Dyssomnias are those sleep disorders which are characterized by disturbances in the amount, quality or timing of sleep. These are the commonest disorders of sleep.

A. Insomnia

Insomnia is also known as DIMS (Disorder of initiation and/or maintenance of sleep). Insomnia means one or more of the following:

1. Difficulty in initiating sleep (going off to sleep).
2. Difficulty in maintaining sleep (remaining asleep).

   This includes both:

   a. frequent awakenings during the night, and
   b. early morning awakening.
3. Non-restorative sleep, i.e. despite adequate duration of sleep, feeling of not having rested present (poor quality sleep).

Insomnia is very common, with nearly 15-30% of general population complaining of a period of insomnia per year requiring treatment. It is required for the diagnosis that the sleep disturbance occurs at least 3 times a week for at least 1 month, and that it causes either marked distress or interferes with social and occupational functioning.

TABLE 11.2. COMMON CAUSES OF INSOMNIA

1. Medical illnesses
   i. Any painful or uncomfortable condition
   ii. Heart diseases
   iii. Respiratory diseases
   iv. Rheumatic & musculo-skeletal disease
   v. Old age
   vi. Brain stem or hypothalamic lesions
   vii. Delirium
   viii. PMS (Periodic movements in sleep)

2. Alcohol and drug use
   i. Drug or alcohol withdrawal syndrome
   ii. Delirium tremens
   iii. Amphetamine or other stimulants, e.g. caffeine
   iv. Chronic alcoholism

3. Current medication, e.g. fluoxetine, steroids, theophylline, propranolol

4. Psychiatric disorders
   i. Mania (may not complain of decrease in sleep, as there is often a decreased need for sleep)
   ii. Major depression (difficulty in maintenance of sleep is more prominent, although difficulty in initiating sleep is also present)
   iii. Dysthymia (difficulty in initiating sleep is characteristic)
   iv. Anxiety disorder (difficulty in initiating sleep is common)
   v. Stressful life situation (may cause temporary insomnia).

5. Idiopathic insomnia

Causes

The common causes of insomnia are listed in Table 11.2.

Insomnia should be differentiated from short-sleeper, who needs less than 6 hours of sleep per night and has no symptoms or dysfunction. A short-sleeper does not need treatment.

One cause of insomnia, PMS *(periodic movements in sleep)* needs elucidation. It actually consists of two different syndromes:

1. Periodic Limb Movement Disorder (PLMD), and
2. 'Restless legs' syndrome (or Ekbom syndrome), which often occur together.

1. Periodic Limb Movement Disorder (PLMD)

It is characterized by sudden, repeated contraction of one or more of muscle groups (usually of the legs) during sleep. Often occurring bilaterally, it is followed by partial (most commonly) or complete arousal. Since each individual contraction lasts for a few seconds and is repeated at an interval of 20-60 sec. during a long sleep-period, partial or complete awakenings occur many times in one night sleep.

The patient is usually not aware of myoclonus. He usually complains of non-restorative sleep or of frequent awakenings. Myoclonus is observed, if at all, by the bed partner. This is commonly seen in middle-aged and elderly people. Due to night-time insomnia, daytime hypersomnia can occur and at times may be the only presenting symptom.

2. 'Restless legs' syndrome (Ekbom syndrome)

It is a condition in which the person experiences, during waking, an extremely uncomfortable feeling in the leg muscles. Sometimes it may resemble painful creeping sensations deep inside the calf muscles.

Classically, these abnormal sensations occur while sitting or lying down and cause an irresistible urge to move the legs. Moving about or standing provides immediate, temporary relief. This is often associated with periodic limb movement disorder (PLMD) (during night sleep). Daily, regular exercises can lead to marked improvement in certain cases.

TABLE 11.3. SLEEP HYGIENE

Some components of sleep hygiene are:

1. Regular, daily physical exercises.
2. Avoid fluid intake and heavy meals just before bedtime.
3. Avoid caffeine intake (e.g. tea, coffee, cola drinks) before sleeping hours.
4. Avoid regular use of alcohol (especially avoid use of alcohol as a hypnotic for promoting sleep).
5. Avoid reading or watching television while in bed.
6. Sleep in a dark, quiet, and comfortable environment.

Treatment

1. A thorough medical and psychiatric assessment.
2. Polysomnography (Table 11.1) may be needed in some patients to reach a diagnosis.
3. Treatment of underlying physical and/or psychiatric disorder, if present.
4. Withdrawal of current medications, if any.
5. Relaxation techniques before sleep time and education regarding *sleep hygiene* (Table 11.3). Sleep hygiene consists of general guidelines for promoting good sleep. In itself, it is not a treatment for insomnia.
6. Psychotherapy.
7. Benzodiazepines may be used, either alone, e.g. in primary insomnia, or may be used with treatment of underlying physical or psychiatric disorder(s). The use of benzodiazepines should only be for short-term periods, not more than for 4-6 weeks at one time.

If the difficulty in initiating sleep is the main symptom, then a benzodiazepine with short half life should be used, e.g. temazepam, oxazepam or lorazepam. If the difficulty in maintaining sleep is the predominant symptom then a longer acting benzodiazepine, e.g. nitrazepam, flurazepam or even diazepam, should be used. Physicians should be careful to avoid benzodiazepine abuse or dependence in patients with insomnia.

Non-benzodiazepine hypnotics (e.g. zopiclone, zolpidem) are useful alternatives (see Chapter 15).

8. L-tryptophan, an amino-acid present in many vegetables, is an apparently non-dependence producing hypnotic. Usual dose is 0.5 g. at night time.

B. Hypersomnia

Hypersomnia is also known as *DOES* (disorder of excessive somnolence). Hypersomnia means one or more of the following:

1. Excessive day time sleepiness.
2. 'Sleep attacks' during day time (falling asleep unintentionally).
3. 'Sleep drunkenness' (person needs much more time to awaken and during this period is confused or disoriented).

Hypersomnia is seen in 1-2% of general population at any given time. As insomnia and hypersomnia may be present at the same time, the underlying causes may be common to both. It is required for the diagnosis that the sleep disturbance occurs daily for at least 1 month or for recurrent periods of shorter duration, and that it causes either marked distress or interferes with social and occupational functioning.

Causes

The common causes of hypersomnia are listed in Table 11.4.

TABLE 11.4. CAUSES OF HYPERSOMNIA

1. Medical illnesses
- i. Narcolepsy (in about 25% of all patients with hypersomnia)
- ii. Sleep apnea (in about 50% of all patients with hypersomnia)
- iii. Kleine-Levin syndrome
- iv. Menstrual-associated somnolence
- v. Sleep deprivation
- vi. Following or with insomnia
- vii. Encephalitis
- viii. Hypothyroidism
- ix. Head Injury
- x. Cerebral tumors in the region of mid-brain
- xi. Hypothalamic lesions
- xii. Trypanosomiasis
- xiii. PMS (Periodic movements in sleep); in about 10% of all patients with hypersomnia.

2. Alcohol and drug use
- i. Stimulant withdrawal
- ii. Alcohol intoxication
- iii. Use of CNS depressant medications.

3. Psychiatric disorders
- i. Dysthymia
- ii. Atypical depression
- iii. Seasonal mood disorder.

4. Idiopathic hypersomnia.

A hypersomnic should be differentiated from long-sleeper, who *needs* more than 9 hours of sleep per night and has no symptoms or dysfunction. A long-sleeper does not need treatment.

A few important causes are discussed below.

1. Narcolepsy

This is a disorder characterized by excessive daytime sleepiness, often disturbed night-time sleep and disturbances in REM sleep. The hallmark of this disorder is decreased REM latency, i.e. decreased latent period before the first REM period occurs. Normal REM latency is 90-100 minutes. In narcolepsy, REM sleep occurs within 10 minutes of the onset of sleep.

The common age of onset is 15-25 years with a stable course throughout life. The prevalence rate is 4 per 10,000.

The classical tetrad of symptoms is:

i. *Sleep attacks* (most common): The person is unable to resist a sleep attack or 'nap', from which he awakens refreshed. These 'attacks' can occur during any time of the day, even while driving. Usually, there is a gap of 2-3 hours between the two attacks.
ii. *Cataplexy:* This is characterized by a loss of muscle tone in the various parts of body, e.g. jaw drop, or paresis of all skeletal muscles of body resulting in a fall. This may be precipitated by sudden emotion. The consciousness is usually clear and memory is normal, unless sleep attacks supervene.
iii. *Hypnagogic hallucinations:* These are vivid perceptions, usually dream-like, which occur at the onset of sleep and are associated with fearfulness. When these occur at awakening, they are called hypnopompic hallucinations.
iv. *Sleep paralysis* (least common): This occurs either at awakening in morning (usually) or at sleep onset. The person is conscious but unable to move his body. The episode may last from 30 seconds to a few minutes and may cause significant distress.

Not all symptoms of tetrad are present in one person. Other associated symptoms are fugue states, blackouts, blurring of vision. Polysomnography helps in making a diagnosis in doubtful cases, showing decreased REM latency.

The treatment consists of forced naps at regular times in the day, stimulant medication (e.g. amphetamines) in some patients, and/or antidepressants (particularly when cataplexy is a prominent symptom).

2. Sleep Apnea

This is characterized by repeated episodes of apnea during sleep. In this context, apnea is defined as cessation of airflow at the nostrils (and mouth) for 10 seconds or longer. The apnea can be of central type, obstructive type or mixed type. It is commoner in elderly and obese (*Pickwickian syndrome*). Typically, there are 5 or more apneic episodes per hour of sleep and the total number of apneic episodes exceed 30 during one night sleep. In severe cases, the number of episodes may be in hundreds.

The patients are usually not aware of the occurrence of apnea. Instead, they complain of an inability to stay awake in the day time and non-restorative sleep at the night. The bed partner may report of loud snoring, restless sleep or of periodic absence of breathing.

The diagnosis can be established in doubtful cases using polysomnography, with the respiratory tracings included.

Sleep apnea, can be a dangerous condition. It can cause cardiac arrhythmias pulmonary and systemic hypertension and death.

The treatment consists of avoidance of alcohol and depressant medications, use of stimulants like caffeine, regular exercises and losing excess weight, teaching correct sleeping posture, and corrective procedures for obstructive sleep apnea (e.g. mechanical tongue retaining device). Very severe obstructive sleep apnea may necessitate tracheostomy (func-tional only at night), CPAP (Continuous positive airway pressure) through nasal mesh, or even pharyngoplasty.

3. Kleine-Levin Syndrome

This is a rare syndrome characterized by:

1. Hypersomnia (always present), occurring recurrently for long periods of time.
2. Hyperphagia (usually present), with a voracious appetite.

3. Hypersexuality (associated at times), consisting of sexual disinhibition, masturbatory activity, exhibitionism, and/or inappropriate sexual advances.

The associated features include apathy, irritable behavior, confusion, social withdrawal, bizarre behavior, psychotic symptoms like delusions and hallucinations, and disorientation. One or more of these symptoms may occur during the episode. EEG abnormalities, usually showing intermittent non-specific slowing, are common but are not diagnostic.

A typical episode lasts for one to several weeks followed usually by a complete remission. Common age of onset is the second decade of life. Apparently this disorder has a finite course with a large majority of patients recovering completely before the fifth decade of life. The disorder is almost always seen in males.

No specific treatment is available, although lithium and occasionally carbamazepine have been reported to be successful.

Treatment

1. A thorough physical and psychiatric assessment.
2. Treatment of the underlying cause is the most important method.
3. Associated or underlying insomnia should be looked for and treated.
4. Withdrawal of current medication causing hypersomnia, especially depressant medication.
5. Benzodiazepines at night may paradoxically decrease hypersomnia by correcting night time insomnia.

C. Disorders of Sleep-Wake Schedule

These are characterized by a disturbance in the timing of sleep. The person with this disorder is not able to sleep when he wishes to, although at other times he is able to sleep adequately. This is due to a mismatch between the person's circadian rhythm and the normal sleep-wake schedule demanded by the environment.

Causes

The common causes are listed below.

1. *'Jet lag'* or rapid change of time zone: This typically occurs during international flights crossing many 'time zones'. At the new place, person's internal time of sleep and the sleep time of surroundings are different, leading to insomnia during the new sleep time and somnolescence in the new daytime, thus causing impairment of functioning.
2. *'Work-shift'* from day to night or vice-versa.
3. *Unusual sleep phases*: Some persons are unable to sleep early. They typically sleep late at night and get up late in the morning. They are called *'owls'*. Others are similarly unable to remain awake at night. They typically sleep early at night and get up early in the morning. They are called *'larks'*. Some others have a longer-than 24 hour sleep-wake cycle (usually of 25 hours).

Treatment

No specific treatment is usually needed. Benzodiazepines may be needed for short-term correction of insomnia. Changes in 'work-shifts' may be needed for persons with unusual sleep phases.

Exposure to sunlight during outdoor activity (instead of staying indoors), and adopting the local (new) hours for sleeping (and working) can help in combating jet lag.

II. Parasomnias

Parasomnias are dysfunctions or episodic nocturnal events occurring with sleep, sleep stages or partial arousals. Most parasomnias are common in childhood though they may persist into adulthood.

A. Stage 4 Sleep Disorders

These are disorders occurring during deep sleep, i.e. stage 3 and 4 of NREM sleep. The common stage 4 parasomnias are:

1. *Sleep-walking* (*somnambulism*): The patient carries out automatic motor activities that range from simple to complex. He may leave the bed, walk about or leave the house. Arousal is difficult and accidents may occur during sleep-walking.
2. *Sleep-terrors* or *night terrors* (*pavor nocturnus*): The patient suddenly gets up screaming, with autonomic arousal (tachycardia, sweating, and hyperventilation). He may be difficult to arouse and rarely recalls the episode on awakening. In contrast, nightmares (which occur during REM sleep) are clearly remembered in the morning.
3. *Sleep-related enuresis* (bedwetting): This is discussed in Chapter 14.
4. *Bruxism* (tooth-grinding): The patient has an involuntary, and forceful grinding of teeth during sleep. Though the bed partner reports the loud sound produced by the grinding of teeth and the destruction of the tooth enamel is obvious, the patient remains completely unaware of the episode.
5. *Sleep-talking* (*somniloquy*): The patient talks during the stage 3 and 4 of sleep but does not remember anything about it in the morning on awakening.

These disorders are often coexistent. As they occur during stage 4 (and 3) of NREM sleep, they are more common during the first one-third of the night. Arousal is difficult and on waking up, there is a complete amnesia for the event(s).

Treatment

Since benzodiazepines suppress stage 4 of NREM sleep, a single dose at bedtime usually provides relief from stage 4 parasomnias.

B. Other Sleep Disorders

Nightmares (dream anxiety disorder) occur during REM sleep. They are characterized by fearful dreams occurring most commonly in the last one-third of night sleep. The person wakes up very frightened and remembers the dream vividly.

This is in contrast to *night terrors* which occur early in the night, are a stage 4 NREM disorder, and are characterized by complete amnesia. In both conditions, the observer finds the person frightened during the episode.

Other sleep disorders include nocturnal angina, nocturnal asthma, nocturnal seizures, paroxysmal nocturnal hemoglobinuria, nocturnal head banging, and familial sleep paralysis.

Treatment

There is no specific treatment. Treatment of the underlying condition is the most important step. The treatment of nightmares is by suppression of REM sleep e.g. by bedtime dose of a benzodiazepine. However on stopping the drug, a rebound increase in symptoms may occur.

12

Behavioral Syndromes Associated With Psychological Disturbances and Physiological Factors

EATING DISORDERS

The eating disorders in ICD-10 include the following disorders:

Anorexia Nervosa

Anorexia nervosa is an *eating disorder* characterized by the following clinical features:

1. It occurs much more often in females as compared to males. The common age of onset is adolescence (13-19 years of age).
2. There is an intense fear of becoming obese. This fear does not decrease even if body becomes very thin and underweight.
3. There is a *body-image disturbance*. The person is unable to perceive the body size accurately. However, the body image disturbances may (sometimes) not be seen in Indian patients.
4. There is a refusal to maintain the body weight above a minimum normal weight for that age, sex and height.
5. Significant loss of weight occurs, usually more than 25% of the original weight. The final weight is usually 15% less than the minimum limit of normal weight (for that age, sex and height) or a Quetelet's body-mass index of 17.5 or less (Quetelet's body-mass index = weight in kg. divided by square of height in meters).
6. No known medical illness, which can account for the weight loss, is present.
7. Absence of any other psychiatric disorder.
8. Amenorrhea, primary or secondary, is often present in females.

In addition to these typical clinical features, other associated features are often present. The patient imposes on herself dietary restrictions; has peculiar patterns of handling food, like breaking food into small bits, hiding food; and involves herself in vigorous exercises.

'Anorexia' is a misnomer, as there is never a decrease in appetite initially. In fact the patient is often preoccupied with food. A lot of time may be spent in collecting recipes and cooking food for the significant others.

Depressive symptoms are common and so are obsessive-compulsive personality traits. Psychomotor activity is usually increased. In severe cases, fine *lanugo hair* may develop all over the body.

The women with anorexia nervosa, usually have poor sexual adjustment. There are often conflicts about being a female and fear of pregnancy. Many patients are unconsciously unable to accept a 'female role'.

A large number (up to 50%) of anorectics also have bulimic episodes. These are characterized by rapid consumption of large amounts of food in a relatively short period of time, occurring usually when alone. This is known as *eating binges*. The binges are followed by intense guilt and attempts to remove eaten food, e.g. by self-induced vomiting, laxative abuse, diuretic abuse.

If untreated, the weight loss becomes marked. Death may occur due to hypokalemia (caused by self-induced vomiting), dehydration, malnutrition or congestive cardiac failure (caused by anemia).

Anorexia nervosa should be differentiated from other conditions capable of causing significant weight loss. These include medical illnesses (like hypopituitarism, lateral hypothalamic lesion, debilitating systemic illnesses, e.g. disseminated tuberculosis), and psychiatric disorders (like depressive episode, schizophrenia). Another differential diagnosis is *bulimia nervosa*. Although bulimic episodes are common in anorexia nervosa (binge eating followed by vomiting), patients of pure bulimia nervosa maintain a near normal body weight, in sharp contrast to anorexia nervosa patients.

Treatment

The treatment is in two phases which merge into each other.

A. Short term treatment, to ensure weight gain and correct nutritional deficiencies, if any.
B. Long term treatment, aimed at maintaining the near normal weight achieved in short term treatment and preventing relapses.

The various treatment modalities used include:

1. *Behavior therapy*: This is based on providing positive reinforcements (and at times negative reinforcements) contingent on weight gain by the patient. The positive reinforcements are provided every day. It is not desirable to have too rapid a weight gain. The gain in weight should not exceed 1.5 kg - 2 kg in a fortnight. As patients are unable to take a large meal, especially in the initial part of treatment, it is advisable to give more number of meals (usually about 6) per day. Occasionally, forceful Ryle's tube feeding may be needed initially, in resistant patients.
2. *Individual psychotherapy* is not often successful.
3. *Hospitalization*, with adequate nursing care for food intake and weight gain, has been helpful in short term treatment. However this method does not necessarily ensure long term improvement.
4. *Drugs* are an important adjunct to other modes of therapy. The drugs used include:
   i. Chlorpromazine.
   ii. Tricyclic antidepressants (e.g. fluoxetine, amitriptyline, clomipramine) for anorexia nervosa and/or for associated depression.
   iii. Cyproheptadine (This is particularly helpful in inducing weight gain, decreasing depressive symptoms and increasing appetite, if anorexia is actually present). The usual dose is 8-32 mg/day, in divided doses.
5. *Group therapy and family therapy*: These methods are used to educate the patient and her family about anorexia nervosa and its treatment. Education also includes loosening of current social norms of slimming and fitness, since there is evidence to suggest that anorexia nervosa is far more common in countries with social pressures for slimming, e.g. America. India is fast catching up with similar social pressures.

The prognosis is better, if

1. The age of onset is younger,
2. The number of previous hospitalizations is very low, and
3. There are no bulimic episodes.

The weight gain and improvement in mental attitude often precede the return of menstrual function.

Bulimia Nervosa

Bulimia nervosa is an *eating disorder* characterized by following clinical features:

1. It occurs in early teens or adolescence.
2. There is an intense fear of becoming obese. There may be an earlier history of anorexia nervosa.
3. There is a body-image disturbance. The person is unable to perceive the body size accurately.
4. There is a persistent preoccupation with eating, and an irresistible craving for food. There are episodes of overeating in which large amounts of food are consumed with in short periods of time *(eating binges)*.
5. There are attempts to 'counteract' the effects of overeating by one or more of the following: self-induced vomitings, purgative abuse, periods of starvation, and use of drugs like appetite suppressants.
6. No known medical illness is present which can account for the disorder.
7. Absence of any other psychiatric disorder.

Treatment

The various treatment modalities used include:

1. Behavior therapy: This is based on providing positive reinforcements (and at times negative reinforcements) contingent on the control of binge eating by the patient.
2. Individual psychotherapy.
3. Drugs are an important adjunct to other modes of therapy. The drugs used include tricyclic antidepressants, e.g. imipramine. Fluoxetine (in doses of 20-60 mg) is particularly useful as it causes a loss of appetite along with its antidepressant effect.
4. Group therapy and family therapy: These methods are used to educate the patient and the family about bulimia nervosa and its treatment.

Obesity (Overeating Associated With Other Psychological Disturbances)

Obesity caused by a reaction to distressing events is included here. Obesity caused by drugs or endocrinal factors, or due to constitutional factors is not included here.

Treatment depends on the underlying cause, e.g. psychotherapy (for stressful life conditions), and antidepressants (for depression).

Binge Eating Disorders

In binge eating disorder, large amounts of food are consumed in a relatively short period, followed by severe discomfort and feelings of self-denigration. There is a sense of lack of control over eating during the episode.

Additionally, there also may be eating of large amounts of food throughout the day with no planned meal times, eating alone because of being embarrassed, and feeling guilty and depressed after overeating.

The disorder is not listed separately in ICD-10 and the symptoms of binge-eating are also seen in bulimia nervosa.

Treatment is similar to bulimia nervosa, though the role of drug treatment in binge eating disorder is not so clear.

Psychogenic Vomiting

This is a clinical syndrome in which psychobiosocial factors interact to produce the symptoms which are often mistaken for upper gastrointestinal tract disease, anorexia nervosa, dissociative (conversion) disorder, somatization disorder, or malingering.

The characteristic clinical features are:

1. Repeated vomitings, which typically occur soon after the meal has begun or just after it has been completed.
2. Vomitings often occur in complete absence of nausea or retching. (Patients say that food just seems to come back up).
3. Vomitings are often self-induced and can be suppressed, if necessary.
4. Despite repeated vomitings, the weight loss is not significant.
5. The course of the illness is usually chronic with frequent remissions and relapses.

Treatment

1. Identification of psychosocial stressor.
2. Environmental manipulation to deal with stress.
3. Teaching coping skills.
4. Psychotherapy.

NON-ORGANIC SLEEP DISORDERS

The non-organic sleep disorders are discussed in Chapter 11.

SEXUAL DYSFUNCTIONS, NOT CAUSED BY ORGANIC DISORDERS OR DISEASE

The non-organic sexual dysfunctions are discussed in Chapter 10.

POST PARTUM PSYCHIATRIC DISORDERS (MENTAL AND BEHAVIORAL DISORDERS ASSOCIATED WITH PUERPERIUM, NOT CLASSIFIED ELSEWHERE)

Pregnancy and puerperium are highly stressful periods in a woman's life. The person is threatened by:

1. Physical changes, physiological changes and endocrinal changes occurring in one's body,
2. Reorganization of psyche in accordance with the new 'mother-role' (especially in the first pregnancy),
3. Body image changes, and
4. Unconscious intrapsychic conflicts relating to pregnancy, childbirth and motherhood become activated.

It is no wonder then, that 25-50% of all women develop mild psychological symptoms in the puerperal period. The commonest type of picture is mild depression and irritability, known as *post-natal blues*. These 'blues' pass off within a few days and usually need no active management.

But, in 1.5-4.6/1,000 deliveries (average 2/1000 deliveries), the mother develops severe psychiatric symptoms or become psychotic. This is known as *post partum psychosis* (PPP).

The post partum psychosis can be:

1. Depressive episode (most common), or
2. Schizophrenia, or
3. Manic episode, or
4. Delirium (least common).

Typically, the onset of symptoms occurs 3-7 days after delivery. Onset before 3rd day postpartum is rare. The symptoms usually peak by the end of 4th week, and often necessitate admission in a hospital.

As the puerperium lasts for 6 weeks, the relevant postpartum period for psychiatric symptomatology to appear is *6 weeks* (according to ICD-10). Hence, any psychiatric symptoms appearing within 6-week period after delivery are called post partum psychiatric disorder(s), if they do not fulfill the criteria of the major psychiatric disorders.

It was earlier believed that schizophreniform disorder is the commonest PPP in the developing countries (including India) in contrast to the developed countries where depression is more common. But, recent studies negate this hypothesis. Even in India, depressive episode is the most common type of PPP encountered in clinical practice.

The factors involved in causation are biological (changes in endocrine status especially steroid withdrawal, sleep disturbances, amine disturbances), and psychosocial (intrapsychic conflicts relating to motherhood, family and interpersonal conflicts in light of new 'role').

Presently, it is believed that PPP is not a special or separate category, but only a residual category in ICD-10. Depressive episode or schizophreniform disorder occurring separately or as a part of PPP are very similar, except presence of confusion as a prominent and common symptom in PPP. Childbirth merely acts as a stressful event precipitating the illness. However, postpartum psychoses have a better prognosis as compared to similar disorders occurring in a non-postpartum setting.

15-25% of PPP patients have a recurrence, usually of the same type, during the next puerperium. During an episode, presence of folate deficiency can prolong the duration of psychiatric disorder and may make it chronic.

Treatment

1. Treatment of the type of PPP, e.g. tricyclic antidepressants and/or ECTs for depressive episode; antipsychotics and/or lithium for manic episode; antipsychotics for schizophreniform disorder.
2. Psychotherapy for minor psychological problems, especially after recovery from psychosis has occurred.
3. General care of the puerperium.

TABLE 12.1. CLASSICAL PSYCHOSOMATIC DISORDERS

The 7 classical psychosomatic disorders are:

1. Bronchial asthma
2. Ulcerative colitis
3. Peptic ulcer
4. Neurodermatitis
5. Thyrotoxicosis
6. Rheumatoid arthritis
7. Essential hypertension.

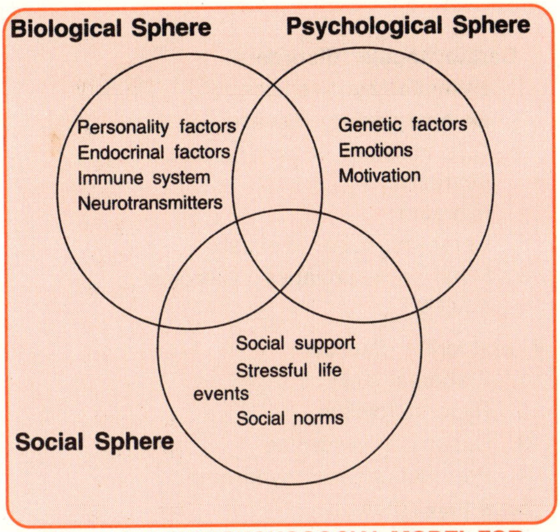

FIG. 12.1. A BIOPSYCHOSOCIAL MODEL FOR PSYCHOSOMATIC ILLNESS

4. Lithium, antipsychotics and antidepressants are excreted in milk and may be dangerous to the infant. A judicious decision has to be made regarding feeding of the infant, depending on the dose being given, social support available and risks of keeping the infant and mother separate.
5. As patients often lack insight, have poor judgement, are unable to care for themselves and the infants, and are receiving psychotropic medication, it is not uncommon that the infant has to be given top feeds (supplementary feeds). In that case, it is essential to extract milk from breast daily (or more often) either manually or with a breast-pump. It is more practical to give oral stilbesterol or pyridoxine (100 mg/day) to inhibit lactation.

PSYCHOSOMATIC DISORDERS (PSYCHOLOGICAL OR BEHAVIORAL FACTORS ASSOCIATED WITH DISORDERS OR DISEASES CLASSIFIED ELSEWHERE)

Psychosomatic disorders (a term coined by Heinroth, 1918) are those disorders in which psychosocial factors are important. Broadly

TABLE 12.2. COMMON EXAMPLES OF PSYCHOSOMATIC DISORDERS

I. Cardiovascular disorders
1. Essential hypertension
2. Coronary artery disease
3. CCU delirium or post-cardiac surgery delirium
4. Migraine
5. Cerebrovascular disease
6. Mitral valve prolapse syndrome (MVPS)

II. Endocrine disorders
1. Diabetes mellitus
2. Hyperthyroidism
3. Cushing's syndrome
4. Peri-menopausal syndrome
5. Amenorrhea
6. Menorrhagia

III. Gastro-intestinal disorders
1. Esophageal reflux
2. Peptic ulcer
3. Ulcerative colitis
4. Crohn's disease

IV. Immune disorders (These overlap with other disorders mentioned in this table)
1. Auto-immune disorders, like Ulcerative colitis, Systemic lupus erythematosis (SLE)
2. Allergic disorders, like Bronchial asthma and Hay fever
3. Viral infections

V. Musculo-skeletal disorders
1. Rheumatoid arthritis
2. SLE

VI. Respiratory disorders
1. Bronchial asthma
2. Hay fever
3. Vasomotor (allergic) rhinitis

VII. Skin disorders
1. Psoriasis
2. Pruritus
3. Urticaria
4. Alopecia areata
5. Acne vulgaris
6. Psychogenic purpura
7. Trichotillomania
8. Dermatitis artifacta
9. Lichen planus
10. Warts.

applied, this term can encompass all physical illnesses. A narrow but more practical definition would include those physical disorders which are either initiated or exacerbated by the presence of meaningful psychosocial environmental stressors. ICD-10 lists these disorders under (Psychological or behavioral factors associated with disorders or diseases classified elsewhere).

Franz Alexander, the Father of psychosomatic medicine, described the seven classical psychosomatic illnesses (Table 12.1).

He gave his *specificity hypothesis*, which said that if a specific environmental stressor or emotional conflict occurs, it results in a specific illness in a genetically predetermined organ.

George Engel, in 1977, gave a *biopsychosocial model* to explain the complex interaction between biological, psychological and social spheres resulting in a psychosomatic illness. This viewpoint has become very popular. It can be depicted in a diagram, which is given below (Fig. 12.1).

Beginning from the 7 classical psychosomatic illnesses of Alexander, the number of these illnesses has continued to increase by leaps and bounds, as the evidence for their biopsychosocial causation became more evident. At present, the list of psychosomatic illnesses is virtually endless. The important and common psychosomatic illnesses are mentioned in Table 12.2.

It is not the purpose of this book to go into the details of these physical disorders. However, certain important aspects and conditions are discussed, which are often not available in detail in the medical textbooks.

Type A Personality

When the personality characteristics of a coronary artery disease (CAD) patient are examined, it is found that there is preponderance of certain type of personality traits, known collectively as *coronary prone type A behavior* (Friedman and Rosenman).

This type A behavior is characterized by:

1. Time Urgency

There is always a hurry to finish the task at hand. This is extended even to day-to-day routine activities like eating, bathing. Speech is usually hurried and psychomotor activity is often increased.

2. Excessive Competitiveness and Hostility

There is a need to win always, with a mistrust for other people's motives. Rage ensues if interrupted in achieving an objective.

Overall, there is a chronic struggle to achieve or complete a large number of tasks, working against the limits of time available and/or other people in the surrounding environment.

In contrast, type B behavior is just the opposite, characterized by a relaxed unhurried attitude and less vigorous attempts to achieve a goal. Some studies report that persons with type B personality are paradoxically more successful than those with type A personality.

Treatment

As the person with type A behavior is usually aware of the presence of these personality traits, he may come for treatment himself, or may need treatment after CAD has occurred. One or more of the following methods may be used.

1. Relaxation techniques: This is one of the most important methods aimed at reducing the basal generalized anxiety or restlessness. The techniques include:
   i. Jacobson's progressive relaxation technique
   ii. Yoga
   iii. Autohypnosis
   iv. Transcendental meditation
   v. Biofeedback.
2. Behavior modification techniques.
3. Individual therapy.
4. Group therapy.

Post Cardiac Surgery Delirium

This is a condition similar to ICU (Intensive care unit) syndrome. A fairly common disorder, its onset typically occurs after 24-48 hours of surgery. The patients who develop post surgery delirium are often the ones who are most fearful before surgery.

Many causes have been attributed for delirium, which include:

1. Cardiac status.
2. Presence of pre-operative, subclinical organic brain disease.
3. Restrictive environment of the ICU/CCU, with isolation.
4. Electrolyte imbalance.
5. Pre-operative anxiety, fearfulness, depression or denial.

Probably the condition is etiologically multifactorial.

Treatment

1. Preoperative measures.
   i. Allaying the anxiety and fears of the patient.
   ii. Treatment of depression.
   iii. Confrontation of denial.
   iv. Providing clocks and windows in ICU/CCU, to keep the patient oriented in time.
   v. Allowing a family member to stay near the patient.
2. Post-delirium measures

Since delirium can be life threatening, as patients can take out the IV lines, catheter or

TABLE 12.3. PHYSICAL ILLNESS AND PSYCHOPATHOLOGY

Physical Illness	Psychiatric Symptomatology (Not all symptoms are present in one patient)
1. Hyperthyroidism (Thyrotoxicosis)	Anxiety, depression (with apathetic hyperthyroidism), impairment of higher mental functions, paranoid disorder, delirium (with thyroid storm), mania, schizophreniform disorder, organic mental disorder.
2. Hypothyroidism (Myxedema)	Apathy and lethargy, memory impairment, slow thinking, poor attention span, irritable mood, paranoid ideation, severe depressive episode, dementia, *myxedema madness*.
3. Hyperadrenalism (Cushing's syndrome)	Depression, with paranoid ideation, generalized anxiety, psychosis with somatic delusions.
4. Adrenal cortical deficiency (Addison's disease)	Depression, with paranoid ideation, delirium (toxic psychosis), stupor.
5. Hyperpituitarism (Acromegaly)	Apathy, depression, anxiety.
6. Hypopituitarism (Simmond's disease)	Depression with memory disturbances, hypersomnia, delirium, stupor or coma.
7. Hyperparathyroidism	Depression, delirium (with 'parathyroid crisis'), coma (following recurrent seizures), early dementia.
8. Hypoparathyroidism	Delirium (particularly in post-operative cases), dementia (in idiopathic hypoparathyroidism), depression (with 'partial parathyroid insufficiency'), mental retardation (especially in pseudo-hypoparathyroidism and pseudo-pseudo-hypoparathyroidism), 'pseudoneurosis'.
9. Pheochromocytoma	Anxiety and panic attacks.
10. Acute intermittent porphyria	Acute anxiety, severe excitement or psychomotor withdrawal, conversion symptoms, schizophreniform disorder (rare), stupor or coma (rare).
11. AIDS (Acquired immunodeficiency syndrome)	Anxiety, depression, delirium, dementia (AIDS-dementia complex), organic catatonia, adjustment disorder, suicidal behavior, delusional disorder.
12. Systemic lupus erythematosus (SLE)	Depression, delirium (toxic psychosis), steroid psychosis (iatrogenic), schizophreniform disorder (uncommon).
13. Hepatolenticular degeneration (Wilson's disease)	Personality changes (slow and (slow and insidious), mental retardation (in early onset), dementia (in late onset), schizophreniform disorder (can become chronic), antisocial behavior, with rapid mood swings, poor impulse control and aggressive behavior.
14. Multiple sclerosis	Euphoria or depression, histrionic personality traits, conversion and/or dissociation symptoms, dementia (if of long duration).
15. Parkinsonism	Depression, dementia, paranoid features.
16. Pancreatic carcinoma	Severe depression.
17. Progressive supra-nuclear palsy (PSP)	Depression, dementia.

other 'life-lines' and can jump down from balcony or window, urgent treatment is often needed.

i. IV diazepam 10-20 mg, or
ii. IV haloperidol 5-10 mg,

are the drugs of choice. The parenteral injection should be repeated every 30 minutes till agitation is controlled. Later, the patient can be switched to low dose oral haloperidol (1-5 mg/day) till recovery from delirium occurs. Anticholinergic medication should not be routinely added to haloperidol, as it may worsen delirium.

PSYCHIATRY IN MEDICINE

About one-third to two-third of medical outpatients have primary or associated psychiatric disorders. If minor psychological and social problems are also taken into consideration, this number would be even larger. Since these patients are benefited by a psychiatric referral, psychiatrists are becoming increasingly involved in treatment of medical and surgical patients. In fact a whole new branch of *consultation-liaison psychiatry* has sprung up.

Consultation-liaison psychiatry is an area of clinical psychiatry which includes diagnostic, therapeutic, teaching and research activities of psychiatrists in the non-psychiatric parts of the hospital.

The common reasons for a psychiatric referral are:

1. Suicidal attempt or ideation or threat.
2. Grossly abnormal behavior disturbing the ward atmosphere.
3. Presence of drug or alcohol abuse or dependence.
4. Organic brain syndromes.
5. Psychosomatic disorders.
6. Psychological reaction to medical illness.
7. Uncertain diagnosis (No medical illness can be found despite the presence of symptoms).
8. Manipulative or difficult or hostile patient; or presence of patient-doctor conflict.
9. Psychiatric side-effects of drugs.
10. Patient has nowhere to go or is unable to manage his or her own affairs.

A large number of medical illnesses can present with psychiatric symptomatology. It is important to keep in mind the possibility of a secondary mental disorder, i.e. a psychiatric disorder which is caused by an underlying physical disease. Some important physical illnesses with their commonly presenting psychiatric symptoms are listed in Table 12.3.

In addition, a large number of physical disorders like auto-immune disorders; infections; nutritional deficiencies (particularly pellagra, pernicious anemia, beriberi); malignancies; alcohol and drug abuse; side-effects or toxicity of many medications; metabolic and water and electrolyte disturbances (and many others) may present with psychiatric symptomatology either alone (especially in initial stages) or with other physical signs and symptoms. Some of these have been mentioned under the causes of organic mental disorders.

GRIEF

Grief is the normal response of an individual to the loss of a loved object, e.g. a close relative or a friend, material values or non-material things such as reputation and self-esteem.

Grief is a universal phenomenon which is usually transient and self-limiting. Uncomplicated grief is not a psychiatric disorder and does not usually require psychiatric treatment. However, as physicians (and psychiatrists) are sometimes called to intervene in cases with complications, the condition is discussed under this chapter.

Bowlby (1961) described three phases of the behavior response to loss of a loved object: *protest*, *despair*, and *detachment*. Following the loss, there is often a *state of shock*.

TABLE 12.4. GRIEF AND DEPRESSION

Features	Grief	Depression*
1. Identification with deceased	Normal	Abnormal
2. Ambivalence	Less	More
3. Suicidal ideas	Rare	Common
4. Global worthlessness	Rare	Common
5. Self-blame	Limited to loss	Global
6. Response evoked from others	Empathy; Sympahty	Annoyance; Irritation
7. Self-limited	Usually	May not be
8. Response to assurance	Good	Poor
9. Vulnerability to physical illness	Increased	Increased
10. Response to TCAs	Poor	Good

*Depression means here *severe depression*

The grieved person feels a sense of bewilderment or numbness, or he may completely deny the loss. Although most commonly this state lasts for a few hours, sometimes it may extend up to 2 weeks.

When the full extent of loss is realized, *various physical and mental symptoms* appear. These include repeated sighing and crying, difficulty in breathing, choking sensation, weakness, poor concentration and poor appetite. These symptoms usually last for 4-6 weeks but may sometimes extend up to 6 months.

Preoccupation with the memory of the deceased is a characteristic feature. This is associated with vivid mental images, vivid dreams and idealization of the deceased (ignoring his negative qualities). These preoccupations are of a comforting nature. This is often associated with a 'sense of presence' of the deceased in the surroundings and a misinterpretation of voices and faces of others as that of the lost person. Rarely, fleeting hallucinations may occur.

The grieved person often becomes depressed (see Table 12.4) and becomes slightly withdrawn socially. Guilt feelings, hostility towards others, panic attacks, sense of futility, tiredness, neglect of work and self, insomnia and suicidal ideas may occur. The person may *identify* with the deceased, taking on his qualities, mannerisms and characteristics.

Finally, a period of reorganization sets in and readjustment to the environment occurs.

Grief has been classified in to *normal grief* and *morbid grief reaction* (Gurmeet Singh). Morbid grief has been further divided in to pathological and complicated grief reactions.

Pathological Grief Reaction

When there is an exaggeration of one or more symptoms of normal grief, or the duration becomes prolonged beyond 6 months without spontaneous recovery, grief becomes morbid.

The various subtypes are chronic grief (duration more than 6 months); delayed grief (onset after 2 weeks of loss); inhibited grief (denial of loss); excessive anxiety, guilt, anger or religiosity grief; identification with the deceased; over-idealization of deceased and anniversary reactions (grief reaction on death anniversary).

Complicated Grief Reaction

Here, grief is complicated by specific neurotic or psychotic illness, in addition to grief reaction symptoms. The various subtypes are hysterical, phobic, obsessive-compulsive, manic or acute psychotic episode.

Treatment

1. Normal grief does not require psychiatric treatment. Occasionally, mild anxiolytic or hypnotic may be needed for short-term use.
2. In morbid and (especially) complicated grief, medication may be needed depending on the presenting clinical features.
3. The emphasis should be on:
   i. Making the person face the loss by counteracting denial.

ii. Ventilation of feelings (catharsis).
iii. Ensuring the presence of significant others.
iv. Bringing together similarly grieved persons, to encourage communication, share experiences of the loss and to offer companionship, and social and emotional support.
v. Reinforcement of goal-directed activities.

13
Mental Retardation

NORMAL CHILD DEVELOPMENT

For an understanding of the behavioral and psychological problems of childhood, it is essential to know the normal patterns of child development. Although no two children are alike, there are general similarities in the mental and physical development of all normal children. A newborn human infant is probably the most helpless of all mammalian infants, and needs much more time to become self-dependent.

The normal development of a child can be divided into four major areas (these are modified after Denver Development Screening Test, DDST).

1. Motor behavior.
2. Adaptive behavior.
3. Language.
4. Personal and social behavior.

As normal children cross these milestones or developmental levels at nearly expected age limits (within a few months' range), it is best to describe these developmental changes as milestones.

In addition to these milestones, there are other developmental parameters like height, weight, activity level and general health which have an important bearing on the development of a child.

As mentioned earlier, slight delay from these milestone dates is not abnormal. Statistically only those values, which are beyond two standard deviation from mean, are abnormal in a normal population.

INTELLECTUAL DEVELOPMENT

Intellectual development goes hand-in-hand with the development of physical and behavioral characteristics. It can be divided into following stages, according to Jean Piaget:

1. Sensori-Motor Stage

This stage extends from birth to 2 years of age, and is characterized by:

i. Actions related to sucking, orality and assimilation of objects.
ii. Ability to think of only one thought at a time.
iii. Inanimate objects are given human qualities.
iv. 'Out of sight' means ceasing to exist.

2. Concrete Thinking Stage

This stage lasts from 2 years to 7 years of life, and is characterized by:

i. Egocentric thought with a unique logic of its own, involving a limited point of view and lacking introspection.
ii. Inability to generalize from specific events and to specify from general events.

3. Abstract or Conceptual Thinking Stage

This stage begins at 7 years of age and lasts till 11 years, although it may be said to

TABLE 13.1. NORMAL DEVELOPMENTAL MILESTONES

Age	Developmental Milestones
1. Motor Behavior	
< 4 weeks	Moves head laterally in prone position.
4 weeks	Momentarily lifts head when prone.
3 months	Head-holding; Lifts head to 90° when prone.
5 months	Sits with support; Rolls over.
6 months	Lifts head and upper chest with the support of extended arms.
8 months	Sits steadily with straight back; Crawls; Early stepping movements when feet are placed on ground, with support.
10 months	Pulls from supine to sitting and sitting to standing; Stands holding furniture; Cruises around; Stands without support momentarily; Creeps on ground without support of abdomen.
14-15 months	Walks well without support; Walks backwards and sideways
2 years	Runs well; Climbs stairs alone; Kicks a large ball; Throws a ball overhead.
2½ years	Walks on tip-toes.
3 years	Climbs stairs in a coordinated manner, with alternate feet going up the staircase; Rides a tricycle; Makes a broad jump; Jumps in place.
4 years	Stands on one foot for 5 seconds.
5 years	Heel-to-toe walk; Jumps on one foot.
2. Adaptive Behavior (includes fine motor movements)	
4 weeks	Momentarily regards close moving objects, close to mid-line.
3 months	Follows the moving objects, even away from mid-line; converges and focuses.
4-5 months	Grasps objects crudely; Reaches to grasp.
6 months	Transfers objects from one hand to other.
9-10 months	Claps hands and matches two hand-held objects in mid line; Thumb-finger grasp.
1 year	Gives hand-held objects to mother, when asked; Turns 2-3 pages of a book at one time.
1½ years	Makes a tower of 3-4 cubes; Scribbles spontaneously, imitating writing; Sometimes may draw a vertical line.
2 years	Turns one page of a book at one time; Makes a tower of 6-7 cubes; Draws (copies) a horizontal line.
3 years	Makes a tower of 9-10 cubes; Makes a 3-cube bridge; Draws (copies) a circle.
4 years	Draws (copies) a cross.
5 years	Draws (copies) a square; Draws (copies) a recognizable man.
6 years	Draws (copies) a triangle.
7 years	Draws (copies) a diamond (Fig. 3:1).
8 years	Draws (copies) the following figures.
9 years	Draws (copies) the following figure.
3. Language	
4 weeks	Turns head and responds to sound of a bell. Vocalizes (apart from crying).
3 months	Laughs aloud.
9 months	Speaks mama, dada, m-m-m, ah (and other vowel sounds); Responds to name.
10 months	Understands spoken speech to some extent, e.g. where is 'mama'?
1-1¼ years	Uses 3-5 words meaningfully.
18 months	About 10 words spoken including name.
2 years	Combines 2 different words; Names at least one object in picture; Points to at least one named body part; Simple sentences made.
3 years	Uses plurals; Has a fairly good vocabulary.
5 years	Color naming accurately (primary colors); Defines words.

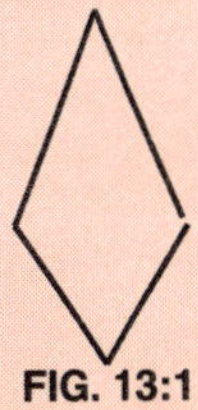

FIG. 13:1

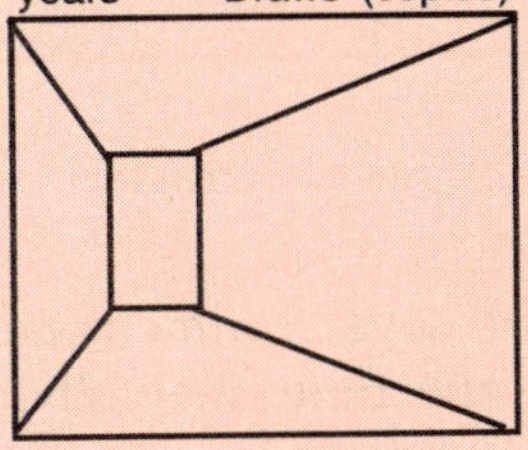

FIG. 13:2

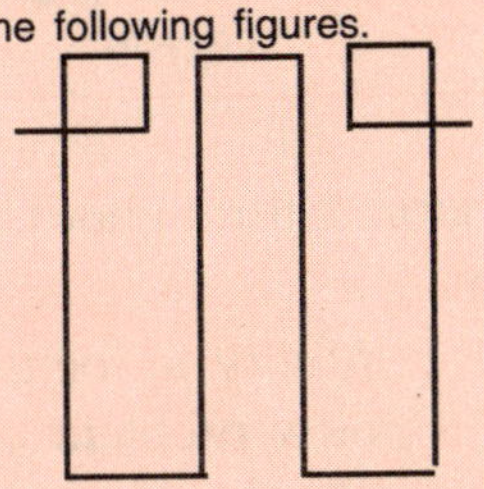

FIG. 13:3

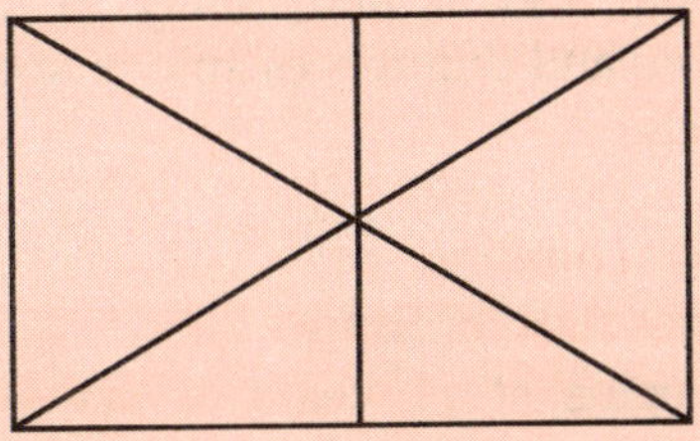

FIG. 13:4

TABLE 13.1. NORMAL DEVELOPMENTAL MILESTONES

Age	Developmental Milestones	Age	Developmental Milestones
4. Personal and Social Behavior		1½ years	Feeds oneself with a spoon, with little spill ing; Mimics actions of others; Pulls a toy with a string; Toilet training started.
4 weeks	Regards face intently.	2 years	Wears simple garments, socks and shoes.
2-3 months	Social smile.	3 years	Unbuttons buttons; Buckles shoes; Can dress and undress, with help.
3 months	Recognizes mother.	4 years	Buttons the dress well; Washes own face; Plays with other children easily; Separates from mother with little difficulty.
6 months	Takes foot to mouth; Smiles back at mirror-image of self.	5 years	Dresses without supervision.
9 months	Responds to social play; Resists pulling away of toy and tries to reach for it; Holds milk-bottle and eats a biscuit all by oneself.		

continue throughout life. This is characterized by:

i. Ability to focus on several dimensions of a problem at one time, mentally.
ii. The thought process is flexible and reversible.
iii. Ability of abstraction, i.e. ability to generalize from specific and ability to find similarities and differences among specific objects.

4. Adolescent Thinking or Formal Operational Stage

This stages begins at 11 years of age and continues life-long. This is characterized by:

i. Ability to imagine the possibilities inherent in a situation, thus making the thought comprehensive.
ii. Ability to develop complete abstract hypotheses and to test them.

By the end of adolescence, the individual's intellectual structures are nearly completely developed, although learning and intellectual growth go on throughout the life span of individual.

MENTAL RETARDATION

One to three percent of the general population is mentally retarded.

Mental retardation is defined as significantly subaverage general intellectual functioning, associated with significant deficit or impairment in adaptive functioning, which manifests during the developmental period (before 18 years of age).

In this definition, general intellectual functioning means, the result of a standardized intelligence test(s); significantly-subaverage means 2 standard deviations below the mean (usually an IQ of below 70); while adaptive behavior is the person's ability to meet the responsibilities of social, personal, occupational and interpersonal areas of life according to his or her age and sociocultural and educational background. Adaptive behavior is measured by clinical interview and standardized assessment scales.

Very often, it is assumed that the mentally retarded persons constitute a homogenous group. This is not true. The mentally retarded persons vary in their behavioral, psychological, physical and social characteristics as much as normal general population does.

Another common error is taking the IQ score as the measure of intelligence. It should be remembered that a mentally retarded person must have a deficit in both general intellectual functioning and adaptive behavior.

TABLE 13.2. CLASSIFICATION OF MENTAL RETARDATION BY IQ

Mental Retardation Level	IQ Range
1. Mild	50-70 *
2. Moderate	35-50 *
3. Severe	20-35 *
4. Profound	<20 *

(*As intelligence tests employed to measure IQ generally have an error of measurement of about 5 points, each figure means ± 5 points, e.g. 50 IQ means an IQ of 50 ± 5, depending on the adaptive behavior).

A classification of mental retardation on the basis of IQ (Intelligence Quotient, which is equal to mental age, i.e. MA, divided by chronological age, i.e. CA, multiplied by 100, i.e. IQ = MA/CA x 100), is provided in Table 13.2.

1. Mild Mental Retardation

This is the commonest type of mental retardation, accounting for 85-90% of all cases. The diagnosis is made usually later than in other types of mental retardation.

In the pre-school period (before 5 years of age), these children often develop like other normal children with very little deficit. Later, they often progress up to 6th class (grade) in school and can achieve vocational and social self-sufficiency with a little support. Only under stressful conditions or in the presence of an associated disease, supervised care is needed.

This group has been referred to as '*educable*' in a previous educational classification of mental retardation.

2. Moderate Mental Retardation

About 10% of all mentally retarded have an IQ between 35 to 50. In the educational

TABLE 13.3. SOME CAUSES OF MENTAL RETARDATION

1. **Genetic** (probably in 5% of cases)
   - i. ***Chromosomal abnormalities***
     e.g. Down's syndrome, Fragile-X syndrome, Turner's syndrome, Klinefelter's syndrome.
   - ii. ***Inborn errors of metabolism***, involving
     amino-acids (phenylketonuria, homo-cystinuria, Hartnup's disease),
     lipids (Tay-Sachs disease, Gaucher's disease, Niemann-Pick disease),
     carbohydrates (galactosemia, glycogen storage diseases),
     purines (Lesch Nyhan syndrome), and
     mucopolysaccharides (Hurler's disease, Hunter's disease, Sanfillipo's disease).
   - iii. ***Single-gene disorders***
     e.g. tuberous sclerosis, neurofibromatosis, dystrophia myotonica.
   - iv. ***Cranial anomalies***
     e.g. microcephaly.
2. **Peri-natal causes** (probably in 10% of cases)
   - i. ***Infections***
     e.g. rubella, syphilis, toxoplasmosis, cytomegalo-inclusion body disease
   - ii. Prematurity
   - iii. Birth trauma
   - iv. Hypoxia
   - v. Intrauterine growth retardation (IUGR)
   - vi. Kernicterus
   - vii. Placental abnormalities
   - viii. Drugs during first trimester.
3. **Acquired physical disorders in childhood** (probably in 2-5% of cases)
   - i. Infections, especially encephalopathies
   - ii. Cretinism
   - iii. Trauma
   - iv. Lead poisoning
   - v. Cerebral palsy.
4. **Sociocultural causes** (probably in 15% of cases)
   - i. Deprivation of sociocultural stimulation.
5. **Psychiatric disorders** (probably in 1-2% of cases)
   - i. ***Pervasive developmental disorders***
     e.g. Infantile autism
   - ii. Childhood onset schizophrenia.

classification, this group was earlier called *'trainable'* although many of these persons can also be educated.

In the early years, despite a poor social awareness, these children can learn to speak. Often, they drop out of school after the 2nd class (grade). They can be trained to support themselves by performing semi-skilled or unskilled work under supervision. A mild stress may destabilize them from their adaptation, thus they work best in supervised occupational settings.

3. Severe Mental Retardation

Severe mental retardation is often recognized early in life with poor motor development (significantly delayed developmental milestones) and absent or markedly delayed speech and other communication skills.

Later in life, elementary training in personal health care can be given and they can be taught to talk. At best, they can perform simple tasks under close supervision. In the earlier educational classification, they were called *'dependent'*.

4. Profound Mental Retardation

This group accounts for 1-2% of all mentally retarded. The associated physical disorders which often contribute to mental retardation are common.

The achievement of developmental milestones is markedly delayed. They often need nursing care or *'life support'* under a carefully planned and structured environment-like-group homes.

Etiology

Mental retardation is a condition which is caused not only by biological factors but also by psychosocial factors. In more than one third of cases, no cause can be found despite an extensive search.

Some of the causes of mental retardation are listed in Table 13.3. There appears to be a preponderance of males among the mentally retarded.

Some important causes of mental retardation are discussed below.

1. Phenylketonuria

An inborn error of metabolism, it accounts for 0.5-1% of all cases of mental retardation. It is an autosomal recessive (AR) disorder, most prevalent in North Europe.

The basic defect is the absence or inactivity of phenylalanine hydroxylase, a hepatic enzyme, responsible for catalysis of phenylalanine to paratyrosine conversion (Fig. 13.1). It results in marked increase in blood phenylalanine levels and its metabolites. There is also a decrease in 5-HT, epinephrine and norepinephrine levels in brain.

The majority of patients with phenylketonuria have severe mental retardation. The associated features may include short stature, fair complexion but coarse features, widely spaced upper incisors, eczematous dermatitis, epilepsy, hyperactivity, poor communication skills and poor motor coordination. EEG may be abnormal in up to 80% of cases.

However, the physical appearance may be normal and diagnosis made only after investigations, which are:

1. *Ferric chloride test:* Addition of $FeCl_3$ to urine gives a green color in patients of phenylketonuria. This results from the presence of phenylpyruvic acid in urine. This test may be positive in other aminoacidurias as well.

2. *Guthrie's test:* This involves a bacteriological procedure aimed at measurement of phenylalanine levels in blood.

3. *Chromatography*: An early diagnosis is of paramount importance, since mental retardation of phenylketonuria is *preventable*.

The *treatment* consists of a low phenylalanine diet, best started before the age of 6 months and usually continued up to 5-6 years of age. The diet should not be completely devoid of phenylalanine, as it is an essential amino-acid and its absence may itself be hazardous.

Other disorders which cause mental retardation and are preventable by dietary treatment, include:

1. *Homocystinuria*: The treatment is with methionine-free diet.
2. *Galactosemia*: The treatment is with lactose and galactose-free diet.
3. *Maple syrup urine disease* (*Menkes' disease*): The treatment is with a diet low in leucine, isoleucine and valine.
4. *Hyperprolinemia*: The treatment is with low proline diet.
5. *Leucine-sensitive hypoglycemia*: The treatment is with low-protein, leucine-deficient diet.
6. *Fructose intolerance*: Fructose, sucrose and other sugars should be replaced in diet.

2. Down's Syndrome

The Down's syndrome or *mongolism* occurs in 1 out of every 700 births. It accounts for about 10% of moderate to severe mentally retarded children.

There are 3 types of chromosomal aberrations in Down's syndrome:

1. Trisomy-21 is the commonest. The karyotype of mother is normal.
2. Mosaicism, with both normal and trisomic cells present.

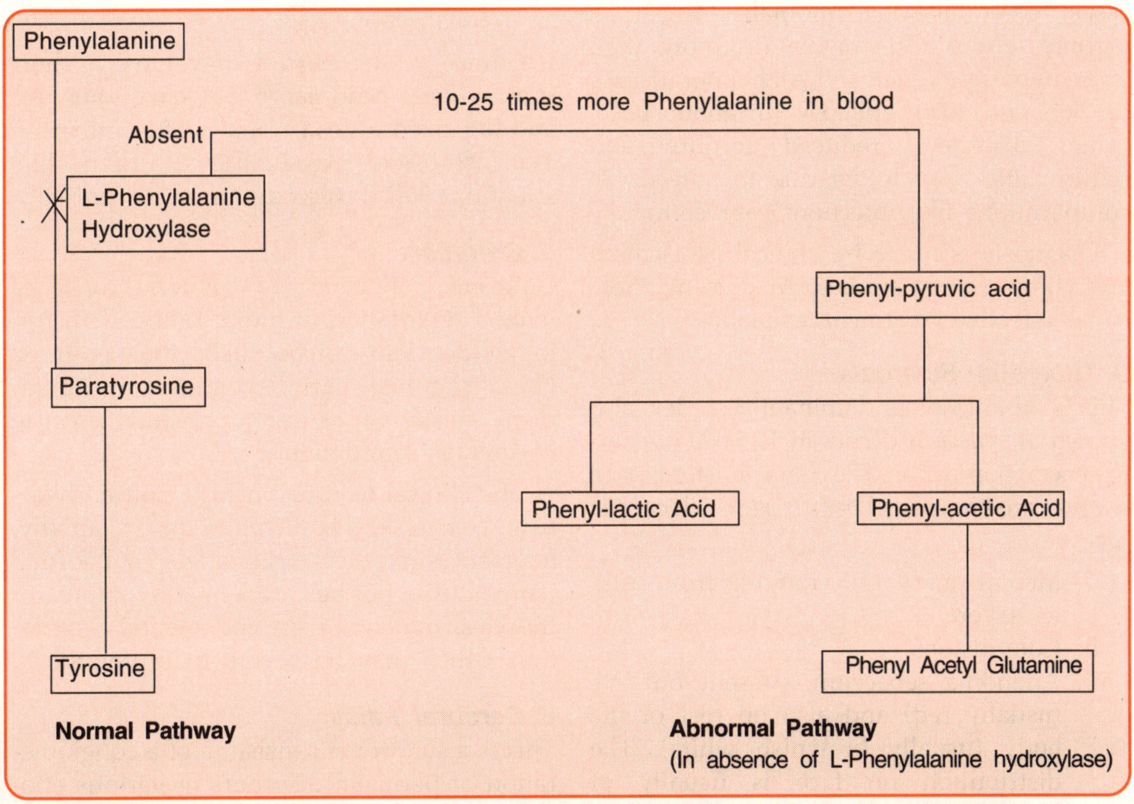

FIG 13.1. METABOLIC PATHWAYS OF PHENYLALANINE: NORMAL AND ABNORMAL

3. Translocation between chromosome 21 and 15. Thus, the total number of chromosomes is 46, in spite of 3 chromosomes at 21. The translocation is inherited, with asymptomatic carriers containing only 45 chromosomes.

The most important risk factor is higher maternal age (> 35 years), with a risk of 1:50 after the age of 45.

The clinical features may include generalized hypotonia, hyperflexibility, round face, oblique palpebral fissures, a flat nasal bridge, short ears, loose skin folds at the nape of neck, persistent epicanthic folds, single palmar crease, high arched palate, thick tongue, incurved little fingers and Brushfield spots on irides.

Congenital heart disease (in about 35% of cases), gastrointestinal anomalies (in 10%), chronic serous otitis media (in more than 50%), hypothyroidism and Alzheimer disease (in 30's and 40's), epilepsy (in about 10%), ocular disorders, reduced fertility and reduced life span (often due to antecedent complications like infections) are common.

Diagnosis is made by clinical assessment and chromosomal studies. At present, there is no effective treatment available.

3. Tuberous Sclerosis

This is an autosomal dominant disorder, also known as *epiloia.* It occurs in 1:15,000 persons in general population. The characteristic clinical features are known as *Vogt's triad* which consist of:

i. Mental retardation, ranging from mild to severe.
ii. Convulsions.
iii. Adenoma sebaceum, present on face (usually red) and also on rest of the body (usually brownish white). The distribution on face is usually of butterfly type.

Multiple glial nodules appear throughout the cerebral cortex and cerebellum. Tumors in the various other parts of body (e.g. rhabdomyoma of heart, mixed tumors of kidney, retinal nerve tumors) may occur. In addition, periosteal thickening, pulmonary fibrosis, renal failure and cardiac failure can be manifested.

There is no effective treatment except symptomatic management of seizures and other systemic manifestations.

4. Fragile-X Syndrome

This is the second commonest chromosomal aberration causing mental retardation. Occurring in 1 out of 1000 live births, it is diagnosed on chromosomal studies. The characteristic presence of a fragile site at the tip of the long arm of X chromosome appears as a constriction.

Clinically, the person may have a short stature, large head, large 'bat' ears, long face and big sized testes (in males after puberty). The associated psychiatric disorders like attention deficit disorder may be present.

5. Cretinism

Goitrous cretinism is a common cause of mental retardation in India. It is endemic in iodine-deficient areas like the goitrous Himalayan belt. Early recognition and treatment is essential as it is a preventable cause of mental retardation.

The clinical features include goitre, dwarfism, coarse skin, ossification delays, apathy, hoarseness of voice, large tongue, subnormal temperature, pot belly, anemia, hypotonia of muscles, hypertelorism and mental retardation which may be severe to profound.

6. Cerebral Palsy

This is a syndrome consisting of a conglomeration of perinatal disorders of various etiologies, presenting with a common feature of paralysis of limbs. The paralysis may be monoplegia, hemiplegia, paraplegia, triplegia or quadriplegia. It is usually of upper motor neuron type, presenting with spasticity.

The extrapyramidal symptoms may be present and seizures occur often. Mental retardation is present in about 70% of all cases, and ranges from mild to severe.

Diagnosis

The diagnosis is made by the following steps:

1. History.
2. General physical examination.
3. Detailed neurological examination.
4. Mental status examination, for assessment of associated psychiatric disorders and clinical assessment of level of intelligence.
5. Investigations.
   i. Routine investigations.
   ii. Urine test, e.g. for phenylketonuria, maple syrup urine disease.
   iii. EEG, especially in presence of seizures.
   iv. Blood levels, for inborn errors of metabolism.
   v. Chromosomal studies, e.g. in Down's syndrome, prenatal (by amniocentesis or chorionic villus biopsy) and postnatal.
   vi. CT scan or MRI brain, e.g. in tuberous sclerosis, focal seizures, unexplained neurological syndromes, anomalies of skull configuration, severe or profound mental retardation without any apparent cause, toxoplasmosis.
   vii. Thyroid function tests, particularly when cretinism is suspected.
   viii. Liver function tests, e.g. in mucopolysaccharidosis.
6. Psychological tests
   The commonly used tests for measurement of *intelligence* are:
   i. Seguin form board test.
   ii. Stanford-Binet, Binet-Simon or Binet-Kamath tests.
   iii. Wechsler Intelligence Scale for Children (WISC) for 6½ to 16 years of age.
   iv. Wechsler's Preschool and Primary Scale of Intelligence (WPPSI) for 4 to 6½ years of age.
   v. Bhatia's battery of performance tests.
   vi. Raven's progressive matrices (colored, standard and advanced).

   The tests used for the assessment of *adaptive behavior* include:
   i. Vineland Social Maturity Scale (VSMS).
   ii. Denver Development Screening Test (DDST).
   iii. Gessell's Development Scale.

Differential Diagnosis

The diagnosis of mental retardation is usually simple. However, while making this diagnosis, following conditions must be kept in mind, as they can be and are many times mistaken for mental retardation, with disastrous results.

1. Deaf and dumb (This possibility must always be ruled out either by clinical examination or by audiometry).
2. Deprived children with inadequate social stimulation (Although this can also cause mental retardation, many children become normal intellectually on providing adequate stimulation).
3. Isolated speech defects.
4. Psychiatric disorders, like infantile autism, childhood onset schizophrenia.
5. Systemic disorders (without mental retardation but with physical debilitation).
6. Epilepsy.

Management

The management of mental retardation can be discussed under *prevention* at primary, secondary and tertiary levels.

1. Primary Prevention

This consists of:

i. Improvement in *socio-economic condition* of society at large, aiming at elimination of understimulation, malnutrition, prematurity and perinatal factors.

ii. *Education* of lay public, aiming at removal of misconceptions about mentally retarded individuals.

iii. Medical measures for good *perinatal medical care* to prevent infections, trauma, excessive use of medications, malnutrition, obstetric complications and diseases of pregnancy.

v. Universal *immunization* of children with BCG, polio, DPT, and MMR.

v. Facilitating research activities to study the causes of mental retardation and their treatment.

vi. *Genetic counseling* in at-risk parents, e.g. in phenylketonuria, Down's syndrome.

2. Secondary Prevention

i. Early detection and treatment of preventable disorders, e.g. phenylketonuria (low phenylalanine diet), maple syrup urine disease (low branched amino-acid diet) and others as discussed earlier; hypothyroidism (thyroxin).

ii. Early detection of handicaps in sensory, motor or behavioral areas with early remedial measures and treatment.

iii. Early treatment of correctable disorders, e.g. infections (antibiotics), skull configuration anomalies (surgical correction).

iv. Early recognition of presence of mental retardation. A delay in diagnosis may cause unfortunate delay in rehabilitation.

v. As far as possible, individuals with mental retardation should be *integrated* with normal individuals in society, and any kind of segregation or discrimination should be actively avoided. They should be provided with facilities to enable them to reach their own full potential. However, their is a role of special schools for those with more severe mental retardation.

3. Tertiary Prevention

i. Adequate treatment of psychological and behavioral problems.

ii. *Behavior modification*, using the principles of positive and negative reinforcement.

iii. *Rehabilitation* in vocational, physical, and social areas commensurate with the level of handicap.

iv. *Parental counseling* is extremely important to lessen the levels of stress, teaching them to adapt to the situation, enlisting them (especially parents) as co-therapists, and encouraging formation of parents' organiztion(s) and self-help groups.

v. *Institutionalization* or *residential care* may be needed for individuals with profound mental retardation.

vi. *Legislation*: In 1995, the '*Persons with Disability Act*' came in to being in India. This act envisages mandatory support for prevention, early detection, education, employment, and other facilities for the welfare of persons with disbilities in general, and mental retardation in particular. This Act provides for affirmative action and non-descrimination of persons with disabilities.

In 1999, the '*National Trust Act*' came in to force. This Act proposes to involve the parents of mentally challenged persons and voluntary organizations in setting up and running a variety of services and facilities with governmental funding.

14 Child Psychiatry

CLASSIFICATION IN CHILD PSYCHIATRY

The various psychiatric disorders seen in childhood (*'disorders of psychological development'* and *'behavioral and emotional disorders with onset usually occurring in childhood and adolescence'*) are discussed under the following headings:

1. Mental retardation
2. Specific developmental disorders
3. Pervasive developmental disorders
4. Hyperkinetic disorders
5. Conduct disorders
6. Tic disorders
7. Enuresis and encopresis
8. Speech disorders
9. Habit disorders
10. Other disorders.

MENTAL RETARDATION

Mental retardation is discussed in Chapter 13.

SPECIFIC DEVELOPMENTAL DISORDERS

Mental retardation is a generalized impairment in nearly all areas of functioning. In contrast, the specific developmental disorders (SDD) are characterized by an inadequate development in usually one specific area of functioning.

The deficit in functioning may be in scholastic skills, speech and language, and motor skills. These may include reading (developmental reading disorder), language (developmental language disorder), arithmetic or mathematics (developmental arithmetic or mathematics disorder), articulation (developmental articulation disorder or phonological disorder), or coordination (developmental coordination disorder). Sometimes, more than one developmental disorder is present.

All the developmental disorders either cause an impairment in academic functioning at school especially when language is affected or an impairment in the daily activities.

A large majority of these children have an underlying cerebral disorder. Boys are more affected than girls.

Before making a diagnosis of SDD, it is important to keep in mind the mental age, IQ, socio-cultural background, schooling, impairment(s) in vision and hearing, or any neurological deficit.

1. Specific Reading Disorder

It is also called as *dyslexia* or developmental reading disorder.

The child presents with a serious delay in learning to read that is evident from the early years. The problems may include omissions, distortions, or substitutions of words, long hesitations, reversal of words, or simply slow reading.

Writing and spelling are also impaired. It is important to differentiate the disorder from scholastic backwardness; therfore proper assessment is mandatory.

2. Specific Arithmetic Disorder

It is also called as developmental arithmetic or mathematic disorder or *dyscalculia*.

The child presents with arithmetic abilities well below the level expected for the mental age (below par).

The problems may include failure to understand simple mathematical concepts, failure to recognize mathematical signs or numerical symbols, difficulty in carrying out mathematical manipulations, and difficulty in learning mathematical tables.

3. Specific Developmental Disorder of Speech and Language

It is also called as communication disorder, developmental language disorder or *dysphasia*.

There are three types:

i. *Phonological disorder:* Also called as *dyslalia*, it is characterized by below par accuracy in the use of speech sounds despite normal language skills.

   The problems include severe articulation errors that make it difficult for others to understand the speech. Speech sounds or phonemes are omitted, distorted or substituted (e.g. wabbit for rabbit, ca for car, bu for blue).

ii. *Expressive language disorder:* It is characterized by a below par ability of using the expressive speech.

   The problems include restricted vocabulary, difficulty in selecting appropriate words, and immature grammatical usage. Cluttering of speech may also be present.

iii. *Receptive language disorder:* The disorder often presents as receptive-expressive language disorder, i.e. both receptive and expressive impairments are present together. The disorder is characterized by a below par understanding of language.

   Problems include failure to respond to simple instructions, provided deafness and pervasive developmental disorder are ruled out.

4. Specific Developmental Disorder of Motor Function

It is also called as motor skills disorder, developmental coordination disorder, *clumsy child syndrome* or *motor dyspraxia*.

It is characterized by poor coordination in daily activities of life, e.g. in dressing, walking, feeding, playing. There is an inability to perform fine or gross motor tasks.

Treatment

The *treatment* of specific developmental disorders is based on the learning theory principles and is behavioral in approach. It involves the use of *special remedial teaching*, focusing on the underlying deficit (e.g. perceptual motor training in motor skills disorder).

The treatment of common co-morbid emotional problems is often necessary. Parental education and counseling is an important prerequisite for proper management.

PERVASIVE DEVELOPMENTAL DISORDERS

Infantile autism was described for the first time by Leo Kanner in 1943 as 'autistic disturbances of affective contact'.

This syndrome has variously been described as autistic disorder, pervasive developmental disorder, childhood autism, childhood psychosis and pseudo-defective psychosis.

This syndrome is more common (3-4 times) in males and has a prevalence rate of 0.4-0.5 per 1000 population. Although earlier it was thought to be commoner in upper socio-economic classes, the recent studies have failed to prove this finding.

Typically, the onset occurs before the age of 2½ years. In some cases, the onset may occur later in childhood. Such cases are called as 'childhood onset autism' or 'childhood onset pervasive developmental disorder'. Autism occurring before or after 2½ years of age is not very different clinically.

Clinical Features

The characteristic features are:

1. ***Autism*** (i.e. marked impairment in reciprocal social and interpersonal interaction):
   - i. Absent social smile.
   - ii. Lack of eye-to-eye-contact.
   - iii. Lack of awareness of others' existence or feelings; treats people as furniture.
   - iv. Lack of attachment to parents and absence of separation anxiety.
   - v. No or abnormal social play; prefers solitary games.
   - vi. Marked impairment in making friends.
   - vii. Lack of imitative behavior.
   - viii. Absence of fear in presence of danger.
2. ***Marked impairment in language and nonverbal communication***
   - i. Lack of verbal or facial response to sounds or voices; might be thought as deaf initially.
   - ii. In infancy, absence of communicative sounds like babbling.
   - iii. Absent or delayed speech (about half of autistic children never develop useful speech).
   - iv. Abnormal speech patterns and content. Presence of echolalia, perseveration, poor articulation and *pronominal reversal* (I-You) is common.
   - v. Rote memory is usually good.
   - vi. Abstract thinking is impaired.
3. *Abnormal behavioral characteristics*
   - i. Mannerisms.
   - ii. Stereotyped behaviors like head-banging, body-spinning, hand-flicking, lining-up objects, rocking, clapping, twirling, etc.
   - iii. Ritualistic and compulsive behavior.
   - iv. Resistance to even the slightest change in the environment.
   - v. Attachment may develop to inanimate objects.
   - vi. Hyperkinesis is commonly associated.
4. *Mental retardation*

   Only about 25% of all autistic children have an IQ of more than 70. A large majority (more than 50%) of these children have moderate to profound mental retardation. There is a direct correlation between severity of mental retardation, absence of speech and epilepsy in autism.
5. Other features
   - i. Many autistic children enjoy music particularly.
   - ii. *'Idiot savant syndrome'*: In spite of a pervasive impairment of functions, certain islets of precocity or splinter functions may remain. Examples of such splinter functions are prodigious rote memory or calculating ability, and musical abilities.
   - iii. Epilepsy is common in children with an IQ of less than 50.

The course of infantile autism is usually chronic and only 1-2% become near normal in marital, social and occupational functioning. A large majority (about 70%) lead dependent lives.

Etiology

Presently the cause of infantile autism seems to be predominantly biological. Earlier reports of cold, 'refrigerator' mothers causing autism in their children have not been substantiated.

The evidence for biological causation includes a higher than average history of perinatal

CNS insult, EEG abnormalities, epilepsy, ventricular dilatation on CT scan brain, increased serotonin (5-HT) levels in brain and/or neurophysiological abnormalities in some patients.

Treatment

The treatment consists of three modes of intervention which are often used together.

1. Behavior Therapy
   i. Development of a regular routine with as few changes as possible.
   ii. Structured class room training, aiming at learning new material and maintenance of acquired learning.
   iii. Positive reinforcements to teach self-care skills.
   iv. Speech therapy and/or sign language teaching.
   v. Behavioral techniques to encourage interpersonal interactions.
2. Psychotherapy
   Psychotherapy, per se, is not effective in treatment of infantile autism. However, parental counseling and supportive therapy are useful in allaying parental anxiety and guilt, and ensuring their active involvement in therapy.
   Overstimulation should be avoided during treatment.
3. Pharmacotherapy
   Drug treatment is used for the treatment of autism and for the treatment of associated epilepsy.
   i. Fenfluramine decreases 5-HT levels in brain. It has been reported to be helpful in increasing IQ and decreasing behavioral symptoms.
   ii. Haloperidol decreases dopamine levels in brain. It is believed to decrease hyperactivity and abnormal behavioral symptoms.
   iii. Other drugs like chlorpromazine, amphetamines, methysergide, imipramine, multi-vitamins and triiodothyronine have been tried without much success.
   iv. Anti-epileptic medication is used for generalized or other seizures.

OTHER PERVASIVE DEVELOPMENTAL DISORDERS

Childhood psychosis is a vague term which includes all psychotic illnesses occurring in childhood, like,

1. Infantile and childhood onset autism,
2. Childhood schizophrenia,
3. Mood disorders, and
4. Organic psychiatric disorders.

This term has frequently been misused in the past, meaning at times infantile autism alone. This is a term which can be best dispensed with.

Schizophrenia, mood disorders and organic psychiatric disorders have a nearly similar picture in children as in adulthood. Sometimes childhood onset schizophrenia may be mistaken for autism. The most important differentiating features are:

1. Delusions, formal thought disorder and hallucinations may be present in childhood-onset schizophrenia while they are always absent in infantile autism.
2. Typical age of onset of symptoms is before 2½ years in infantile autism while it is after 5-6 years in childhood onset schizophrenia.
3. Moderate to severe mental retardation and epilepsy are common in infantile autism while they are rare in childhood-onset schizophrenia. Mental retardation, if present, is usually of mild type.

Another type of childhood psychosis, called *Heller's syndrome* or *disintegrative psychosis*, has been often described in literature. Typically, the age of onset is between 3 to 5 years and the syndrome is characterized by rapid downhill course leading to deterioration and development of neurological deficits. This is a 'rag-bag' category containing diverse organic brain syndromes of varying etiologies (e.g. some are caused by lipoid degeneration of ganglia in central nervous system). Prognosis is usually poor.

Two other syndromes with autistic features have been described, namely Asperger's syndrome and Rett's syndrome. *Asperger's syndrome* is characterized by autism without any significant delay in language or cognitive development (including intelligence). This syndrome occurs predominantly in boys (male: female ratio = 8:1). It probably represents mild cases of autism.

Rett's syndrome is a disorder which is only reported in girls so far. After an apparently normal early development and normal head circumference at birth, there is a deceleration of head growth between the age of 5 months and 30 months. There is also a loss of purposive hand movements and acquired fine motor manipulative skills between the same ages, with subsequent development of stereotyped hand movements (e.g. hand-wringing). Later, other movement disorders also develop and severe mental handicap is invariable.

HYPERKINETIC DISORDER (ATTENTION DEFICIT DISORDER)

This is a syndrome first described by Heinrich Hoff in 1854. Since then, it has been known by a variety of names like minimal brain dysfunction (MBD), hyperkinetic syndrome, Strauss syndrome, organic drivenness and minimal brain damage.

A common disorder, it occurs in about 3% of school age children. Males are 6-8 times more often affected. The onset occurs before the age of 7 years and a large majority of patients exhibit symptoms by the 4th year of age.

Attention deficit disorder is of 4 clinical types: with hyperactivity, without hyperactivity, residual type, and with conduct disorder.

1. ***Attention deficit disorder with hyperactivity*** (hyperkinetic disorder) is the commonest type. The characteristic clinical features are:

A. *Poor attention span with distractibility*
   i. Fails to finish the things started.
   ii. Shifts from one uncompleted activity to other.
   iii. Doesn't seem to listen.
   iv. Easily distracted by external stimuli.
   v. Often loses things.

B. *Hyperactivity*
   i. Fidgety.
   ii. Difficulty in sitting still at one place for long.
   iii. Moving about here and there.
   iv. Talks excessively.
   v. Interference in other people's activities.

C. *Impulsivity*
   i. Acts before thinking, on the spur of the moment.
   ii. Difficulty in waiting for turn at work or play.

2. ***Attention deficit disorder without hyperactivity*** is a rare disorder with similar clinical features, except hyperactivity.
3. ***Residual type*** is diagnosed in a patient with a past history of ADD and presence of a few residual features in adulthood.
4. ***Hyperkinetic disorder with conduct disorder*** (hyperkinetic conduct disorder).

Diagnosis

The diagnosis is made on the basis of:

1. Teacher's school report (often the most reliable).
2. Parent's report.
3. Clinical examination (many children with hyperactivity may be able to sit still in the new setting of hospital and thus the diagnosis may be missed).

Hyperactivity is a common clinical symptom in mental retardation. Thus, mental retardation should always be excluded before making a diagnosis of ADD.

Etiology

Many factors, like minimal brain damage, maturational lag, genetics, neurotransmitters (norepinephrine and dopamine) and early developmental psychodynamic factors, have been incriminated. The cause is not yet known but it is more likely to be a biological factor than a purely psychosocial one.

Course

A large majority (about 80%) of patients improve on their own by puberty. A few (15-20%) may have persistent symptoms even in adulthood.

Impulsivity and inattention are the most common residual features after puberty while hyperactivity often remits.

Treatment

The management consists of following methods:

1. Pharmacotherapy

i. Stimulant medication

Dextro-amphetamine (10-40 mg/day) and methylphenidate (10-60 mg/day) are the drugs of choice in treatment of hyperkinetic disorder, with a response rate of nearly 90%. They act on the reticular activating system causing stimulation of inhibitory influences on the cerebral cortex, thus decreasing hyperactivity and/or distractibility.

ii. Others

When stimulant medication is not available or is not effective, other drugs can be used. These include clonidine, imipramine, bupropion, venlafaxine, chlorpromazine, thioridazine, and lithium carbonate.

Barbiturates are *contraindicated* as they increase hyperactivity.

2. Behavior therapy

3. Counseling and supportive psychotherapy

These two are not usually effective alone, but are used along with drug therapy.

CONDUCT DISORDERS

Conduct disorder is characterized by a persistent and significant pattern of conduct in which the basic rights of others are violated or rules of society are not followed. The diagnosis is only made when the conduct is far in excess of the routine mischief of children and adolescents. The onset occurs much before 18 years of age, usually even before puberty.

The disorder is much more (about 5-10 times) common in males. In United States of America, about 10% of all male children have conduct disorder, before 18 years of age.

According to ICD-10, there are 4 subtypes of this disorder:

1. Conduct disorder confined to the family context.
2. Unsocialized conduct disorder
3. Socialized conduct disorder.
4. Oppositional defiant disorder.

The characteristic clinical features include:

1. Frequent lying.
2. Stealing or robbery.

3. Running away from home and school.
4. Physical violence like rape, fire-setting, assault or breaking-in, use of weapons.
5. Cruelty towards other people and animals.

In the more common socialized (group) type of conduct disorder, the person claims loyalty to his or her group. The unsocialized (solitary) type is a more serious disorder with usually a severe underlying psychopathology.

Earlier, the patients of conduct disorder were called as *juvenile delinquents*.

Many patients of conduct disorder, especially socialized (group) type, go on to improve markedly and may lead well adjusted lives. Some others, especially those with severe symptomatology, have a chronic course and may be diagnosed as antisocial personality disorder or trait after 18 years of age.

In addition to the typical symptoms of conduct disorder, secondary complications often develop like drug abuse and dependence, unwanted pregnancies, syphilis, AIDS, criminal record, suicidal and homicidal behavior.

The *treatment* is difficult. The most common mode of management is placement in a corrective institution, often after the child has had legal difficulties. Behavioral, educational and psychotherapeutic measures are employed for changing the behavior.

Drug treatment may be needed in presence of epilepsy (anticonvulsants), hyperactivity (stimulant medication), impulse control disorder and episodic aggressive behavior (lithium, carbamazepine), and psychotic symptoms (antipsychotics).

TIC DISORDERS

Tic disorders are characterized by the presence of tics. *Tic* is an abnormal involuntary movement (AIM) which occurs suddenly, repetitively, rapidly and is purposeless in nature. It is of 2 types:

1. Motor Tic, characterized by repetitive motor movements.
2. Vocal Tic, characterized by repetitive vocalizations.

Tic disorders can be either transient or chronic. A special type of chronic tic disorder is Gilles de la Tourette's syndrome or Tourette's disorder.

Tourette's Disorder

Tourette's disorder is characterized by:

1. Multiple motor tics.
2. Multiple vocal tics.
3. Duration of more than 1 year.
4. Onset usually before 11 years of age and almost always before 21 years of age.

The disorder is more common (about 3 times) in males and has a prevalence rate of about 0.5 per 1000 people.

1. Motor Tics

The motor tics present can be simple or complex.

i. *Simple motor tics:* These may include eye-blinking, grimacing, shrugging of shoulders, tongue protrusion.
ii. *Complex motor tics:* These are facial gestures, stamping, jumping, hitting self, squatting, twirling, *echokinesis* (repetition of observed acts), *copropraxia* (obscene acts).

Motor tics are often the earliest to appear, beginning in the head region and progressing downwards. These are followed by vocal tics.

2. Vocal Tics

The vocal tics also can be simple or complex.

i. *Simple vocal tics:* Simple vocal tics include coughing, barking, throat-clearing, sniffing, clicking.
ii. *Complex vocal tics:* These include some very characteristic, though not always present,

symptoms of Tourette syndrome. For example, *echolalia* (repetition of heard phrases), *palilalia* (repetition of heard words), *coprolalia* (use of obscene words), and *mental coprolalia* (thinking of obscene words).

3. ***Obsessions*** and ***compulsions*** are often associated symptoms. These are usually the last symptoms to appear.

Etiology

The etiology of Tourette syndrome is not known but the presence of learning difficulties, neurological soft signs, hyperactivity, abnormal EEG record, abnormal evoked potentials and abnormal CT Brain findings in some patients point towards a biological basis. There is some evidence to suggest that Tourette syndrome may be inherited as autosomal dominant disorder with variable penetrance.

Treatment

Pharmacotherapy is the preferred mode of treatment. The drug of choice is *haloperidol*. In resistant cases or in case of severe side-effects, pimozide or clonidine can be used.

Behavior therapy may be used, sometimes, as an adjunct.

NON-ORGANIC ENURESIS

Enuresis is repetitive voiding of urine, either during the day or night, at inappropriate places. This state of affairs is normal in infancy. Most children achieve bladder control by the age of 3 years. By the age of 5 years, there are still about 7% of children who wet their bed. Technically, enuresis is diagnosed only after 5 years of age (and at least 4 years of mental age).

Enuresis can be:

1. Primary type, where bladder control has never been achieved.
2. Secondary type, where enuresis emerges after a period of bladder control (at least one year).

The majority (about 80%) of enuretics have nocturnal bed wetting only. Non-organic enuresis is more common (two times) in males.

Etiology

The exact cause of enuresis is not known. The variety of factors, which are implicated in its causation, are biopsychosocial. About 75% of enuretics have a first degree relative with history of enuresis.

The most commonly occurring factor is psychosocial, e.g. emotional disturbances, insecurity, sibling rivalry, death of a parent.

Organic cause must be looked for in diurnal enuretics (15% of all cases of diurnal enuretics) and adolescent enuretics. The organic causes are present in about 5% of cases and include worm infestation, spina bifida, neurogenic bladder, urinary tract infection, diabetes mellitus, seizure disorder.

In secondary enuresis, the age of onset is 5-8 years. Enuresis tends to remit spontaneously and only 1% of enuretics continue to have the disorder in adulthood.

Treatment

The management consists of one or more of the following measures:

1. Restriction of fluid intake after 8 PM, in nocturnal enuresis.
2. Bladder training during daytime, aimed at increasing the holding-time of bladder. This is carried out in a step-by-step manner using positive reinforcements.
3. Interruption of sleep before the expected time of bed wetting. The child should be fully woken up and made aware of passing of urine.
4. Conditioning devices which cause an alarm to sound as soon as the voided urine

touches the bedsheet (check child's hearing before starting treatment). It causes inhibition of further micturition and the child awakens. Properly used, it is an effective method of therapy.

5. Supportive psychotherapy to the child, parents and the whole family is often needed.
6. Pharmacotherapy: The drug of choice is a tricyclic antidepressant, usually imipramine (25-75 mg/day). It probably acts by its anticholinergic effect as well as by decreasing the deep sleep (stage 4 NREM sleep) period. Intranasal desmopressin has been found useful in some patients.

   The other drugs used for this purpose include diazepam, anticholinergics, amphetamines, placebos, but none has shown a good therapeutic response.

NON-ORGANIC ENCOPRESIS

Encopresis is repetitive passage of feces at inappropriate time and/or place, after bowel control is physiologically possible. This is not due to the presence of any organic cause, which is called as fecal incontinence.

Normally, toilet training is achieved between the ages of 2 and 3. Encopresis is defined as occurring after the age of 4 years.

Encopresis can be:

1. Primary type, where toilet training has never been achieved.
2. Secondary type, where encopresis emerges after a period of fecal continence.

This type typically occurs between the ages of 4 and 8.

Encopresis is more common (3-4 times) in males. By the age of 5 years, 1-1.5% of children are encopretic. It tends to remit spontaneously with increasing age and by the age of 16, there are virtually no encopretics. 25% of these patients have associated enuresis.

Etiology

The factors implicated in causation of encopresis are:

1. Inadequate, inconsistent toilet training.
2. Sibling rivalry.
3. Maturational lag.
4. Underlying hyperkinetic disorder.
5. Emotional disturbances.
6. Mental retardation.
7. Childhood schizophrenia.
8. Autistic disorder.

Whenever presented with a patient of encopresis, organic causes (fecal incontinence) must be ruled out (e.g. Hirschsprung's disease, overflow diarrhea with constipation, hypothyroidism, inflammatory bowel disease and neurological lesions).

Treatment

The best treatment is *preventive*. The toilet training period should be made as consistent and smooth as possible. The family environment should be warm and understanding. The emotional disturbances of the child should not be ignored and should be dealt with at the earliest. The communication between the family members should be direct.

After encopresis has developed, the treatment of choice is *behavior therapy*, using reinforcements (both positive and negative). The other treatments include psychotherapy, biofeedback and imipramine (in non-retentive encopresis).

SPEECH DISORDERS

Stuttering is a disorder of speech, characterized by the following features:

1. Disturbed fluency and rhythm of speech.
2. Intermittent blocking.
3. Repetition of words rapidly.
4. Prolongation of sounds.
5. Associated anxiety or distress.

Earlier *stammering* and stuttering were differentiated on the basis of minor differences.

At present, they are thought to be synonymous.

The disorder is a fairly common one, affecting 2-5% of all children and 0.5-1% of all adults. Males are more commonly (about 3 times) affected.

Differential diagnosis is from *cluttering*, which is characterized by erratic and dysarrhythmic pattern of speech with jerky and rapid spurting of words. Unlike in stuttering (where the person is aware of the difficulty in speech), the affected person in cluttering is usually unaware of the abnormal speech pattern.

Treatment

Treatment is by behavior modification techniques like desensitization, biofeedback and stammer suppresser; and by techniques to diminish anxiety like relaxation therapy, drug therapy, individual or group psychotherapy.

HABIT DISORDERS

These are stereotyped disorders which are intentionally and repetitively produced but serve no constructive or socially acceptable function.

The *common* habit disorders include thumb sucking, nail biting, pulling out of hair (trichotillomania), head banging, masturbation, teeth grinding, picking of nose, biting parts of the body, skin-scratching, body rocking, breath-holding, and swallowing of air (aerophagia).

These habits range from normal to abnormal, depending on the severity of occurrence and the time of presentation during the developmental period (what is normal in infancy, may be abnormal in later childhood).

Many of the habit disorders, particularly those which are self-stimulating in nature, are called as *gratification habits* and are considered by some as masturbatory equivalents. Also, these habit disorders tend to be commoner in mentally retarded individuals.

Treatment

The treatment is by behavior modification techniques and treatment of underlying psychopathology, if present.

ELECTIVE (SELECTIVE) MUTISM

Elective mutism is characterized by the presence of marked emotionally determined selectivity in speaking, despite the presence of language competence in at least some situations.

Typically, it is first manifested in early childhood and is seen more often in girls. It is estimated to be present in 3-8/10,000 children. It may be associated with temperamental traits involving social anxiety, withdrawal, sensitivity or resistance. The child is often mute in front of strangers or at school. Other socio-emotional disturbances may also be present.

Elective mutism should be differentiated from shyness in normal children, mental retardation, pervasive developmental disorder, expressive language disorder, and conversion disorder. Most cases improve with passage of time, though some children may require pharmacotherapy (e.g. fluoxetine) and/or psychosocial management.

OTHER DISORDERS

The other child psychiatric disorders include separation anxiety disorder, phobic anxiety disorder of childhood, social anxiety disorder of childhood, sibling rivalry disorder, mixed disorders of conduct and emotions, and reactive attachment disorder of childhood.

15 Psychopharmacology

HISTORY OF TREATMENT IN PSYCHIATRY

The treatment of psychiatric disorders in the past had often constituted of merely institutionalization (i.e. admission in an asylum or mental hospital), sometimes along with the use of treatment which now seems either ridiculous or fantastic or mostly both.

The advent of psychopharmacology in the last fifty years has brought the treatment of psychiatric disorders with in the realm of scientific medicine.

Some important milestones in the treatment of psychiatric disorders are summarized in Table 15.1.

CLASSIFICATION OF PSYCHOTROPIC DRUGS

The drugs which have a significant effect on higher mental functions, are called as *psychoactive* or *psychotropic drugs*. These psychotropic drugs can be classified as follows:

1. Antipsychotics
2. Antidepressants
3. Mood stabilizing drugs
4. Anti-anxiety and hypnosedatives
5. Anti-epileptics
6. Alcohol and drugs of dependence (discussed in Chapter 4)
7. Antiparkinsonians
8. Miscellaneous drugs, e.g. stimulants, drugs used in eating disorders, drugs used in de-addiction, anesthetics, drugs used in dementia, drugs used in child psychiatry, vitamins, calcium channel blockers, and other drugs.

An Ideal Psychotropic Drug

An *ideal* psychotropic drug should have the following characteristics (modified after Hollister, 1983):

1. It should cure the underlying pathology causing the disorder or symptom(s) under focus, so that the drug can be stopped after some time.
2. It should benefit all the patients suffering from that disorder.
3. It should have no side-effects or toxicity in the therapeutic range.
4. It should have rapid onset of action.
5. There should be no dependence on the drug and no withdrawal symptoms on stopping the drug.
6. There should be no tolerance to the drug so that same dose is effective for long duration of time.
7. It should not be lethal in overdoses.
8. It can be given in both inpatient and outpatient settings.

Although the psychotropic drugs available at present are far from ideal, they still do a lot to alleviate symptoms and suffering. With increasing research, the new emerging products appear to be better in efficacy and have fewer side-effects.

ANTIPSYCHOTIC DRUGS

Antipsychotics are psychotropic drugs which are used in the treatment of psychotic

TABLE 15.1. A BRIEF HISTORY OF PSYCHOPHARMACOLOGY

<4000 BC: Ayurveda describes treatment of psychiatric patients with sympathy and kindness. The methods of treatment included *dhatura* and roots of 'serpentina' plant mixed with oil (*ghee*).

1853: Bromide used as a sedative-hypnotic.

1869: Chloral hydrate used in the treatment of melancholia and mania.

1882: Paraldehyde used as a hypnotic.

1883 (Bernthsen): Phenothiazines synthesized during synthesis of methylene blue.

1903: Barbiturates (barbital) used for sedation in 1903; phenobarbital introduced in 1912.

1917 (Julius von Wagner Jauregg): Malarial treatment for General Paralysis of Insane (GPI) received a Nobel prize!

1922 (Jacob Klaesi): Barbiturate-induced coma introduced for the treatment of psychoses.

1927 (Manfred Sakel): Insulin-shock treatment introduced for schizophrenia.

1931 (Ganesh Sen & Kartik Bose): First report of successful treatment of psychoses (from India); using *Rauwolfia serpentina* extract (reserpine). Report ignored till Nathan Kline (1958) confirmed the finding.

1934 (Laszlo von Meduna): Metrazol-induced convulsions used for the treatment of psychoses.

1936 (Egas Moniz & Almenda Lima): Frontal lobotomy advocated for treatment of psychiatric disorders.

1937 (C Bradley): Amphetamines used in the treatment of behavior disorders of children.

1938 (Ugo Cerletti & Lucio Bini): Electroconvulsive therapy used for the treatment of psychoses.

1940 (Tracy Putnam): Phenytoin used as an anticonvulsant.

1943 (Albert Hofmann): LSD synthesized.

1949 (John F. Cade): Lithium used in mania; did not receive much attention even in Australia.

1950 (Charpentier): Chlorpromazine synthesized while making a better antihistaminic than promethazine.

1950: Methylphenidate used in treatment of ADHD, then known as Minimal Brain Dysfunction (MBD).

1951 (Laborit): Lytic cocktail used; Chlorpromazine earlier used (as '456 ORP') in artificial hibernation.

1951: Isoniazid (INH) and iproniazid, its derivative, found to have mood elevating properties in patients with tuberculosis. Iproniazid, a MAOI, was later (1958) introduced for treatment of depression.

1952 (Jean Delay & Pierre Deniker): The revolution in psychopharmacology came with introduction of chlorpromazine. The number of admissions in mental hospitals show a sudden decrease after introduction of chlorpromazine.

1955: Meprobamate was introduced as an anti-anxiety agent.

1958 (Thomas Kuhn): Imipramine, a tricyclic antidepressant (TCA) synthesized by Haflinger & Schindler in the late 1940's, was introduced for treatment of depression in 1958.

1958 (Nathan Kline): MAOIs, like iproniazid, introduced for treatment of depression.

1958 (Janssen): Haloperidol synthesized in Belgium.

1960 (Sternbach): Chlordiazepoxide used as an anti-anxiety agent in 1960-1961 (Synthesized in 1957).

1966 (Lambert): Valpromide (Valproate) used in bipolar disorder

1968 (Janssen): Pimozide used for treatment of schizophrenia.

1967 (Fernandez & Lopez-Ibor): Clomipramine used in OCD.

1971 (Takezaki & Hanoaka): Carbamazepine used in bipolar disorder (Synthesized in 1953 by Schindler).

1986: Buspirone introduced in US market as an non-benzodiazepine anti-anxiety agent.

1988 (Kane et al): Clozapine re-discovered in US as an effective treatment for refractory schizophrenia (Synthesized in 1959). Approved by US FDA in 1990 and introduced in Indian market in 1995.

disorders and psychotic symptoms. These are also known as major tranquilizers, neuroleptics, ataractics, antischizophrenic drugs and D_2-receptor (dopamine receptor) blockers, but the term *antipsychotic* is the most appropriate.

Indications

Although used earlier as urinary antiseptic and antihelminthic (use stopped due to toxicity), the current *indications* for the use of antipsychotics include the following:

A. Organic Psychiatric Disorders

1. Delirium (in small doses; e.g. haloperidol, risperidone)
2. Dementia (for psychotic features, and severe agitation)
3. Delirium tremens (and psychoses occurring in drug and alcohol withdrawal states; e.g. haloperidol)
4. Drug induced psychosis (e.g. haloperidol in amphetamine-induced psychosis)
5. Other organic mental disorders (e.g. organic hallucinosis; organic delusional disorder; secondary mania)

B. Non-Organic Psychotic Disorders

1. Schizophrenia
2. Schizo-affective disorder
3. Acute psychoses
4. Mania (with or without mood stabilizer)
5. Major depression (for psychotic features, agitation, and melancholic features; along with antidepressants)
6. Delusional disorder, including MHP (mono-symptomatic hypochondriacal psychosis) (e.g. pimozide)

C. Child Psychiatric Disorders

1. Attention deficit disorder with hyperactivity (in low doses, when stimulant medication is either not available or is contraindicated; e.g. thioridazine) (rarely used)
2. Infantile autism and other pervasive developmental disorders (e.g. haloperidol)
3. Conduct disorders in children (presenting with aggression) (rarely used)

D. Neurotic and Other Psychiatric Disorders

1. Severe, intractable, and disabling anxiety (e.g. rarely, low doses of thioridazine)
2. Treatment refractory obsessive compulsive disorder (e.g. low doses of olanzapine)
3. Anorexia nervosa

E. Medical Disorders

1. Huntington's chorea (e.g. haloperidol)
2. Intractable hiccups (e.g. chlorpromazine in low doses) (rarely used)
3. Nausea and vomiting (sometimes, in low doses): ondansetron, an anti-emetic drug, is a weak antipsychotic
4. Neuroleptanesthesia (droperidol with fentanyl, a meperidine-like drug) (rarely used)
5. Tic disorders, e.g. Gilles de la Tourette syndrome (e.g. haloperidol)
6. Ecclampsia (chlorpromazine, promethazine and pethidine are given together as *lytic cocktail*) (rarely used)
7. Heat stroke (e.g. chlorpromazine) (rarely used)
8. Tetanus (e.g. chlorpromazine) (rarely used)
9. Intractable pruritis (rarely used)
10. Severe pain in malignancies (e.g. chlorpro-mazine) (rarely used)
11. Pre-anesthetic medication (e.g. chlorpromazine) (rarely used)

Pharmacokinetics

The orally administered antipsychotics are absorbed erratically and variably from the gastrointestinal tract, with uneven blood levels. Intramuscular and intravenous administration provide much more reliable blood levels. On an average, the oral liquid dose produces a peak level at 1½ hours, while the intramuscular dose peaks at 30 minutes.

The antipsychotics are highly lipophilic and highly protein-bound. They easily enter areas with good blood supply like brain, lung, kidneys and fetus, and accumulate there. They are not dialyzable.

The half-lives of all antipsychotics are long and theoretically a single dose administration per day is enough to produce sustained therapeutic blood levels. However in practice, divided doses are given initially to avoid side effects. Later, an attempt is made to give the whole dose or a major part of total daily dose at night. Steady state plasma levels are usually reached in 5-10 days. Once the drug is withdrawn, it may remain in body for many days to many months.

The main metabolic pathway is through liver (hepatic microsomal enzymes). Oxidation and conjugation are the most important methods of metabolism for phenothiazines. Many of the metabolites, e.g. mesoridazine (for thioridazine) and reduced haloperidol (for haloperidol), are also active. Chlorpromazine has more than 150 metabolites, some of which are active. The excretion of the metabolites is through kidneys and liver (entero-hepatic circulation).

Most of the antipsychotics tend to have a *therapeutic window*. If the blood level is below this 'window', the drug is ineffective. If the blood level is higher than the upper limit of the 'window', there is toxicity or the drug is again ineffective.

Classification

The currently available antipsychotic drugs can be classified as given in Table 15.2.

Mechanism of Action

The exact mechanism of action of antipsychotics is unknown. But, most probably, one of the major mechanisms is the *antidopaminergic activity* of these drugs.

Antipsychotic drugs block D_2-receptors, the dopamine receptors which are mainly present in the mesolimbic system (mesolimbic system is concerned with emotional reactions) and extrapyramidal system. The relative potencies of these drugs in competing for D_2 receptors parallel quite closely their clinical potencies.

It is currently believed that the antipsychotic drugs are effective in treating psychosis due to their action on D_2 receptors located in limbic system, while the extrapyramidal symptoms (EPS) are caused by blockade of D_2 receptors situated in extrapyramidal system.

However, other neurotransmitters (e.g. 5-HT, acetylcholine) are clearly implicated. The newer or *atypical antipsychotics* (called as *SDAs* or *serotonin-dopamine antagonists*), like risperidone and olanzapine, particularly act on the 5-HT_2 receptors.

Sedation is caused by histaminergic blockade, which is maximum for drugs like chlorpromazine and thioridazine.

The antipsychotics possibly correct the disordered thinking, impairment in attention and concentration, and abnormalities in perception in a psychotic patient. In addition, the psychomotor activity becomes normal in both excited and withdrawn patients.

Atypical antipsychotics (e.g. risperidone, clozapine, olanzapine, ziprasidone), in addition to the above actions, are believed to be effective in the treatment of negative symptoms (like apathy, decreased sociality, anhedonia) of chronic schizophrenia. Clozapine in particular is effective in the management of treatment-resistant schizophrenia.

Side Effects

The antipsychotics are safe drugs with a high therapeutic index and wide margin of safety in dosages. In spite of this safety, a wide range of side-effects do occur with the use of antipsychotics even in the therapeutic doses.

The side-effects are listed in Table 15.4 with their mechanisms of causation and management.

TABLE 15.2. CLASSIFICATION AND PROPERTIES OF ANTIPSYCHOTICS

Class and Examples of Drugs	*Oral Dose (mg/day)*	*Parenteral Dose (mg)*	*Equivalent# Dose (Equal to 100 mg CPZ)*	*Common Side Effects***		
				Sedation	*Hypo-tension*	*EPS**
I. PHENOTHIAZINES						
A. *Aliphatics*						
1. Chlorpromazine (CPZ)	300-1500	50-100 IM	100	+++	+++	+
2. Triflupromazine	100-400	30-60 IM	25	++	++	++
B. *Piperidines*						
1. Thioridazine	300-800	——	100	+++	++	+
2. Mesoridazine	100-400	——	50	++	+	+
C. *Piperazines*						
1. Trifluoperazine	15-60	1-5 IM	5	+	+	+++
2. Prochlorperazine	45-150	40-80 IM	15	+	+	+++
3. Fluphenazine	2-20	——	2	+	+	+++
4. Fluphenazine decanoate	——	25-50 IM every 2 weeks	***	+	+	+++
II. THIOXANTHENES						
A. *Aliphatics*						
1. Chlorprothixene	75-600	25-75 IM	50	+++	++	++
B. *Piperazines*						
1. Thiothixene	6-60	2-6 IM	5	+	++	++
2. Zuclopenthixol	25-150	50-100 IM	——			
3. Zuclopenthixol decanoate	——	200-400 IM every 2-4 weeks	****			
4. Flupenthixol	3-40	——	——	±	±	+
5. Flupenthixol decanoate	——	20-40 IM every 2-4 weeks	*****	±	±	+
III. BUTYROPHENONES						
1. Haloperidol	5-100	5-20 IM	2	+	+	+++
2. Haloperidol decanoate	——	25-250 IM every 2-4 weeks	******	+	+	+++
3. Trifluperidol	0.5-8.0	2.5-5.0 IM	0.6	±	±	+++
IV. DIPHENYLBUTYLPIPERIDINES						
1. Pimozide	4-20	——	2	+	+	++
2. Penfluridol	20-60 mg once every week	——	3.5 (Probably for 20 mg.given every week)	+	+	++

TABLE 15.2. CONTD..

Class and Examples of Drugs	Oral Dose (mg/day)	Parenteral Dose (mg)	Equivalent[#] Dose (Equal to 100 mg CPZ)	Common Side Effects** Sedation	Hypo-tension	EPS*
V. INDOLIC DERIVATIVES (DIHYDROINDOLONES)						
1. Molindone	50-225	——	10	++	0	+
VI. DIBENZOXAZEPINES						
1. Loxapine	25-100	——	10	+	+	++
VII. ATYPICAL ANTIPSYCHOTICS						
A. Dibenzodiazepines						
1. Clozapine	50-450	——	50	+	+	0
B. Substituted Benzamides						
1. Sulpiride	400-1800	——	——	+	+	0
2. Amisulpride	400-1200	——	——	-	+	±
C. Benzisoxales						
1. Risperidone	2-10	——	1-2	±	+	±
D. Benzisothiazolyl						
1. Ziprasidone	40-160	——	20	±	+	0
E. Thienobenzodiazepine						
1. Olanzepine	5-20	——	2-3	+	++	0
F. Dibenzothiazepine						
1. Quetiapine	300-500	——	50-100	+	+	±

\# *Equivalent doses* mentioned in Table 15.2 and Table 15.5 are a very rough guideline to the clinical use of antipsychotics/antidepressants. Most of this data has either come from animal data or is emperical. The drug dosage in each patient needs to be individualized based on the clinical symptoms, their severity, response to treatment and several other factors.

* EPS means Extrapyramidal symptoms.

** 0 = Absent; ± = Probable/Very Little; + = Mild; ++ = Moderate; +++ = Severe.

*** 25 mg of fluphenazine decanoate every 2 weeks = 300 mg CPZ/day

**** 200 mg of zuclopenthixol decanoate every 2 weeks = 25 mg/day of oral clopixol

***** 40 mg of flupenthixol decanoate every 2 weeks = 25 mg of fluphenazine decanoate every 2 weeks.

****** 100 mg of haloperidol decanoate every 4 weeks = 5 mg/day of oral haloperidol.

Other Comments

A large number of psychotic patients are uncooperative and have a poor drug compliance. So, it may be at times difficult to ensure proper administration of antipsychotics on an outpatient (OPD) basis. Since discontinuation of antipsychotic medication often leads to relapse, long-acting preparations of antipsychotics are valuable in the treatment. They may be given in a depot form, either intramuscularly or administered orally.

There are about 20 different preparations available in the international market but the following are used most often:

TABLE 15.3. SIDE EFFECTS OF ANTIPSYCHOTICS

Category and Side-effect	*Probable Cause*	*Maximum with (For example)*	*Minimum with (For example)*	*Management*
I. AUTONOMIC SIDE-EFFECTS				
1. Dry Mouth	Muscarinic Cholinergic Blockade	Chlorpromazine (CPZ)	Haloperidol Risperidone	Usually none. Tolerance develops Occasionally Pilocarpine 2%.
2. Constipation	—do—	—do—	—do—	Usually none. Tolerance develops. Bulk laxatives. Occasionally other laxatives.
3. Cycloplegia	—do—	—do—	—do—	Usually none. Tolerance occurs. Sometimes Pilocarpine 2%.
4. Mydriasis	—do—	Thioridazine (CPZ: miosis)	—do—	Usually none. Tolerance occurs. Sometimes Pilocarpine 2%.
5. Urinary Retention	—do—	Chlorpromazine	—do—	Usually none, if only hesitancy occurs. Tolerance develops.Rule out BHP. Bethanethol or Catheterization for retention.
6. Central Anti-cholinergic Syndrome (Delirium)	—do—	—do—	—do—	Physostigmine (Neostigmine does not enter CNS). Diazepam sometimes. General supportive care.
7. Orthostatic Hypotension	α_1 Adrenergic Blockade	—do—	—do—	Usually none. Tolerance develops. Change in posture slowly. When severe, use plasma expanders, raise leg, supportive measures.
8. Impotence	—do—	—do—	—do—	Decrease dose. If severe, change medication.
9. Impaired Ejaculation	—do—	Thioridazine	—do—	Decrease dose. If severe, change medication.
II. EXTRA-PYRAMIDAL SIDE EFFECTS (EPSE)				
1. Parkinsonian syndrome (esp. tremor)	Dopaminergic (D_2) receptor blockade in striatal areas	Haloperidol	Clozapine	Antiparkinsonian medication for treatment and many times also for prevention of EPS.
2. Akathisia (Motor restless-ness)	—do—	—do—	—do—	Change of medication or reduction of dose; b-blockers, like propranolol; Benzodiazepines
3. Acute Dystonia	—do—	—do—	—do—	Antiparkinsonian medication; Rule out hypercalcemia
4. Rabbit Syndrome (Peri-oral tremor)	—do—	—do—	—do—	Antiparkinsonian medication
5. Tardive Dys-kinesia (late onset oro-facial dyskinesia)	Dopaminergic gic (D_2) receptor super-sensitivity	Not known	Clozapine	Treatment unsatisfactory, though several drugs are available. Prevention best.
6. Neuroleptic Malignant Syn-drome (Fever, EPS, High CPK,	Not known	Probably haloperidol	Not known	Bromocriptine, Dantrolene, Baclofen, General supportive care. Add-on lorazepam, Occasionally ECT.

Contd.

TABLE 15.3. CONTD.

Category and Side-effect	*Probable Cause*	*Maximum with (For example)*	*Minimum with (For example)*	*Management*
catatonic symptoms and autonomic dysfunction)				
III. OTHER CENTTRAL NERVOUS SYSTEM EFFECTS				
1. Seizures	Decreased seizure threshold	Clozapine, Chlorpromazine (High doses)	Trifluoperazine	Decrease dose. Change to a safer antipsychotic.
2. Sedation	Histaminergic blockade	—do—	Haloperidol	This side-effect may be beneficial Otherwise decrease dose. Change drug. Give single dose only at night.
3. Depression or Pseudo-depression	Decreased catecholamine levels in brain	Not known	SDAs (e.g. ziprasidone)	Decrease dose. Change drug. Occasionally antidepressants or ECT.
IV. METABOLIC AND ENDOCRINE SIDE-EFFECTS				
1. Weight gain	H_1 blockade	Almost all antipsychotics esp. Olanzapine	Molindone	Change drug. Dietary control. Exercises.
2. Diabetes	Not known	Olanzapine Clozapine	Haloperidol	Change drug. Dietary control.
3. Galactorrhea with/without Amenorrhea	Increased Prolactin released due to dopaminergic blockade in hypothalamus	Haloperidol	Thioridazine	None. Change drug.
V. ALLERGIC SIDE-EFFECTS				
1. Cholestatic Jaundice	Hypersensitivity reaction	Chlorpromazine	Haloperidol	Change drug. Benign course. Supportive care.
2. Agranulocytosis (very rare)	—do—	Clozapine	—do—	Stop drug immediately. Treat infection. Isolation. General supportive care. Figastrim may be useful.
VI. CARDIAC SIDE-EFFECTS				
1. EKG Changes (e.g. QTc prolongation)	Anticholinergic effect Calcium channel blocking effect	Thioridazine Pimozide	—do—	None . Change drug, if severe.
2. Sudden Death (very rare)	Probably ventricular fibrillation	Not known	Not known	None.
VII. OCULAR SIDE-EFFECTS				
1. Granular deposits	Not known	Chlorpromazine	Haloperidol	Change drug.

Contd.

TABLE 15.3. CONTD.

Category and Side-effect	Probable Cause	Maximum with (For example)	Minimum with (For example)	Management
in cornea and lens	(Probably photo-sensitivity	(High doses for long duration)		
2. Pigmentary retinopathy resembling retinitis pigmentosa	Not known	Thioridazine only (Dose-related)	All other antipsychotics	Never give more than 800 mg/ day of thioridazine. Prevention only.
VIII. DERMATOLOGICAL SIDE-EFFECTS				
1. Contact dermatitis	Allergic	Chlorpromazine (By handling)	—do—	Avoid handling. Symptomatic treatment.
2. Photosensitive reaction	Probably photosensitive	—do— (High doses)	—do—	Avoid sunlight. Use sunscreen.
3. Blue-gray metallic discoloration	—do—	—do— (High doses for long duration)	—do—	Change drug.

1. Fluphenazine decanoate (25-50 mg IM every 2-3 weeks).
2. Haloperidol decanoate (50-100 mg IM every 4 weeks).
3. Flupenthixol decanoate (20-40 mg IM every 2-3 weeks)
4. Zuclopenthixol decanoate (50-100 mg IM every 2 weeks)
5. Penfluridol (20-40 mg oral every 1 week).
6. Pimozide (8-40 mg oral every 24 hours).

A search for an antipsychotic drug, which acts only on the limbic system but has no effect on the extrapyramidal system, has led to the development of a heterogeneous group of drugs, collectively known as *atypical* or *newer antipsychotics*.

By definition, these drugs are effective antipsychotics without producing undesirable extrapyramidal side-effects (i.e. *antipsychotics without neuroleptic effect*), and do not cause

TABLE 15.4. SOME FACTORS IN POOR DRUG COMPLIANCE

I. Drug Related Factors
   i. Adverse Effects (particularly their early appearance and persistence)
   ii. Slow onset of desirable effects
   iii. Complexity of regimen (e.g. several doses/day)
   iv. Route of administration (IM/IV as opposed to oral)

II. Patient Related Factors
   i. Poor education regarding illness and medication
   ii. Denial of illness/absent insight
   iii. Perceived stigma of mental disorder, medication, or visible side-effects (e.g. dystonia)
   iv. Treatment access problems (e.g. poverty, cost of medications, distance from hospital)
   v. Low IQ and/or low educational level
   vi. Poor social support
   vii. Specific psychopathology, e.g. persecutory ideation, hopelessness
   viii. Poor doctor-patient relationship.

elevation of the serum prolactin levels. These are characterized by a selective limbic dopamine blockade, D_4 receptor blockade, or a combination of potent 5-HT_2 and weak D_2 antagonism. Such a drug ideally will not have serious side-effects like tardive dyskinesia and neuroleptic malignant syndrome, and will be much safer.

Clozapine is one such drug but it causes significant agranulocytosis and seizures. Risperidone, olanzapine ans ziprasidone are currently being used widely as atypical antipsychotics, while quetiapine is about to be launched in Indian market.

ANTIDEPRESSANT DRUGS

Antidepressants are those psychotropic drugs which are used for the treatment of depressive illness. These are also called as mood-elevators and thymoleptics.

The first antidepressant to be discovered was *imipramine* in 1958 by Thomas Kuhn. It was different from phenothiazines in only a replacement of sulphur with an ethylene linkage. After this small structural difference (discovered by chance), imipramine was no longer effective as an antipsychotic but instead was quite beneficial in depressed patients. Since 1958, the number of antidepressants has been gradually increasing.

Antidepressants have no euphoriant effect when administered to normal, non-depressed individuals.

Indications

Presently, the indications for the use of antidepressants are:

A. Depression

1. Depressive episode (also called as major depression, MDP depression, and endogenous depression)
2. Depressive episode with melancholia (used with or without ECTs)
3. Depressive episode with psychotic features (used with antipsychotics or ECTs)
4. Dysthymia (used with psychotherapy)
5. Reactive depression (used, sometimes, with psychotherapy)
6. Depressive equivalents and masked depression (sometimes)
7. Atypical depression (MAOI drugs)
8. Secondary depression (e.g. in hypothyroidism, Cushing's syndrome)
9. Abnormal grief reaction

B. Child Psychiatric Disorders

1. Enuresis (used with or without behavior therapy)
2. Attention deficit disorder with hyperactivity (used in low doses, after 6 years of age, when stimulant medication is not available)
3. School phobia (sometimes, in low doses)
4. Separation anxiety disorder (in children)
5. Somnambulism
6. Night terrors

C. Other Psychiatric Disorders

1. Panic attacks (e.g. SSRIs, imipramine)
2. Agoraphobia, and social phobia (especially MAOIs)
3. Obsessive compulsive disorder with or without depression (e.g. clomipramine; fluoxetine; fluvoxamine, paroxetine)
4. Cataplexy (associated with narcolepsy)
5. Aggression in elderly (trazodone)
6. Eating disorders (e.g. fluoxetine in bulimia nervosa)
7. Borderline personality disorder (when depression is a prominent clinical feature)
8. Trichotillomania (e.g. clomipramine; fluoxetine)
9. Depersonalization syndrome
10. Post-traumatic stress disorder (PTSD)
11. Generalized anxiety disorder (e.g. doxepine)
12. Nicotine dependence (e.g. bupropion is sometimes used for treatment of craving)

13. Alcohol dependence (e.g. fluoxetine is sometimes used for treatment of craving)

D. Medical Disorders

1. Chronic pain (in low doses)
2. Migraine (as an adjuvant)
3. Peptic ulcer disease (e.g. doxepine has marked antihistaminic properties).

Classification

See Table 15.5.

Pharmacokinetics

The oral dose of tricyclic antidepressants is incompletely, though adequately absorbed. As they are highly anticholinergic in nature, they delay the gastric emptying and slow the gastro-intestinal motility. SSRIs are well absorbed from the gastro-intestinal tract.

These antidepressants, like antipsychotics, are highly lipophilic and are highly protein bound. Thus, they have a large volume of distribution and tend to accumulate in areas with good blood supply. Like antipsychotics, they are also not dialyzable.

Their other pharmacokinetic properties are similar to those of phenothiazines. The half-life is long, usually more than 24 hours. Although, tricyclics can be given in a single night-time dose, the routine in clinical practice is to give divided doses, at least in the initial days of treatment, to prevent accumulated side-effects.

The metabolism of tricyclic antidepressants is by oxidation (hepatic microsomal enzymes) followed by conjugation (glucoronic acid). The major metabolites of imipramine and amitriptyline (desipramine and nortriptyline respectively) are active antidepressants themselves. Fluoxetine is demethylated in liver to norfluoxetine.

With the regular administration of tricyclic antidepressants, a constant blood level is achieved usually by the end of two weeks. Although routine monitoring of blood levels is not indicated, it is important in cases of toxicity. Also, some antidepressants like nortriptyline and protriptyline have a *therapeutic window.*

Antidepressants (especially SSRIs e.g. fluoxetine) also cause inhibition of cytochrome P450 enzymes in liver (e.g. P450-2D6 and P450-3A).

The MAOIs are absorbed well by the oral route, and are predominantly metabolized in liver by acetylation.

Mechanism of Action

The exact mechanism of action is not known. It seems from the clinical studies that the predominant action of antidepressants is to increase the catecholamine levels in brain (*Amine hypothesis*).

The tricyclic antidepressants are also called as *Mono-Amine Reuptake Inhibitors* (MARIs). Their main modes of action are:

1. Blocking the reuptake of norepinephrine (NE), serotonin (5HT) and/or dopamine (DA) at the nerve terminals, thus increasing the NE, 5HT and/or DA levels at the receptor site.
2. Down-regulation of the β-adrenergic receptors.

The *Mono-Amine Oxidase Inhibitors* (MAOIs), instead, act on MAO (mono-amine oxidase) which is responsible for the degradation of catecholamines after reuptake. The final effect is the same, i.e. a functional increase in the NE and/or 5HT levels at the receptor site.

The increase in the brain amine levels is probably responsible for the antidepressant action.

Another important clinical point is that it takes 5-10 days before a MAOI, and 2-3 weeks before a tricyclic antidepressant drug has any evident action on depression (although sleep and agitation may respond earlier). The

TABLE 15.5. CLASSIFICATION AND PROPERTIES OF ANTIDEPRESSANTS

Class and Examples of Drugs		Oral Dose (mg/day)	Equivalent# Dose (to 75 mg of IMI)	Common Side Effects* Sedation	Orthostatic Hypotension	Anticholinergic
I.	**CYCLIC ANTIDEPRESSANTS**					
A.	**Tricyclic Tertiary Amines**					
1.	Imipramine (IMI)	75-300	75	++	++	++
2.	Amitriptyline	75-300	75	+++	+++	+++
3.	Doxepine	75-300	75-100	+++	+++	+
4.	Tri-imipramine	75-300	75	++	++	++
5.	Clomipramine	75-250	75	++	++	++
6.	Dotheipin	75-300	75	+++	+++	++
B.	**Tricyclic Secondary Amines**					
1.	Nortriptyline	75-200	75	++	++	+
2.	Protriptyline	15-60	20	0	++	++
3.	Desipramine	75-300	75	±	+	++
C.	**Tetracyclic Antidepressants**					
1.	Mianserin	30-120	30	+++	±	±
2.	Maprotiline	75-225	75	++	++	++
3.	Amoxapine	150-400	150	+	+	++
D.	**Bicyclic Antidepressants**					
1.	Viloxazine	100-300	100	±	±	±
II.	**SELECTIVE SEROTONIN REUPTAKE INHIBITORS (SSRIs)**					
1.	Fluoxetine	10-60	——	Activating	0	0
2.	Paroxetine	10-40	——	+	0	0
3.	Fluvoxamine	50-300	——	±	±	±
4.	Sertraline	50-200	——	±	±	0
5.	Citalopram	10-40	——	+	±	0
III.	**SEROTONIN NOREPINEPHRINE REUPTAKE INHIBITORS (SNRIs)**					
1.	Venlafaxine	75-375	——	+	±	±
IV.	**NOREPINEPHRINE SEROTONIN REUPTAKE ENHANCERS (NSREs)**					
1.	Tianeptin	37.5	——	±	0	±
V.	**NORADRENERGIC AND SPECIFIC SEROTONERGIC ANTIDEPRESSANTS (NaSSA)**					
1.	Mirtazapine	15-45	——	+++	+	±
VI.	**NOREPINEPHRINE DOPAMINE REUPTAKE INHIBITORS (NDRIs)**					
1.	Bupropion	150-450	——	Activating	0	0
VII.	**SEROTONIN ANTAGONISTS AND REUPTAKE INHIBITORS (SARIs)**					
1.	Trazodone	150-600	150	+++	±	±
2.	Nefazodone	200-600	150	++	+	±

Contd.

TABLE 15.5. CONTD.

Class and Examples of Drugs		Oral Dose (mg/day)	Equivalent# Dose (to 75 mg of IMI)	Common Side Effects* Sedation	Orthostatic Hypotension	Anticholinergic
VIII. NORADRENERGIC REUPTAKE INHIBITORS (NARIs)						
1. Reboxetine		8-10	——	±	±	±
IX. MONO-AMINE OXIDASE INHIBITORS (MAOIs)						
A. Irreversible Non-selective and Selective MAOIs						
Not Avaialble in India						
B. Reversible Selective MAOIs						
MAOI-B						
1. Selegiline	Jumax	5-10	Not equal	Useful in Parkinsonism		
MAOI-A (Reversible Inhibitors of MAO-A: Called as RIMAs)						
1. Moclobemide	Rimarex	300-600	——	Activating	0	0

** 0 = Absent; ± = Very Little; + = Mild; ++ = Moderate; +++ = Severe #See Table 15.2

reason for this is not fully clear. Therefore, it is useless to give antidepressants on a SOS ('whenever needed') basis. They must be administered regularly in sufficient doses to achieve the desired effect.

After remission of symptoms, it is essential to continue the antidepressant for a period of 6-12 months in the first episode of depressive disorder (and for longer duration in subsequent episodes) to prevent recurrence of symptoms.

Only when sufficient doses (150-300 mg imipramine equivalent) have been given for sufficient time (at least 6 weeks), the drug should be called ineffective for a particular patient. Another drug, usually from a different class or group, or ECT may then be used.

Side Effects

The common side-effects with their management are listed in Table 15.6.

Refractory Depression

About 20-35% of patients do not respond to the antidepressant therapy. The major reasons for this non-response are:

1. Poor drug compliance.
2. Inadequate dosage.
3. Insufficient treatment duration.
4. Low plasma antidepressant levels.
5. Incorrect diagnosis.

Even when these important reasons are excluded, there still remains a group (15%) of depressed patients who are non-responders or poor-responders.

Such patients should be given a trial of another antidepressant from a different group (e.g. tetracyclic) for sufficient time or should be treated with MAOI drugs. In case the patient still does not respond, the treatment of choice of refractory depression is electroconvulsive therapy (ECT).

LITHIUM AND OTHER MOOD STABILIZING DRUGS

Lithium (Li) is an element (Atomic number 3 and Atomic weight 7) which is the smallest alkali ion. The element was discovered in 1817 by Arfuedson. Since then, it was used for treatment of gout and for salt replacement in cardiac disease, but its use was restricted due to fatal toxicity.

It was re-discovered in 1949 by Cade, for use in treatment of mania but its potential went unrecognized. Schou, in 1957, had to rediscover it yet again before it became popular as a treatment of mania.

As it is very effective in treatment of mania, the word *antimanic* is often used to describe it. But, since it is equally effective in preventing mood swings in bipolar disorders, the better term is *mood-stabilizing agent*.

The most commonly used mood-stabilizing agents are lithium, valproate, and carbamazepine, though there are several other experimental mood stabilizers like lamotrigine and topiramate.

Indications

Although lithium salts are used in treatment of a myriad of psychiatric and non-psychiatric disorders, the established *indications* are only the following ones:

1. Treatment of acute mania
2. Prophylaxis of bipolar mood disorder.

In addition, the following may also constitute *possible clinical indications* of lithium use.

3. Treatment of schizo-affective disorder
4. Prophylaxis of unipolar mood disorder
5. Treatment of cyclothymia
6. Treatment of acute depression
7. Treatment of chronic alcoholism (in presence of significant depressive symptoms) and psychoactive use disorders (e.g. cocaine dependence)
8. Treatment of impulsive aggression
9. Treatment of Kleine Levin syndrome
10. Treatment of miscellaneous medical disorders like cluster headaches, cyclical vomiting, hyperthyroidism, Huntington's chorea, neutropenia in Felty's syndrome, periodic hypokalemic paralysis (rarely used in these conditions).

Pharmacokinetics

Lithium is very rapidly absorbed from the gastrointestinal tract. The peak serum levels occur between 30 minutes to 3 hours. The absorption is virtually complete in about 8 hours.

The distribution is in total body water with a slow entry into the intracellular compartment. Lithium is not protein bound. The maximum levels occur in thyroid (3-5 times serum level), saliva (2 times), milk (0.3-1.0 times) and CSF (0.4 times). The steady state levels are achieved in about 7 days.

There is no metabolism of lithium in body. It is excreted almost entirely by kidneys. As proximal reabsorption is influenced by sodium balance, depletion of sodium results in retention, causing higher blood levels of lithium.

Mechanism of Action

The exact mechanism of action is not known. The following mechanisms of action of lithium have been hypothesized:

1. It affects the Na^+-K^+ ATP-ase and accumulates intracellularly as a substitute of Na^+.
2. It inhibits the adenylate cyclase and thus decreases cAMP (II messenger) intracellularly.
3. It accelerates the presynaptic reuptake and destruction of catecholamines, like norepinephrine.
4. It inhibits the release of catecholamines at the synapse.
5. It decreases the postsynaptic serotonin 5-HT_2 receptor sensitivity.
6. It stabilizes the cell membrane, along with Ca^{++} and Mg^{++}.
7. It decreases the Ca^{++} mobilization from the intracellular pools by inositol-triphosphate dependent Ca^{++} channels (*II messenger system*).
8. It interferes with the phosphatidyl-inositol cycle by blocking the conversion of inositol monophosphate (IMP) to inositol by

TABLE 15.6. SIDE-EFFECTS OF ANTIDEPRESSANTS

Category and Side Effect	*Probable Cause*	*Maximum with (For example)*	*Minimum with (For example)*	*Management*
I. AUTONOMIC SIDE-EFFECTS				
1. Dry mouth	Muscarinic	Amitriptyline	Trazodone	See Table for 'Side Effects of Antipsychotics' (Table 15.3)
2. Constipation	Cholinergic	Amitriptyline	Fluoxetine	
3. Cycloplegia	Blockade	Amitriptyline	Fluoxetine	
4. Mydriasis	- do -	Amitriptyline	Fluoxetine	
5. Urinary retention	- do -	Amitriptyline	Fluoxetine	
6. Delirium	- do -	Amitriptyline	Fluoxetine	
7. Aggravation of glaucoma (Narrow angle)	- do -	Amitriptyline	Fluoxetine	Don't use in elderly and in patients with past history. Change or stop drug.
8. Orthostatic hypotension	α_1 Adrenergic Blockade	Amitriptyline	Trazodone Fluoxetine	See Table for 'Side Effects of Antipsychotics' (Table 15.3)
II. SEXUAL SIDE-EFFECTS				
1. Impotence	α_1 Adrenergic Blockade	Amitriptyline	Mirtazapine Bupropion	
2. Impaired/retarded ejaculation	- do -	Amitriptyline Paroxetine	Mirtazapine Bupropion	Cyproheptadine given 1 hour before, can reverse anorgasmia and retarded ejaculation caused by SSRIs.
3. Anorgasmia	5-HT Blockade	SSRIs TCAa	Bupropion Mirtazapine	
4. Priapism	Not known	Trazodone	Not known	Stop drug. Muscular relaxation. Sometimes surgical procedure needed.
III. CNS EFFECTS				
1. Sedation	α Adrenergic Blockade	Amitriptyline	Protriptyline Fluoxetine	This side-effect may be beneficial. otherwise decrease dose. Change drug. Give single dose only at night
2. Tremor and other EPS	Not known	Amoxapine	Not known	Decrease dose. Change drug
3. Jitteriness syndrome	Adrenergic; Serotonergic	Imipramine Fluoxetine	MAOI	This is very common in first week of therapy. Add diazepam for first 1-2 weeks. Tolerance occurs.
4. Withdrawal syndrome (mild)	Dependence	Imipramine Paroxetine	Protriptyline Fluoxetine	Slow withdrawal of drug.
5. Seizures	Decreased threshold	Bupropion Amitriptyline	Nomifensine	Decrease dose. Change drug
6. Aggravation of psychosis	Sympatho-mimetic	Not known	Amoxapine	Stop drug. Re-evaluate.
7. Precipitation of mania	Sympatho-mimetic	Tricyclics Fluoxetine	Probably Tetracyclics	Stop drug. Use mood stabilizers.
IV. CARDIAC SIDE EFFECTS				
1. Tachycardia	Anticholinergic	Amitriptyline	Trazodone	Decrease dosage . Use safer drugs in elderly and those with past history or coexisting heart disease.
2. Quinidine-like action (decreased conduction time)	Cardiotoxic	Amitriptyline	Mianserin Fluoxetine	
3. EKG changes	- do -	Amitriptyline	- do -	- do -

TABLE 15.6. CONTD.

Category and Side Effect	*Probable Cause*	*Maximum with (For example)*	*Minimum with (For example)*	*Management*
4. Arrhythmias (in overdoses)	- do -	Dotheipin Amitriptyline	- do -	- do -
5. Direct myocardial depression (in overdoses)	- do -	Amitriptyline	- do -	- do -
V. ALLERGIC SIDE EFFECTS				
1. Agranulocytosis (very rare)	Hypersensitivity	Mianserin Mirtazapine	Not known	See Table for 'Side-Effects of Antipsychotics'(Table. 15.2)
2. Cholestatic jaundice (very rare)	- do -	Not known	Not known	
3. Skin rashes	- do -	Not known	Not known	
4. Systemic vasculitis	Not known	Not known	Not known	
VI. METABOLIC AND ENDOCRINE SIDE EFFECTS				
1. Weight gain	Not known	Amitriptyline	Bupropion	Change drug . Exercise. Diet control. Fluoxetine causes weight loss.
VII. SPECIAL EFFECTS OF MAOI DRUGS				
1. Hypertensive crises	Interaction with tyramine in foods (cheese, red wine, chicken liver) and /or sympathomimetic drugs (e.g. amphetamine)	Tranylcypromine	Non-MAOIs	Prevent use of such agents with MAOI. Carry warning cards. When crisis occurs, use alpha (α) blockers like phentolamine.
2. Severe Hepatic Necrosis (rare)	Toxic or Hypersensitive	Iproniazid	Tranylcypromine	Stop/change drug. Supportive care. Death rate high.
3. Hyperpyrexia	Interaction with tricyclics or meperidine	Not known	Not known	Stop drug. Keep a gap of 1 week between Imipramine and MAOI. Supportive care.
VIII. TOXICITY OF TCAS				
Tricyclics are dangerous medications especially in depressed patients. Features of overdoe include agitation, delirium, paralytic ileus, urinary retention, coma, respiratory depression, seizures, hyperpyrexia, cardiac arrhythmias, conduction defects, mydriasis, and death. Lethal dose is 1-2 g. (40-80 tabs. of 25 mg Imipramine equivalence)				1. Gastric lavage or induce vomiting. 2. Activated charcoal for adsorption. 3. Cardio-respiratory resuscitation. 4. Quinidine-like drugs are contraindicated 5. Antiarrhythmics like Lignocaine. 6. General supportive care for coma. 7. Physostigmine 0.5 mg IV/IM bolus repeated to a total of 3-4 mg/day may be used under careful supervision. 8. Treat seizures. 9. Other symptomatic management. Coma often reverts in less than 24 hours, although toxicity lasts for 5-6 days.

inositol monophosphate phosphatase. The muscarinic acetylcholine (Ach) receptor is among one of the neurotransmitter receptors linked to this system in brain. The anti-manic effects of lithium may be attributed to this effect on Ach, thus affecting the cholinergic-adrenergic balance.

All these actions result in decreased catecholamine activity, thus ameliorating mania. However, these mechanisms do not explain the antidepressant effect and the prophylactic effect in bipolar mood disorder.

There is a lag period of 7-10 days before onset of action occurs, which is probably due to the time taken to achieve steady state levels.

Clinical Use

Lithium is available in market in the form of the following preparations.

1. Lithium carbonate
   300 mg tablets.
   400 mg sustained-release tablets.
2. Lithium citrate
   300 mg/5 ml. liquid.

Before starting treatment, it is essential to make sure of normal functioning of kidneys (most important), thyroid, heart and central nervous system. After starting lithium, it is necessary to investigate these systems at repeated intervals. The usual profile of investigations is as follows:

1. Routine general and systemic physical examination.
2. Routine blood counts (Hb, TC, DC, ESR).
3. Urine-routine and microscopic examination
4. EKG.
5. Renal function tests (blood urea, serum creatinine, 24 hour urine volume, urine specific gravity). GFR with creatinine clearance test, if indicated.
6. Thyroid function tests (TSH, T_3, T_4).

The initial starting dose (per day) of lithium for acute mania is 900-2100 mg/day, given in 2-3 divided doses. Ideally, the treatment is started after serial lithium estimation, done after a loading dose of 600 mg or 900 mg of lithium carbonate, to determine the pharmacokinetics.

During the treatment, it is essential to estimate blood lithium levels at regular intervals. The blood sample for estimation is taken 12 hours after the last lithium dose. If any changes are made in the lithium dosage, the next blood level is estimated after at least 7 days of the last change.

While stopping lithium treatment (except in cases of lithium toxicity), it is desirable to gradually taper the dose of lithium over several days in order to minimize the risk of early relapse.

Side-Effects

The side-effects are common and toxicity occurs easily, if blood levels reach about 2.0 mEq/L. Life-threatening intoxication occurs, if levels reach about 3.5 mEq/L. In acute administration, the toxicity is primarily neurological, while during the maintenance therapy the renal side-effects are the commonest.

The common side-effects are listed below:

I. Neurological

1. Tremor: This is the commonest side effect, occurring in up to 50% of patients. Treatment is by decreasing the dose of lithium or by adding propranolol.
2. Muscular weakness.
3. Cogwheel rigidity (mild).
4. Seizures (decreased threshold).
5. Neurotoxicity: The important features include delirium, cerebellar signs, abnormal involuntary movements. seizures, coma. In some individuals, toxicity may occur within

TABLE 15.7. BLOOD LITHIUM LEVELS

Therapeutic Levels = 0.8-1.2 mEq/L
For treatment of acute mania
Prophylactic Levels = 0.6-1.2 mEq/L
For relapse prevention in bipolar disorder
Toxic Lithium Levels > 2.0 mEq/L

the therapeutic range. The treatment of choice for acute toxicity is hemodialysis.

II. Renal

The renal side-effects occur in 10-50% of all patients on maintenance lithium therapy.

1. Polyuria, polydipsia.
2. Tubular changes.
3. Nephrogenic diabetes insipidus.
4. Nephrotic syndrome.

III. Cardiovascular

The effects on heart are similar to those of hypokalemia. The commonest EKG change is T-wave depression.

IV. Endocrine

1. Goitre.
2. Hypothyroidism.
3. Abnormal thyroid function (30-40%).
4. Weight gain (pedal edema also is common).

V. Gastro-Intestinal

These side-effects are nausea, vomiting, diarrhea, metallic taste and abdominal pain.

VI. Dermatological

These include acneiform eruptions, papular eruptions and exacerbation of psoriasis.

VII. Side-Effects During Pregnancy and Lactation

1. Teratogenic (possibly).
2. Increased incidence of Ebstein's anomaly (distortion and downward displacement of tricuspid valve in right ventricle), when taken in first trimester.
3. Secreted in milk with 30-100% of maternal blood Li levels. Can cause toxicity in infant.

Contraindications of Lithium Use

1. Presence of clear evidence of cardiac, renal, thyroid or neurological dysfunction.
2. Presence of blood dyscrasia.
3. During first trimester of pregnancy and lactation.
4. Concomitant administration of thiazide diuretics, tetracyclines or anesthetics.

VALPROATE

Valproate is rapidly emerging as a first line drug for treatment of mania and also a good drug for prophylaxis of bipolar mood disorder.

Valproic acid was first synthesized by Burton and used as an organic solvent. In 1963, Meunier serendipitously discovered the antiepileptic properties of valproic acid, while Lambert reported in 1966 that valpromide (a valproic acid analogue) might be effective as an anti-manic. It was approved by US FDA as an antiepileptic drug for absence seizures in 1978 and for the treatment of acute mania and (for migraine headache prophylaxis) in 1996.

The term *valproate* is often used to denote all commercial preparations since the common entity in blood is valproic acid. The following preparations of valproate are available in India:

i. Valproate sodium
ii. Divalproex (Enteric-coated stable coordination compound composed of sodium valproate and valproic acid in a 1:1 molar relationship)
iii. Chrono preparations (Enteric-coated compound composed of sodium valproate and valproic acid in a 3:2 ratio).

It is rapidly and completely absorbed after oral administration. The peak plasma levels are reached at 1-4 hours after a single oral dose. The half-life is 8-17 hours.

The dose of valproate is 1000-3000 mg/day orally in divided doses. The therapeutic blood levels are 50-150 μg/ml. Oral loading strategies (20-30 mg/kg/day) are rapidly effective in management of acute mania.

Indications

In addition to its primary indication as an anticonvulsant, Valproate has several other indications in psychiatric and neuropsychiatric disorders.

1. Bipolar Disorder

i. Acute Mania (as a first-line agent for treatment of acute mania in oral and IV forms): Several factors associated with a favorable anti-manic response to valproate (as well as carbamazepine) include:

a. Co-morbid substance abuse or other psychiatric disorders

b. Later age at onset and/or shorter duration of illness

c. History of poor response to lithium Dysphoric mania, mixed affective episodes, or rapid cycling

d. Organic/complicated mania associated with seizure disorder, history of head trauma, EEG abnormalities

e. D-M-I (Depression-Mania-Well Interval) pattern of illness as opposed to M-D-I pattern

There is some suggestion that patients non-responsive to valproate may be responsive to carbamazepine.

ii. Prophylaxis: Valproate is less effective in the maintenance treatment of bipolar disorder than in treatment of acute mania. It has been used alone as well as along with lithium and other mood stabilizers in maintenance treatment.

The addition of valproate to lithium has been recognized as a first-line treatment for mania that is refractory to lithium monotherapy. Conversely, the treatment of choice for acute mania with partial response to valproate is the addition of lithium.

iii. Rapid cycling bipolar disorder and mixed/dysphoric mania: Patients with rapid cycling, mixed affective episodes or dysphoric mania are often resistant to lithium treatment and respond better to valproate. Valproate is also effective in the management of ultra-rapid cycling mood disorders.

iv. Bipolar depression: Valproate appears to be more effective in the treatment of acute mania than in depression.

2. Neurological disorders

i. Migraine and Pain syndromes: Valproate has been used for the prophylaxis of migraine headaches, as well as for aborting an acute attack (IV route). Valproate has also been used in trigeminal neuralgia and neuropathic pain.

ii. Seizure disorders: Valproate is primarily indicated for the treatment of absence seizures (both simple and complex), complex partial seizures, myoclonic seizures, and generalized tonic-clonic seizures, as monotherapy as well as adjunct therapy.

3. Other disorders

Valproate has also been used in behavioral agitation in dementia, severe behavioral symptoms in mental retardation, ADHD and conduct disorder, schizoaffective disorder (bipolar type), alcohol withdrawal, tardive dyskinesia, impulse control disorder, panic disorder and borderline personality disorder.

Side Effects

The side effects are more common with valproate concentrations above 100 microgram/ml.

The common side effects are nausea, sedation, tremor, flushing, weight gain, thrombocytopenia, menstrual disturbances (in women) and hair loss. There are some reports of polycystic ovaries and hyperandrogenism in young women with epilepsy.

The most serious (though uncommon) side-effects are hepatic toxicity (especially in children), acute hemorrhagic pancreatitis, and Steven Johnson syndrome.

The use of valproate in pregnancy and lactation should be best avoided.

In overdose, the amount of drug that is not protein bound is high. Therefore dialysis is useful in the management of an overdose with valproate.

Drug Interactions

Certain drug may *increase* (e.g. aspirin, cimetidine, ibuprofen, erythromycin, fluoxetine, fluvoxamine, phenothiazines) or *decrease* (e.g. carbamazepine, phenytoin, phenobarbital, ethosuximide, rifampicin, mefloquine) the serum levels of valproate.

In addition, valproate *increases* serum levels of other drugs (e.g. lamotrigine, tricyclic antidepressants, zidovudine, tolbutamide).

CARBAMAZEPINE

Like lithium and valproate, carbamazepine too is an anti-manic and mood-stabilizing agent. It is a tricyclic compound synthesized in 1953 by Schindler.

The onset of action is faster as compared to lithium, but slower compared to valproate.

The dose of administration is 600-1600 mg/day orally, in divided doses. The treatment is best monitored with repeated blood levels. The therapeutic blood levels are 6-12 μg/ml. The toxic blood levels are reached at more than 15 μg/ml.

Indications

The *indications* for use of carbamazepine are:

1. Seizures
   i. Complex partial seizures (CPS)
   ii. Generalized tonic clonic seizures
   iii. Alcohol withdrawal seizures (rum fits), if persistent (also used sometimes for treatment of simple alcohol withdrawal syndrome)
2. Psychiatric disorders
   i. Bipolar mood disorder (especially rapid cyclers; lithium-refractory patients; lithium-intolerant patients; for prophylaxis; for treatment of acute mania especially severe and dysphoric mania; for treatment of acute depression, along with antidepressants or even alone)
   ii. Impulse control disorder and aggression
   iii. Psychosis (especially mania) with epilepsy
   iv. Schizo-affective disorder
   v. Borderline personality disorder
   vi. Cocaine withdrawal syndrome
3. Paroxysmal pain syndromes
   i. Trigeminal neuralgia
   ii. Phantom limb pain
   iii. Other paroxysmal pain syndromes (neuralgias)

Side Effects

The major side effects include diplopia, drowsiness, dizziness, nausea, vomiting, ataxia, skin rash, Steven-Johnson syndrome (erythema multiforme major), photosensitivity, cholestatic jaundice, acute oliguria with hypertension, leucopenia and thrombocytopenic purpura.

The most dangerous side-effects are bone marrow depression (causing aplastic anemia) and cardiovascular collapse.

So, it is essential to monitor cardiac, renal, hepatic and bone-marrow functions during carbamazepine treatment.

The use of valproate in pregnancy and lactation should be best avoided.

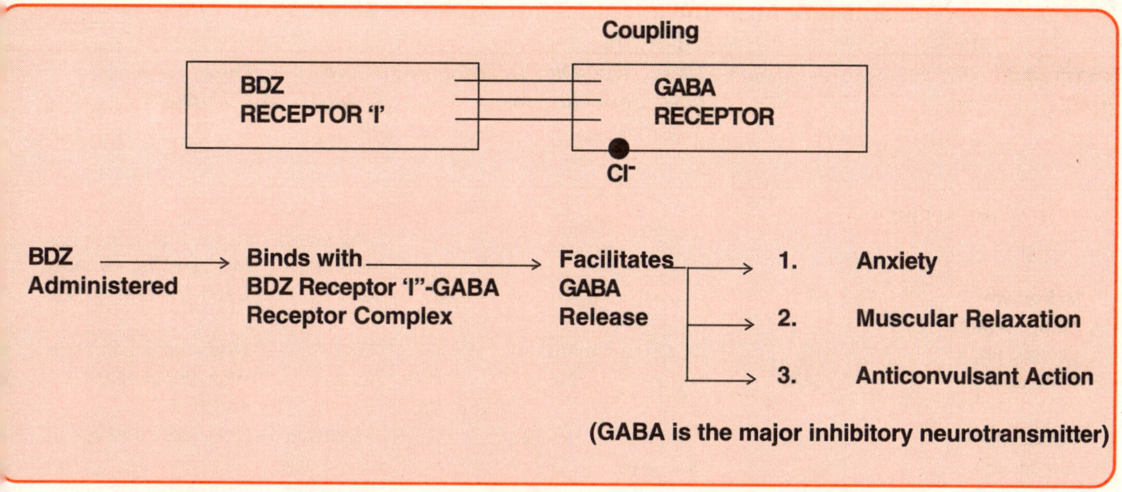

FIG. 15.1. PROBABLE MECHANISM OF ACTION OF BENZODIAZEPINES

ANTI-ANXIETY DRUGS

'he anti-anxiety drugs, also called as minor ranquilizers and anxiolytics, can be classified is follows:

Classification

. Barbiturates

Barbiturates can be divided into 4 main types:

A. Long Acting
Duration of action is more than 8 hours. Example is phenobarbital.

B. Intermediate Acting
Duration of action is 5-8 hours. Examples are mobarbital and pentobarbital.

C. Short Acting
Duration of action is 1-5 hours. Example is ecobarbital.

D. Ultra-Short Acting
Duration of action is less than 1 hour. xamples are thiopentone and methohexital.

The barbiturates are no longer used comnonly as anti-anxiety agents. They produce nultiple side-effects like excessive sedation, respiratory and circulatory depression, hepatic enzyme induction, dependence, withdrawal symptoms, rebound increase in REM sleep on withdrawal, and potential for use in suicide.

II. Non-barbiturate, Non-benzodiazepine Anti-anxiety Agents

These can be further divided into following categories:

A. Carbamates
Examples are meprobamate, tybamate and carisoprodol. Not used commonly due to potential for abuse and dependence.

B. Piperidinediones
Example is glutethimide. This too is not used now, due to dependence potential.

C. Alcohols
Examples include ethanol, chloral hydrate and ethchlorvynol. These drugs are highly dependence producing.

D. Quinazoline Derivatives
Example is methaqualone. Methaqualone had become a street drug, i.e. a drug of abuse, before it was discontinued as an anti-anxiety agent and a hypnotic.

TABLE 15.6. CLASSIFICATION AND PROPERTIES OF BENZODIAZEPINES

Class and Drug	*Elimination Half Life (hours)*	*Usual Hypnotic Dose (mg HS)*	*Oral Dose (mg/day)*	*Parenteral Dose (mg)*	*Active Metabolites*	*Other Comments*
I. Very Short Acting						
1. Triazolam	2-5	0.125-0.25	—	—	α-hydroxy-triazolam	Rapid oral absorption Marketed as hypnotic
2. Midazolam	2-5	—	—	—	—	Used for anesthesia
II. Short Acting						
1. Oxazepam	5-15	15-30	15-120	—	None	Slow oral absorption
2. Lorazepam	10-20	0.5-2	2-6	(2-4 IV or IM)	None	High dependence potential
3. Temazepam	10-20	15-30	15-30	—	Oxazepam	Slow oral absorption
4. Alprazolam	6-20	Not used	0.5-6	—	α-hydroxy-alprazolam	Also an effective anti-depressant,antiphobic and antipanic agent.
5. Estazolam	8-24	1-2	1-2	—	—	—
III. Long Acting						
1. Chlordiazepoxide	25-48	10-25	15-100	(50-100 IV slowly)	Desmethyl-demoxepam	Erratically absorbed after IM injection. If it has to be given, IM injection should be given in deltoid (and
2. Diazepam	14-90	2-10	2-60	2-20 IV or IM slowly	Nordiazepam	in gluteal) muscle as it has a better circulalation
3. Flurazepam	30-100	15-30	15-60	—	Desmethyl - hydroxy-ethyl-flurazepam	Marketed as hypnotic
4. Chlorazepate	30-100	7.5-30	7.5-60	—	Nordiazepam	Hydrolyzed to active form in stomach.
5. Nitrazepam	20-60	5-10	5-20	—	Nordiazepam	Marketed as a hypnotic
6. Prazepam	30-60	10-20	20-60	—	Nordiazepam and diazepam	Slow oral absorption
7. Halazepam	30-60	20-40	40-160	—	Nordiazepam	—
8. Clonazepam	20-40	—	0.5-20	(2-5 IM)	—	Also used in mania.
9. Quazepam	40-160	7.5-30	7.5-15	—	—	Probably selective for benzodiazepine receptor I and may cause less cognitive and motor disturbances.

E. Anti-Histaminics

Examples are diphenhydramine, hydroxyzine and pro-methazine. Diphenhydramine is usually combined with methaqualone or diazepam.

They may be used as a hypnotic-sedative but their use as an anti-anxiety agent is minimal and probably not effective.

F. Cyclic Ethers

Example is paraldehyde. Not used commonly as it is not very effective and is dependence producing.

G. Others

Antipsychotics (e.g. thioridazine) and antidepressants (e.g. doxepine) are sometimes used for treatment of severe, intractable anxiety. However, they are not the drugs of first choice and should be used with discretion, when all other drugs have failed to benefit.

H. Beta-(β) Blockers

Example is propranolol. This is particularly effective in treatment of peripheral somatic manifestations of anxiety. It is also the drug of first choice for treatment of anticipatory anxiety and situational anxiety.

Propranolol can be used either alone or along with benzodiazepines.

The role of β-blockers in the treatment of psychic manifestations of anxiety is still investigational.

Propranolol is contraindicated in patients of bronchial asthma and cardiac conditions. It should be used with caution in patients of age 40 and above.

The dosage are 40-240 mg/day in divided doses.

III. Benzodiazepines

Since the discovery of chlordiazepoxide in 1957 by Sternbach, benzodiazepines have replaced other anti-anxiety drugs. Presently, benzodiazepines are the drugs of first choice in treatment of anxiety and for the treatment of insomnia.

The benzodiazepines can be classified according to their elimination half-lives (Table 15.8).

Indications

The *indications* for use of benzodiazepines are as follows:

1. Generalized anxiety disorder; adjustment disorder with anxious mood.
2. Panic disorder, agoraphobia, and school phobia (particularly alprazolam and clonazepam).
3. Agitated depression (added to antidepressants for first 1-2 weeks); alprazolam probably has an antidepressant effect.
4. Insomnia.
5. Stage 4 NREM sleep disorders like enuresis, somnambulism (diazepam reduces duration of stage 4 NREM sleep).
6. Nightmares (diazepam also reduces REM sleep duration).
7. Premedication in anesthesia (intravenous lorazepam, midazolam, or diazepam).
8. Anticonvulsant use (drugs of choice for status epilepticus, myoclonic seizures and certain infantile spasms).
9. To produce skeletal muscle relaxation (e.g. in tetanus, cerebral palsy).
10. Treatment of alcohol and other drug withdrawal syndromes.
11. For minor surgical, endoscopic or obstetric procedures.
12. Acute mania (clonazepam, either alone or with lithium).
13. Antipsychotic-induced akathisia.
14. Emergency management of acute psychoses (IV lorazepam, along with parenteral antipsychotics).
15. Narcoanalysis or abreaction (IV diazepam).
16. Treatment resistant schizophrenia (experimental use in high doses).
17. Psychosomatic disorders.

Whenever administered, benzodiazepines should not be ordinarily used for more than 6 weeks at one time. Otherwise, the risk of dependence is high, and tolerance occurs.

Mechanism of Action

The exact mechanism of action of benzodiazepines is not clear. The recent discovery

(1977) of benzodiazepine receptors has shed some light on the mode of action (Fig. 15.1).

There are, presently, two known benzodiazepine (BDZ) receptors.

1. BDZ Receptor I, which is linked with GABA (Gamma-Amino-Butyric-Acid) receptor and is probably involved in mediation of sleep.
2. BDZ Receptor II, which is alone and is probably involved in cognition and motor control.

Thus, benzodiazepines probably act by enhancing GABA-transmission in brain.

Benzodiazepine receptor antagonists (e.g. Flumazenil) arc anxiety-provoking agents. Flumazenil has a half life of 60 minutes and administered in a parenteral dose of 0.2 mg-1.0 mg IV given over 1-2 minutes in the treatment of benzodiazepine toxicity.

Side Effects

The side-effects of benzodiazepines include nausea, vomiting, weakness, epigastric pain, diarrhea, vertigo, blurring of vision, body aches, urinary incontinence (rare), impotence, sedation, lassitude, increased reaction time, ataxia (in high doses), dry mouth, retrograde amnesia (rare), impairment of driving skills, severe effects when administered with alcohol, irritability (particularly with flurazepam and chlordiazepoxide), disinhibited behavior (particularly with diazepam), dependence and withdrawal symptoms (on stopping the drug).

Cross-tolerance occurs with barbiturates, methaqualone and ethyl alcohol.

Worsening of depression and pre-existing psychosis with the use of benzodiazepines has been reported.

Since withdrawal symptoms occur, the drug should be withdrawn slowly.

IV. Newer Drugs

1. Buspirone

Buspirone is a new anti-anxiety drug which is not a benzodiazepine. It is a azaspirodecane-dione (azaspirone) derivative and is a 5-HT_{1A} partial agonist and a selective DA autoreceptor antagonist. It also inhibits the spontaneous firing of 5-HT neurons. It does not seem to act on benzodiazepine receptors. It is anxioselective with no sedative action, no anticonvulsant, or muscle-relaxant properties.

It is administered in a dose of 15-30 mg/day, in a thrice daily schedule due to a short half-lef. As it has a slower and more gradual onset of action, it usually takes about two weeks before the anti-anxiety effects of buspirone are evident. It is not useful in the treatment of panic disorder. The side effects include dizziness, headache, lightheadedness and diarrhea.

As it is anxio-selective and lacks any risk of dependence, it may replace the benzodiazepines as the drug of choice in generalized anxiety disorders.

2. Zopiclone

Zopiclone belongs to a new class of non-benzodiazepine drugs, the cyclopyrrolones. Cyclopyrrolone derivatives also act on the GABA receptors, but at a site distinct from that of the benzodiazepines.

Zopiclone has a short duration of action as well as shorter onset. After oral administration, it is absorbed rapidly, with peak plasma concentration occurring in about 60 minute. The elimination half life is 4-6 hours.

The usual dose of zopiclone is 3.75-7.5 mg at bedtime (lower dose in elderly patients and in patients with severe hepatic failure). The side effects include bitter taste, dry mouth, drowsiness, nausea and headache. Its safety in children, and in pregnancy and lactation is not proven.

It is clinically superior to benzodiazepines in subjective awakening quality, well-being, and attention span in the morning.

3. Zolpidem

Zolpidem is an imidazopyridine derivative which is being marketed as a hypnotic. It is administered in a dose of 5-10 mg for hypnotic use. It has a half life of 2-3 hours; therefore it is useful in the treatment of difficulty in initiation of sleep (initial insomnia).

The side-effects include drowsiness, dizziness, headache, depression, nausea, dry mouth, and myalgia. It should not be used for more than 2 weeks at one time. Its safety in children, and in pregnancy and lactation is not proven.

4. Zalpelon

Zalpelon is an pyrazolo-pyrimidine derivative which is being marketed as a hypnotic. Although a non-benzodiazepine drug, it acts on the omega-1 benzodiazepine receptor located on the alpha sub-unit of the GABA-A receptor complex (causing sedation), with very little effect on omega-2 and omega-3 receptors.

It is administered in a dose of 5-10 mg for hypnotic use. It has a half life of one hour with a rapid onset of effect. Therefore, it is useful in treatment of difficulty in initiation of sleep (initial insomnia).

It can be taken again at night if there is more than 4 hours of sleep time remaining. Because of the very short haf life, there is virtually no hangover in the morning.

The side-effects include headache, drowsiness, dizziness, nausea, and myalgia. It should not be used for more than 2 weeks at one time. Its safety in children, and in pregnancy and lactation is not proven.

5. Other Drugs

The other newer, hypno-sedative and anti-anxiety drugs include *suriclone* (a cyclopyrrolone derivative; a hypnotic), *bretazenil* and *imidazenil* (partial benzodiazepine agonists; anxiolytic without sedation; rapid onset of action), *abecarnil* (β-carboline partial agonist at benzodiazepine receptor; anxiolytic and anticonvulsant), and *alpidem* (anxiolytic).

16 Other Biological Methods of Treatment

The last 70 years have seen the development of several biological methods of treatment for the treatment of psychiatric disorders. The earlier modes of treatment, like malarial treatment for general paralysis of insane (GPI), insulin coma therapy, atropine coma therapy, continuous sleep treatment, subconvulsive ECT, chemical convulsive therapy, sleep deprivation, mega-vitamin therapy and hallucinogens (to name a few important methods) are no longer used in the routine clinical practice.

There are two methods which, though were introduced at the same time, have been revised extensively and are still in use presently. These methods are electroconvulsive therapy and psychosurgery.

ELECTROCONVULSIVE THERAPY

Brief History

Von Meduna, in 1934, used 25% camphor in oil intramuscularly to produce convulsions for the first time for therapeutic purposes. Later,

TABLE 16.1. A BRIEF HISTORY OF BIOLOGICAL TREATMENTS IN PSYCHIATRY

Year	Treatment	Started by
1785	Camphor-induced seizures	W Oliver
1917	Malarial treatment of GPI	Julius Wagner von Jauregg
1922	Barbiturate coma therapy	Jacob Klaesi
1931	Reserpine (1st drug treatment in psychosis)	Ganesh Sen and Kartik Bose
1933	Insulin coma therapy	Manfred Sakel
1934	Cardiazol (Metrazol) induced seizures	LLJ von Meduna
1936	Psychosurgery (Prefrontal leucotomy)	Egas Moniz and Almenda Lima
1938	Electroshock (Electroconvulsive therapy)	Ugo Cerletti and Lucio Bini
1949	Lithium (for mania)	John F Cade
1952	Chlorpromazine (1st antipsychotic)	Jean PL Delay and Pierre Deniker
1954	Meprobamate	FM Berger
1958	Iproniazid (1st MAO Inhibitor)	Nathan Kline
1958	Imipramine (1st tricyclic antidepressant)	Thomas Kuhn
1958	Haloperidol (1st non-phenothiazine antipsychotic)	Janssen
1960	Chlordiazepoxide (1st benzodiazepine)	Hugo Sternbach

he used pentylenetetrazol (metrazol) for the same purpose.

A much safer form of convulsive therapy was used by Cerletti and Bini in 1938. They called it EST or electroshock therapy. Later, this method of treatment came to be known as ECT or electroconvulsive therapy.

The 1970s saw widespread criticism of ECT with many legislations passed in the US states (e.g. in California, 1975), restricting the use of ECT. Following this, widespread modifications in the ECT technique made it even safer mode of treatment.

In 1974, American Psychiatric Association's (APA's) Council on Research and Development appointed a Task Force on ECT. *The APA Task Force on ECT*, in 1976, gave its report which provided clear guidelines for use of ECT and declared it to be a safe and effective method of treatment when used by professionals trained in the technique.

The 1990 the APA Task Force Report on ECT redefined the indications, gave guidelines for obtaining consent and set standards for training, treatment and privileging of ECT.

Indications

The indications for electroconvulsive therapy are:

1. Major severe depression
   i. With suicidal risk (This is the first and most important indication for ECT)
   ii. With stupor
   iii. With poor intake of food and fluids
   iv. With melancholia
   v. With psychotic features
   vi. With unsatisfactory response to drug therapy
   vii. Where drugs are contraindicated, or have serious side-effects
   viii. Where speedier recovery is needed.
2. Severe catatonia ("functional")
   i. With stupor
   ii. With poor intake of food and fluids
   iii. With unsatisfactory response to drug therapy
   iv. Where drugs are contraindicated, or have serious side-effects.
   v. Where speedier recovery is needed.
3. Severe psychoses (schizophrenia or mania)
   i. With risk of suicide, homicide or danger of physical assault
   ii. With unsatisfactory response to drug therapy
   iii. Where drugs are contraindicated, or have serious side-effects
   iv. With very prominent depressive features (e.g. schizo-affective disorder).

The use of ECT in mania and schizophrenia is not a treatment of first choice and is employed only in the above-mentioned conditions. A history of good response with ECT and patient preference for ECT also determine the use of ECT.

The 1990 APA Task Force on ECT has also defined as *suggestive indications* (for occasional use) the following disorders:

1. Organic mental disorders (e.g. organic mood syndrome, organic hallucinosis, organic delusional disorder, and delirium).
2. Medical disorders (e.g. organic catatonia, hypopituitarism, intractable seizure disorder, neuroleptic malignant syndrome and parkinsonism).

Pre-Treatment Evaluation

The pre-treatment evaluation consists of the following steps:

1. An *informed consent*, taken from the patient or the guardian (if the patient is not competent to give consent).
2. Detailed medical and psychiatric history taking, which includes the current and past treatment history.

3. General and systemic physical examination.
4. Routine laboratory investigations, like Hb, TC, DC, ESR, urine-routine and microscopic examination, EKG, X-Ray chest, and any other investigations in the light of history and examination.
   Other optional (not done routinely) investigations are EEG and estimation of plasma pseudo-cholinesterase activity (for patients who would receive succinylcholine for general anesthesia).
5. Examination of fundus oculi to rule out papilledema.

Contraindications

A. Absolute

The only absolute contraindication is the presence of *raised intracranial tension* (so examination of fundus oculi is an essential step). However, the 1990 APA Task Force Report on ECT recognizes this too as a relative contraindication.

B. Relative

These include:

1. Recent myocardial infarction (MI)
2. Severe hypertension
3. Cerebrovascular accident (CVA)
4. Severe pulmonary disease
5. Retinal detachment
6. Pheochromocytoma.

Technique

The techniques used for ECT administration are of two types:

i. *Direct ECT*: Here, ECT is given in the absence of muscular relaxation and general anes-thesia. All the other steps are the same as modified ECT. This method of treatment is now very infrequently used.
ii. *Modified ECT*: Here, ECT is modified by drug-induced muscular relaxation and general anesthesia given by an anesthetist.

ECT is usually administered in the morning after an overnight fast. If given at any other time during the day, the patient should be *empty stomach* for at least 4 hours. No oral medication should be given in the morning.

The *bladder* (and bowel) should be emptied just before the treatment, as incontinence can occur during the induced seizure. Dentures, if present, should be removed, and the presence of loose teeth should be ruled out. Tight clothing, and metallic and sharp objects (if any) should be removed from the person's body.

The usual anesthetic precautions are taken. The patient is placed on a hard bed which is well insulated. A slow intravenous drip may be started (though not needed in all patients). Atropine (0.6 mg) is given IV just before the treatment or else is given IM or SC 30 minutes before treatment. Atropine is given to decrease the oral secretions and to prevent vagal stimulation during ECT which can cause cardiac arrest.

This is followed by administration of an anesthetic agent like propofol or thiopentone (150-250 mg, usually individualized dose for each patient) and a muscle relaxant like succinylcholine (0.5-1.5 mg/kg). An anesthetic mask is placed on the face and ventilation with 100% oxygen is given.

As succinylcholine is a depolarizing blocking agent, its administration is followed by muscular fasciculations which move from above downwards. When the fine twitching movements disappear from the lower extremities, it is the time of complete muscular relaxation.

Now a mouth gag is inserted between the teeth, to prevent tongue bite during the convulsion and pressure is applied on the mandible to approximate upper and lower teeth till the convulsions stop.

The electrodes (U-shaped in most equipments) are moistened with saline or 25% bicarbonate solution and are applied on head. According to the position of application of electrodes, ECT is of two types:

i. *Bilateral ECT:* This is the standard form of ECT used most commonly. Each electrode is placed 2.5-4.0 cm. (1-1½") above the midpoint, on a line joining the tragus of the ear and the lateral canthus of the eye.
ii. *Unilateral ECT:* Here, the electrodes are placed only on one side of head, usually the non-dominant side (right side of head in a right-handed individual). There are various positions described for electrode placement.

The unilateral ECT is safer, with much fewer side effects particularly those of memory impairment. However, according to the 1990 APA ECT Task Force Report, bilateral ECT is superior to unilateral ECT in effectiveness.

The place(s) of electrode placement is also cleaned with normal saline or 25% bicarbonate solution, or a conducting gel is applied.

One attendant places one hand each on both thighs near the knee joint, while another attendant holds the shoulders. This is a must in direct ECT, but should also be done in modified ECT. This is to prevent fall from bed and causation of fractures and dislocations due to muscular contractions (which may occasionally occur even in modified ECT).

The therapeutic adequacy of the treatment is gauzed by the occurrence of a generalized tonic-clonic seizure lasting for not less than 25-30 seconds. This is made sure by:

1. Observing the seizure (in direct ECT).
2. EEG recording during ECT (in modified ECT).
3. Occluding the circulation of one extremity with a BP apparatus cuff, before giving succinylcholine. Thus the whole body is paralyzed but one extremity convulses and can be directly observed.
4. Observing plantar extension and eyelid contractions, which may be seen even despite the muscular relaxation (not a very reliable method).

The usual dose for obtaining an adequate seizure response is 90-150 volts (average 110 volts) for 0.1-1.0 seconds (average 0.6 seconds). The usual amount of current passed in an ECT session is 200-1600 mA.

Earlier, the ECT machines used a *'sine wave'* to deliver the current (with a positive and a negative wave constituting a cycle). However with *'sine wave'*, unnecessarily excessive and inefficient electrical stimulus is delivered. The newer ECT machines instead use a *'brief pulse'* wave form that delivers the electrical stimulus, usually in a 1-2 msec. time period at a rate of 30-100 pulses/second. Therefore, the *'brief pulse'* current is more efficacious and safer than the *'sine wave'* current.

After the seizure has occurred, mouth gag is removed, secretions are removed by a suction machine from the oral cavity, and oxygen mask is applied. Till consciousness is regained, the patient is turned to one side to prevent aspiration. The vital parameters are constantly monitored till recovery occurs. The patient is made to rest, for about 30 minutes to 1 hour, on bed after the treatment is over.

Duration of Therapy

The total duration and number of treatments given depends on the diagnosis, presence of side-effects, and the response to treatment.

Usually 6-10 treatments are sufficient, although up to 15 treatments can be given if needed. The treatments should be spaced, so that no more than 3 ECTs are given per week.

Although ECT is very effective in severe depressive disorder (for example), the benefit lasts only till the ECTs are given. There is no residual benefit after the treatment is over. Hence, the patient needs antidepressants (for example) during and after the ECTs are over.

Mechanism of Action

One point is clear that the efficacy of ECT is linked with the production of generalized tonic-clonic seizures lasting at least 25-30 sec.

Although exact mechanism is unclear, one hypothesis states that ECT possibly affects the catecholamine pathways between diencephalon (from where seizure generalization occurs) and limbic system (which may be responsible for mood disorders), also involving the hypothalamus.

As ECT increases the threshold for further seizures, it may paradoxically act as an anticonvulsant. ECT also causes down-regulation of β_1 receptors in cortex and hippocampus.

Side Effects

1. Side-effects associated with general anesthesia: *Deaths* during ECT are due to general anesthesia, succinylcholine (in patients with deficiency of pseudo-cholinesterase) and drug-interactions. The mortality rate is 1:1000 to 1:10,000 which is similar to any operative procedure under anesthesia.
2. *Memory disturbances* (both anterograde and retrograde) are very common. These are usually mild and recovery occurs within 1-6 months after treatment. Unilateral ECTs cause much less memory disturbance than bilateral ECTs.
3. *Confusion* may occur in the post-ictal period. Like memory disturbances, confusion is much commoner with the bilateral ECTs. Usually, no treatment is needed. Parenteral diazepam may be given for excitement during this period.
4. *Other side-effects* include headache (uncommon), prolonged apnea, prolonged seizure, cardiovascular dysfunction, emergent mania, muscle aches and apprehension. ECT does *not* cause brain damage.

PSYCHOSURGERY

Definition

Psychosurgery is defined (by APA's Task Force) as, a surgical intervention, to sever fibers connecting one part of brain with another, or to remove, destroy or stimulate brain tissue, with the intent of modifying, behavior, thought or mood disturbances, for which there is no underlying organic pathology (i.e., the distur-bance is 'functional').

Brief History

Although surgery on skull (trephining) was done for mental illnesses even in primitive times, psychosurgery in this century was introduced as *leucotomy* by Egas Moniz and Almenda Lima in 1936. Egaz Moniz received a Noble prize for this achievement.

Freeman and Watts introduced *prefrontal lobotomy* in 1937 while in India, Govindaswami

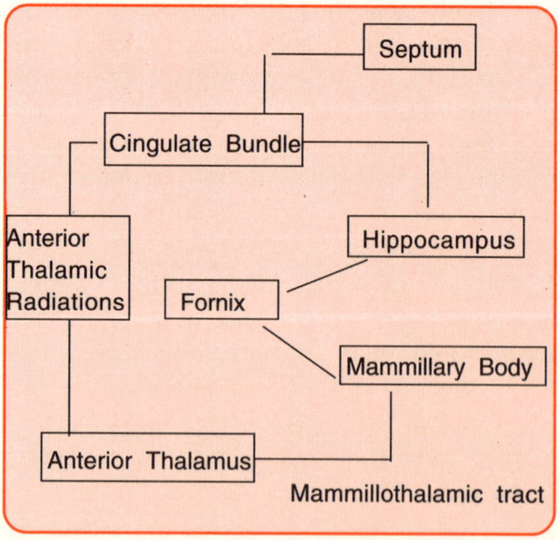

FIG. 16.1. PAPEZ CIRCUIT

and Rao performed the first leucotomies in 1944.

Psychosurgery came in for a severe public criticism in the 1950's when its use decreased. In the last few years, several better methods of treatment have been developed which are safer and more specific. In addition, careful guidelines for the use of psychosurgery have also been laid down.

Anatomical Basis

It is believed that limbic system is closely linked with normal and abnormal emotional reactions. Limbic system (Fig. 16.1) consists mainly of cingulum (cingulate gyrus and cingulate bundle), hippocampus, parahippocampal gyri, fornix, amygdala, parts of thalamus, parts of hypothalamus and posterior part of orbital frontal cortex.

Limbic system is closely connected with the frontal and temporal lobes, midbrain and other parts of brain, by many connecting fibers.

The aim of psychosurgery is to produce surgical lesions in carefully selected parts of limbic system and/or its connecting fibers.

One major part of limbic system, believed to be important in emotional experiences, is *Papez circuit*. This important circuit, which lies within the limbic system, connects cingulate bundle, hippocampus, anterior thalamus, mammillary bodies, fornix and septum (Fig. 16.1).

Indications

The current indications for psychosurgery are (In the past, the list of such indications was virtually endless):

1. Chronic, severe, incapacitating depression, which has not responded to all available treatments.
2. Chronic, severe, incapacitating obsessive-compulsive disorder (OCD), which has not responded to all available treatments.
3. Chronic, severe, incapacitating anxiety disorder, which has not responded to all available treatments.
4. Schizophrenia with severe depressive component, which has not responded to all available treatments.
5. Severe, pathological and uncontrolled aggressive behavior associated with a psychiatric or neurological illness (e.g. temporal lobe epilepsy).

It is believed that the maximum improvement occurs in distress, tension, anxiety and agitation rather than in other symptoms. An intact, well-maintained premorbid personality is a good prognostic sign.

At present, psychosurgery is an extremely uncommonly used procedure in the routine psychiatric practice in India and most of the world.

Techniques

Before any procedure, an *informed consent* must be obtained by the neurosurgeon and the treat-ment team. Currently all techniques use *stereotactic methods*, so that the lesion made is precise and side-effects produced are few. The available procedures include bimedial leucotomy, orbital undercutting, rostral leucotomy, prefrontal leucotomy, anterior or posterior cingulumectomy and stereotactic tractotomy (in addition to those mentioned below).

The lesion is produced by electrocoagulation, freezing, thermocoagulation, ultrasonic method, Yttrium-90 seeds, or laser.

The currently employed procedures are:

1. Stereotactic Subcaudate Tractotomy

A large subcaudate lesion is produced. It is recommended for severe depression, severe anxiety, severe obsessive-compulsive disorder and schizo-affective disorder.

2. Stereotactic Limbic Leucotomy

A small subcaudate lesion is made, in addition to a lesion in cingulate bundle. It is used for treatment of intractable obsessive-compulsive disorder and schizophrenia.

3. Amygdalotomy

This is used for severe, pathological, uncontrolled and intractable aggression associated with neuropsychiatric disorders.

Side-Effects

With the use of stereotactic procedures, side-effects are very rare. These include a less than 1% risk of seizures, a very uncommon risk of personality change (which used to be frequent with earlier procedures) and a 1:1,000 to 1:10,000 mortality risk.

17
Psychoanalysis

The term psychoanalysis denotes:

1. A psychological theory of mind and personality development based primarily on the concept of intrapsychic 'conflict'.
2. A procedure for the investigation of unconscious psychical processes, otherwise inaccessible.
3. A therapeutic technique of treating psychiatric disorders by psychological means.

HISTORICAL OVERVIEW

Although the credit for 'invention' of psychoanalysis belongs to Sigmund Freud (1856-1939), he drew heavily from the work of several prominent researchers including Jean-Martin Charcot (hypnosis), Theodor Meynert (neuroanatomy and psychiatry), Ernst Brucke (physiology and physiochemistry). Hippolyte Bernheim (hypnosis) and Josef Breuer (hysteria), among others.

Although there were several changes, some of them even fundamental, in psychoanalysis, as Freud's thinking evolved over the years, an attempt is made here to illustrate the basic concepts of psychoanalysis as it existed near the end of Freud's career.

BASIC CONCEPTS

A. Topographic Theory of Mind

This theory was advanced in the year 1900 in '*The Interpretation of Dreams*'. Although it was later almost replaced by the structural theory, it is still useful in understanding the mental mechanisms.

The tripartite division of mind included the unconscious, the preconscious and the conscious.

1. The Unconscious

Much of the mental activity lies outside the sphere of consciousness. However this unconscious mental activity influences the conscious thought and behavior even if it is not available to voluntary recall.

The unconscious contains those ideas and affects which have been repressed (by the censor, as repression is known). This repressed material can only reach the consciousness through preconscious when the censor is relaxed (e.g. dreams, abreaction) or overpowered (e.g. slips of tongue, free association).

The unconscious mental activity is characterized by *primary process thinking* which is typically found in young children, severe psychosis, mental retardation and dreams. It is different from normal thinking (*secondary process thinking*) in that it strives for immediate discharge of drive energy, lacks contact with reality, is full of contradictions, lacks organization and logical connections, and is based on *pleasure principle.*

2. The Preconscious

This region of mind lies between the unconscious and the conscious with access to both. The unconscious mental contents can reach the conscious only through the preconscious. It is not present at birth but develops in childhood, paralleling the ego development. The censor lies here maintaining the repressive barrier.

The preconscious mental contents can easily become conscious with the focusing of attention.

3. The Conscious

The conscious constitutes a tiny position of the mind. Freud conceptualized it as a type of special sense organ of attention concerned with registration of stimuli from both within and without. The conscious mental contents are characterized by *secondary process thinking* based on *reality principle.*

In addition to the topographic model of mind, Freud also theorized the concept of *psychic determinism* which means that *all* mental activity is meaningful and purposeful, though unconscious, and is linked with previous life experiences. Hence no mental activity can be accidental or purposeless.

B. Structural Theory of Mind

In 1923, in *'The Ego and The Id'*, Freud divided the mental apparatus into three dynamic structures: the id, the ego and the super-ego (Fig. 17.1).

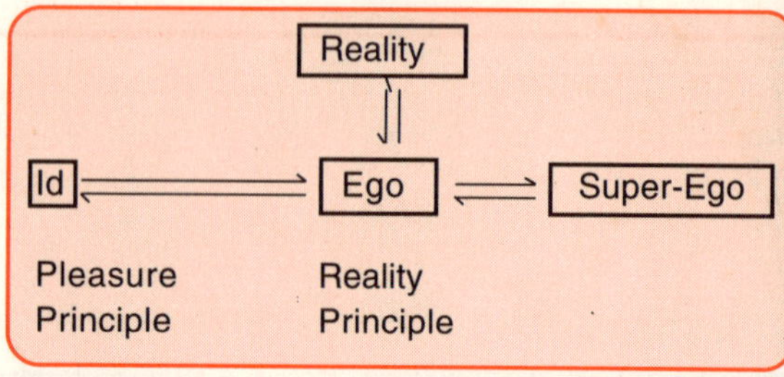

FIG. 17.1. STRUCTURAL THEORY OF MIND

1. The Id

The id is the original state of human mental apparatus with which a newborn baby is born. It is totally unconscious, containing the basic drives and instincts concerned with survival, sexual drive and aggression. It is characterized by primary process thinking and is based on pleasure principle, lacking any direct link with reality. The only urge of these drives is immediate gratification.

2. The Ego

The ego is primarily determined by the experience of reality and is therefore guided by the reality principle. It is predominantly conscious though some parts (like ego defense mechanisms) are unconscious. Ego maintains a balance between the id and the super-ego on one hand and the reality on the other.

For example, the individual observes a pleasurable object surrounded by a barrier. The id wants immediate gratification by obtaining the object, without seeing the reality of a barrier around it. The super-ego, on the other hand, proclaims that it is sinful to derive pleasure from an object surrounded by barrier. The ego strikes a balance between the two, as well as the real world, and decides to wait and find a way to 'climb' the barrier and derive pleasure. Although simplistic, the example illustrates the ego's function of delaying gratification in view of the reality.

The ego is the seat of conscious, intellectual, self preservative and defensive functions of mental apparatus.

3. The Super-ego

The super-ego is predominantly unconscious subdivision of mental apparatus that develops from the ego. It is specially concerned with moral standards and has 2 parts: a punitive conscience and a non-punitive ego ideal. Both derive from the effect of parental influence on the ego. This parental influence not only includes the effect of actual parents but also of the important family members, religion and important people in the surrounding environment. The criticisms, prohibitions,

TABLE 17.1. COMMONLY USED EGO DEFENSE MECHANISMS

Defense mechanism	*Definition*	*Example in normals*	*Clinical illustration*
A. PRIMARY			
1. Repression	Unconsciously excluding from conscious awareness of anxiety provoking ideas and/or feelings	1. 'Forgetting' 2. Slips of the tongue	1. Psychogenic amnesia
B. PSYCHOTIC / NARCISSISTIC			
1. Regression	Reversion to the modes of psychological functioning which are characteristic of earlier life stages, especially childhood years.	1. Dreams 2. *Regression in the service of ego.* (Ability of a mature adult to indulge periodically in playful childlike activities)	1. Neuroses (mild regression) 2. Psychoses (more pervasive regression) 3. Severe, prolonged physical illness
2. Denial	Involuntary exclusion of unpleasant or painful reality from conscious awareness.	1. Grief 2. Children (3-6 year olds)	1. Psychoses 2. Terminal illnesses
3. Projection	Unconscious attribution of one's own attitudes and urges to other person(s), because of intolerance or painful affect aroused by those attitudes and urges.	A universal phenomenon though occurs more commonly in children	1. Persecutory delusions and hallucinations
4. Distortion	Unconscious gross 'reshaping' of external reality to satisfy inner needs	—	1. Hallucinations 2. Delusions, especially of grandiosity
C. NEUROTIC / IMMATURE			
1. Conversion	A repressed, forbidden urge is simultaneously kept out of awareness and also expressed in symbolic/disguised form of some somatic disturbance (usually either motor or sensory)	Sometimes seen in normals when exposed to catastrophic stress; otherwise presence of a clear conversion 'reaction' always implies psychopathology	1. Conversion disorder (Hysteria)
2. Dissociation	Involuntary splitting or suppression of a mental function or a group of mental functions from rest of the personality in a manner that allows expression of forbidden unconscious impulses without having any sense of responsibility for actions	1. Near death experience	1. Dissociative disorders e.g. Psychogenic amnesia, Psychogenic fugue, Multiple personality, Somnambulism, Possession syndrome
3. Displacement	Unconscious shifting of emotions, usually aroused by perceived threat, from an unconscious impulse to a less threatening external object which is then felt to be the source of threat.	1. Normal, day-to-day deflection of 'anger' on a substitute target	1. Phobia (especially in children) 2. Obsessive compulsive disorder

Contd.

TABLE 17.1. (CONTD.)

Defense mechanism	*Definition*	*Example in normals*	*Clinical illustration*
4. Isolation (Isolation of affect)	Separation of the idea of an unconscious impulse from its appropriate affect, thus allowing only the idea and not the associated affect to enter awareness	1. Grief 2. Ability to discuss traumatic events without the associated disturbing emotions, with passage of time	1. Obsessional thoughts
5. Reaction formation	Unconscious transformation of unacceptable impulses into exactly opposite attitudes, impulses, feelings or behaviors	1. Normal character formation in childhood (from 3 years onwards)	1. Obsessive compulsive personality traits and disorder 2. Obsessive compulsive disorder
6. Undoing	Unconsciously motivated acts which magically/symbolically counteract unacceptable thoughts, impulses or acts	1. Checking of gas knobs or the locks to ensure safety 2. Automatically saying 'I am sorry' on bumping into somebody	1. Compulsive acts in Obsessive compulsive disorder 2. Compulsive rituals
7. Rationalization	Providing 'logical' explanations for irrational behavior motivated by unacceptable unconscious wishes.	A universal phenomenon	Usually used to explain behaviors resulting from other defense mechanisms.
8. Intellectualization	Excessive use of intellectual processes ('logic') to avoid affective expression ('emotion')	1. When faced with stressful situation, use of logic to focus closely on external reality and avoiding expression of inner feelings (e.g. fear)	—
9. Acting out	Expression of an unconscious impulse, through action, thereby gratifying the impulse	1. Destruction of property in a fit of rage	1. Impulse control disorders
10. Schizoid fantasy	Withdrawal into self to gratify frustrated wishes by fantasy	1. Seen in adolescence ('wish fulfilling daydreams')	1. Schizoid personality disorder 2. Schizotypal personality disorder
11. Turning against the self (Retroflexion)	Unconscious deflection of hostility towards another person onto oneself resulting in lowered self-esteem, self-criticism and at times injury to self	1. Head banging in children 2. Destruction of property or self in a fit of rage	1. Suicide 2. Severe depression 3. Any form of deliberate self harm (DSH)
12. Introjection	Unconscious internalization of the qualities of an object or person	1. Identification with the aggressor (e.g. sometimes seen in victims kidnapped by terrorists; also known as Stockholm syndrome) 2. Grief reaction	1. Depression

Contd.

TABLE 17.1. (CONTD.)

Defense mechanism	*Definition*	*Example in normals*	*Clinical illustration*
13. Hypochondriasis	Unconscious transformation of unacceptable impulses into inappropriate somatic concern	1. Abnormal illness behavior in physically disordered or normal individuals	1. Hypochondriasis
14. Inhibition	Involuntary decrease or loss of motivation to engage in some goal directed activity to prevent anxiety arising out of conflicts with unacceptable impulses	1. Writing 'blocks' or work 'blocks' 2. Social shyness	1. Obsessive compulsive disorder 2. Phobias
15. Compensation (Counterphobic defense)	Unconscious tendency to deal with a fear or conflict by unusual degree of effort in the opposite direction	1. Involvement in dare-devil activities (e.g. sky diving to counter fear of heights) 2. Excessive pre-occupation with body building to counter feelings of inferiority	1. Nymphomania (to counter a sense of sexual inadequacy) 2. Keeping excessive details in a diary in patients suffering from dementia
16. Splitting	Unconscious viewing of self or others as either good or bad without considering the whole range of qualities	1. Seeing all people without a mustache as feminine 2. Believing personalities to be either 'black' or 'white' without the shades of 'grey' (e.g. in a typical Hindi movie the Hero is all good and the Villain all bad)	Borderline personality disorder
D. MATURE			
1. Sublimation	Unconscious gradual channelization of unacceptable infantile or aggressive impulses into personally satisfying and socially valuable behavior patterns	1. Channelization of sexual or aggressive impulses into creative activities (e.g. diverting forbidden sexual impulses into artistic paintings)	—
2. Suppression (Voluntary)	Voluntary postponement of focusing of attention on an impulse which has reached conscious awareness	1. Voluntary decision not to think about an argument with parents while going for an interview	—
3. Anticipation	Realistic thinking and planning about future unpleasurable events	Anticipation is a universal phenomenon occurring in all intelligent persons	—
4. Humor	Overt expression of unacceptable impulses using humor in a manner which does not produce unpleasantness in self or others	A universal phenomenon	—

* *No ego defense mechanism is psychotic, neurotic, immature, mature or normal per se. Almost all mechanisms of defense are sometimes used in normal individuals. It is an exclusive or abnormally excessive use that makes a defense mechanism neurotic or psychotic.*

TABLE 17.2. PSYCHOSEXUAL STAGES OF DEVELOPMENT (FREUDIAN)

Phase	*Age range*	*Normal development*	*Psychiatric syndromes theorized to result from fixation at the regression to this stage*
1. Oral phase	Birth to 1-1½ years	Major site of gratification is the oral region. It consists of 2 phases : i. Oral erotic phase (sucking) ii. Oral sadistic phase (biting)	1. Dependent personality traits and disorder 2. Schizophrenia (oral and pre-oral phase) 3. Severe mood disorder 4. Alcohol dependence syndrome and drug dependence
2. Anal phase	1-1½ years to 3 years	Major site of gratification is the anal and peri-anal area; major achievement is the toilet training (sphincter control). It consists of 2 phases: i. Anal erotic phase (excretion) ii. Anal sadistic phase ('holding' and 'letting go' at will)	1. Obsessive compulsive personality traits and disorder 2. Obsessive compulsive disorder (Anal sadistic phase)
3. Phallic (Oedipal) phase	3 to 5 years	Major site of gratification is the genital area; genital masturbation is common at this stage. According to Freud, development is different in both sexes. *Male development* The boy develops *castration anxiety* (fear of castration at the hand of his father in retaliation for the boy's desire to replace his father in his mother's affections). This leads to formation of the *Oedipus complex* (aggressive impulses directed towards the father; named after the Greek tragedy *Oedipus rex* in which Oedipus unknowingly kills his father and marries his mother, unaware of their true identities). Oedipus complex is usually resolves by identification with father, attempting to adopt his characteristics *Female development* The girl develops *penis envy* (discontent with female genitalia following a fantasy that they result from loss of penis). This is theorized by Freud to lead to a wish to 'receive' the penis and to bear a child. Resolution occurs by identification with the mother. This phase has been called as *Electra complex*	1. Sexual deviations 2. Sexual dysfunctions 3. Neurotic disorders

Contd.

TABLE 17:2. PSYCHOSEXUAL STAGES OF DEVELOPMENT (FREUDIAN)

Phase	*Age range*	*Normal development*	*Psychiatric syndromes theorized to result from fixation at the regression to this stage*
4. Latency phase	5-6 years to 12 years	Oedipus (and Electra) complex is usually resolved at the beginning of this stage. This is a stage of relative sexual quiescence. *Superego* is formed at this stage. Sexual drive is channelized into socially appropriate goals like development of interpersonal relationships, sports, school work, etc.)	Neurotic disorders
5. Genital phase	12 years onwards)	Adult sexuality develops with capacity for intimacy (Puberty and respect for others. Gradual release from parental controls with more influence of peer group. True self identity develops	Neurotic disorders

* *The normal development described here is a simplified account of Sigmund Freud's theory of psychosexual development. Till date, it remains a theory; there is no empirical evidence for, say, Oedipus complex.*

guilt arousing statements and punishments are introjected as conscience.

On the other hand, the approvals and the rewards become introjected as the ego ideal. The ego ideal is later involved in the setting of goals and aspirations.

C. Mechanism of Ego Defense

The term ego defense mechanism refers to the various automatic, involuntary, and unconsciously instituted psychological activity by which the unacceptable urges or impulses are excluded from conscious awareness. These defense mechanisms are a function of ego.

The defense mechanisms usually operate on an unconscious level (except, for example, suppression which is a voluntary defense mechanism). In contrast, coping mechanisms are voluntary and conscious mechanisms of defense which an individual employs to deal with day-to-day external and conscious fears and conflicts.

There is no 'standard' list of defense mechanisms; however, a few commonly used ego defense mechanisms are listed in Table 17.1, along with definitions, clinical illustrations and examples in normal situations. No ego defense mechanism is psychotic, neurotic, immature, mature or normal. Almost all mechanisms of defense are sometimes used in normal individuals. It is an exclusive or abnormally excessive use that makes a defense mechanism neurotic or psychotic.

D. The Theory of Psychosexual Development

In 1905, in 'three essays on the theory of sexuality', Freud enunciated his theory of infantile sexuality and described the psychosexual stages of development (Table 17.2).

E. Theory of Dreams

Dream interpretation is a major component of psychoanalysis. Beginning with his own dream experiences, Freud analyzed dreams as 'the royal road to the unconscious'. He believed dreams to be conscious expression of unconscious fantasies or impulses which are not accessible to the individual in wakefulness, thereby providing gratification by wish fulfillment.

Since expression of unconscious forbidden fantasies can evoke considerable anxiety, these fantasies are considerably modified so as to preserve sleep on the one hand and provide gratification of the fantasies on the other. This modification is known as dream work. Here the unconscious forbidden fantasies or wishes which threaten to break sleep constitute the latent dream content, whereas the dream content modified by dream work constitutes the manifest dream content. According to Freud, the aim of dream interpretation is to get to the latent dream content from manifest dream content via free association, in order to understand the 'real meaning' of the dream experience.

The dream work consists of the following mechanisms:

1. Symbolism
2. Displacement
3. Condensation
4. Projection
5. Secondary elaboration (since dream content consists of *primary process thinking*, secondary elaboration is used to introduce logical thinking or *secondary process thinking* in the dream content).

In addition to the unconscious impulses, wishes and fantasies, the dream content is also influenced by:

1. Nocturnal sensory stimuli (e.g. thirst, hunger, full bladder).
2. Day residue (residue of day experiences of previous one or several days).

F. Psychoanalysis and Psychoanalytical Psychotherapy

Psychoanalysis and psychoanalytical psychotherapy as treatment methods are briefly discussed in Chapter 18.

18 Psychological Treatments

PSYCHOTHERAPY

Psychotherapy can be defined (modified from Wolberg) as, the treatment by psychological means, of problems of an emotional nature, in which a therapist deliberately establishes a professional relationship with the patient to,

1. Remove, modify or retard existing symptoms,
2. Mediate disturbed patterns of behavior, and/or
3. Promote positive personality growth and development.

Psychotherapy can be conducted by either verbal or non-verbal means.

There are several different kinds of psychotherapies. The important types are (Table 18.1):

1. Psychoanalysis and Psychoanalytical Psychotherapy

These psychotherapeutic methods are based primarily on Sigmund Freud's work, although many other techniques developed by other important workers (like Carl Jung, Alfred Adler, Erich Fromm, Harry Stack Sullivan, Karen Horney, Melanie Klein, Otto Rank, Wilhelm Reich and many others) are also in use.

A detailed discussion of Freudian Psychoanalysis is not attempted here (See Chapter 17). A very brief outline of therapy is presented.

TABLE 18.1. PSYCHOSOCIAL THERAPIES

Therapy/School	Proponent
1. Psychoanalysis	Sigmund Freud
2. Analytical psychology	Carl Gustav Jung
3. Transactional analysis	Eric Berne
4. Client-centered psychotherapy	Carl R Rogers
5. Hypnosis	James Braid
6. Group therapy	Joseph Pratt
7. Cognitive therapy	Aaron T Beck
8. Cognitive behavior therapy	Donald Meichenbaum
9. Behaviorism	John Broadus Watson
10. Classical conditioning	Ivan Petrovich Pavlov
11. Operant conditioning	Burrhus Frederic Skinner
12. Dual sex therapy	William Masters Virginia Johnson
13. Therapeutic community	Maxwell Jones
14. Psychodrama	Jacob L Moreno
15. Rational emotive therapy (RET)	Albert Ellis
16. Primal therapy	Arthur Janov
17. Will therapy	Otto Rank
18. Gestalt therapy	Frederich Perls
19. Existential logotherapy	Victor E Frankl
20. Reciprocal inhibition	Joseph Wolpe
21. Progressive muscular relaxation	E. Jacobson
22. Character analysis	Wilhelm Reich
23. Token economy	Ayllon and Azrin

A. Classical Psychoanalysis

Freudian Psychoanalysis typically needs 3-5 visits/week by the patient for a period of 3-5 years (even longer). No history taking, examination, or diagnosis is attempted. The patient is allowed to communicate unguided, by using '*free association*'.

The therapist remains passive and his approach is non-directive. He constantly challenges the existing 'defenses' and interprets *resistance* (during the therapy) and *transference* (patient's feelings, behavior and relationship with the therapist).

No advice is ever given to the patient. The crux of the therapy is on *interpretation*.

During the therapy, the patient typically lies on the couch, with the therapist sitting just out of vision.

No other therapy is used as adjunct.

B. Psychoanalytically-oriented Psychotherapy

Psychoanalytically oriented psychotherapy is a much more direct form of psychoanalysis. The duration of therapy is much briefer and advice is given to the patient occasionally. The patient and the therapist sit face-to-face. The rest of the method is nearly the same. However, additional modes of treatment, including drug therapy can be used.

The *indications* for both psychoanalysis and psychoanalytically oriented psychotherapy are not based on any psychiatric diagnoses.

The most important indication is the presence of long standing mental conflicts which, although are unconscious, produce symptomatology. The prerequisites of therapy are that the patient should be motivated for therapy, should have strong 'ego-structure' (which can bear frustrations of impulses during therapy), should be psychologically-minded and should not have significant life stressors.

It is usually used for the treatment of neurotic disorders and personality disorders.

2. Behavior Therapy

Behavior therapy is a type of psychotherapy (broadly defined) which is based on theories of learning, and aims at changing maladaptive behavior and substituting it with adaptive behavior.

Although, there are many theories of learning, a majority of behavior therapy techniques are based on operant conditioning model (Skinner) and classical conditioning model (Pavlov). Many of the ideas actually seem like common sense principles. The learning theories assume that all behavior is "learned behavior". The behavior that is followed by a reward is more likely to occur again (operant model), and that behavior is learned more easily if taught in small steps.

Behavior therapy is a short duration therapy, therapists are easy to train and it is cost-effective. The total duration of therapy is usually 6-8 weeks. Initial sessions are given daily but the later sessions are spaced out.

A *behavioral analysis* is usually carried out before planning behavior therapy. One of the simplest methods of behavior analysis is ABC charting, i.e. a close look at the *A*ntecedents (e.g. circumstances under which the behavior began; who, if any, were present; other details), *B*ehavior (description of the behavior in detail) and *C*onsequneces (what happened afterwards; what factors helped to maintain the behavior).

Some of the important behavioral techniques are described briefly.

A. Systematic Desensitization

Systematic desensitization (SD) is based on reciprocal inhibition principle (given by Wolpe). If a response incompatible with anxiety is made to occur at the same time as an anxiety provoking stimulus, then anxiety is reduced by reciprocal inhibition.

SD consists of 3 main steps:

i. Relaxation training (described later).
ii. Hierarchy construction.
Here the patient is asked to list all the conditions which provoke anxiety. Then, he is asked to list them in a descending order of anxiety provocation. Thus, a hierarchy of anxiety producing stimuli is prepared.
iii. Systematic desensitization proper.
This can be done either in Imagery (SD-I) or in reality/in-vivo (SD-R).

At first, the lowest item in hierarchy is confronted (in reality or in imagery). The patient is advised to signal whenever anxiety occurs. With each signal, he is asked to relax (Step-I). After a few trials, patient is able to control his anxiety.

Thus, gradually the hierarchy is climbed till the maximum anxiety provoking stimulus can be faced in the absence of anxiety.

SD is a treatment of choice in phobias and obsessive-compulsive disorders.

B. Aversion Therapy

Aversion therapy is used for the treatment of conditions which are pleasant but undesirable, e.g. alcohol dependence, transvestism, homo-sexuality, other sexual deviations.

The underlying principle is the pairing of the pleasant stimulus (e.g. alcohol) with an unpleasant response (e.g. brief electrical stimulus), so that even in absence of the unpleasant response (after therapy is over), the pleasant stimulus becomes unpleasant by association.

The unpleasant aversion is produced by electric stimulus (low voltage), drugs (like-apomorphine and disulfiram) or even by fantasy (when it is called as covert sensitization).

Typically, 20-40 sessions are given, with each session lasting about 1 hour. After completion of treatment, booster sessions may be given.

C. Operant Conditioning Procedures for Increasing a Behavior

The common methods for augmenting an adaptive behavior are:

i. *Positive reinforcement*. Here, the desirable behavior is reinforced by a reward, material or symbolic.
ii. *Negative reinforcement*. Here, on performance of the desirable behavior, punishment can be avoided.
iii. *Modeling*. The person is exposed to a 'model' behavior and is induced to copy it. This can also be used to avoid certain behaviors.

D. Flooding

This is a method used in treatment of phobias. Here, the person is directly exposed to the phobic stimulus, but escape is made impossible. By prolonged contact with the phobic stimulus, therapist's guidance and encouragement and therapist's modeling behavior, anxiety decreases.

E. Operant Conditioning Procedures for Decreasing a Behavior

These methods include:

i. *Time-out*. Here, the reinforcement is withdrawn for some time, contingent upon the undesired response. This is often used in therapy with children.
ii. *Punishment*. Aversive stimulus is here presented, contingent upon the undesired response (i.e., whenever the undesired response occurs, punishment is given).
iii. *Satiation*. The undesired response is positively reinforced, so that tiring occurs. A similar technique is *negative practice procedure*.

F. Other Behavioral Techniques

Last two decades have seen an explosion in the behavior therapy methodology. Many other techniques like token economy (for hospitalized patients), social-skills training (for patients with social difficulties), family therapy, marital therapy, and cognitive behavioral therapy are available. The interested reader is referred to the Reading List.

3. Cognitive Therapy or Cognitive Behavior Therapy

Cognitive therapy or cognitive behavior therapy (CBT) is a type of psychotherapy which aims at correcting the maladaptive methods of thinking, thus providing relief from symptoms. The therapist plays an active role, unlike in psychoanalysis.

Cognitive therapy is viewed by some as psychotherapy and by others as behavior therapy.

Developed separately by Beck and Meichenbaum, it is used for the treatment of depression, anxiety disorder, panic disorder, phobias, eating disorders, anticipatory anxiety, and also for teaching problem solving methods.

A typical cognitive therapy schedule consists of about 15 visits over a 3 month period.

Some important techniques in cognitive therapy are *cognitive techniques* (recognizing and correcting negative automatic thoughts, teaching reattribution techniques, increasing objectivity in perspectives, identifying and testing maladaptive assumptions, and decentering), *behavioral techniques* (activity scheduling, homework assignments, graded task assignment, behavioral rehearsal, role playing, and diversion techniques), and teaching *problem solving skills*.

4. Supportive Psychotherapy

This is a very direct method of psychotherapy, with the focus clearly on the existing symptoms and/or current life situations.

The aims of the therapy are:

i. Correction of the situational problem.
ii. Symptom rectification.
iii. Restoring or strengthening defenses.
iv. Prevention of emotional breakdown.
v. Teaching new coping skills.

The aim is achieved by a conglomeration of techniques which include guidance, suggestion, environmental manipulation, reassurance, persuasion, development of a doctor-patient relation-ship, diversion, and even hospitalization and medication.

This is a highly skilled method of psychotherapy which can provide excellent results when used judiciously.

5. Family and Marital Therapy

In family therapy and marital therapy (also called as *couples therapy*), the focus of intervention is not on the individual but is instead on the family as a unit or the marital unit.

There are several varieties of family and marital therapies, e.g. based on psychodynamic or behavioral principles. Whenever there are relational problems within a family or marital unit (either primarily or secondary to a psychiatric disorder), family and/or marital therapy is indicated.

For example, in a behavioral marital therapy, the components of therapy may include problem solving, training in communication skills, writing a behavioral marital contract, and home-work assignments.

6. Group Therapy

Group therapy or group psychotherapy is a less time consuming procedure in which usually 8-10 people can be treated at one time. This was first used by Joseph Pratt (an Internist) in 1905, for patients of tuberculosis.

Now, it is known that group therapy is not only time-saving but also especially beneficial for certain group of patients. Group therapy offers patients (and their relatives) an opportunity to realize that many others have and share problems which are very similar to their own problems, and that they are not alone in their suffering.

Typically, sessions are held once or twice a week, with each session lasting 1-2 hours (often 1½ hours). The patients usually sit in a circle.

Group therapy may utilize psychoanalytic, supportive, transactional or behavioral approaches.

Over the years, many types of group therapies have emerged like Self-help groups (Alcoholics Anonymous for alcoholics, Weight Watchers for obese, Phoenix-House for opiate addicts), Transactional Analysis groups (Eric Berne), Training groups (Kurt Lewin), Psychodrama (Jacob Moreno) and the like.

7. Suggestion

Although an integral part of supportive psychotherapy, it is often used alone. It is used by nearly all medical practitioners, without realizing or naming it as such.

It is suggestion, which is largely responsible for the placebo-response. A placebo prescribed confidently by an impressive physician can lead to some improvement in about 33% of patients.

8. Hypnosis

Hypnosis is a state of artificially induced (by self or others) increased suggestibility.

There is a constriction in the peripheral awareness with increased focal concentration on task at hand. Trance phenomena were routinely utilized by Anton Mesmer in 1775 who called this force as *animal magnetism*. The word *hypnotism* was first used by James Braid in the 19th century.

Not everyone can be hypnotized. The capacity for hypnosis is called *hypnotizability*, which can be measured in a person by using tests like the *eye roll sign* or *hand levitation* test. Basically, these tests measure suggestibility.

About 60% of the general population can be hypnotized but only 5-10% reach deep hypnotic trance.

A wide variety of techniques are available for induction of hypnosis.

Following changes occur commonly during hypnotic trance:

i. The person under hypnosis becomes highly suggestible to the commands of hypnotist, without understanding their nature.
ii. Dissociation of a part of body or emotions from the remainder may occur.
iii. There is a partial or complete amnesia for the events occurring during the hypnotic trance.
iv. There is an ability to produce or remove symptoms, perceptions and/or movements.
v. Post-hypnotic suggestion can be given just after the trance and it is followed by the hypnotized person.

Persons who are hypnotizable are in no way abnormal as compared to the rest of the population.

Indications in Psychiatry

i. As an adjunct to psychotherapy.
ii. To abreact past experiences.

The conditions in which hypnosis can help in treatment are many. The most important ones are listed below.

i. Psychosomatic disorders
ii. Conversion disorder (hysteria)
iii. Dissociative disorder (hysteria)
iv. Eating disorders (anorexia nervosa, bulimia nervosa and obesity)

v. Habit disorders (smoking)
vi. Pain
vii. Anxiety disorder.

9. Abreaction

Abreaction is an important procedure which brings to the conscious awareness, for the first time, unconscious conflicts and associated emotions.

The release of emotions is therapeutic. Although abreaction is an integral part of psychoanalysis and hypnosis, it can be used independently also.

Abreaction can be done with or without the use of medication.

Abreaction with Medication

Earlier amphetamines, ether, nitrous oxide and lysergic acid diethylamide (LSD) have been used for abreaction. Particularly, intravenous amphetamines were very successful as they lead to a marked increase in productivity of speech, thus facilitating release of unconscious ideas and emotions.

These agents are no longer commonly used in clinical practice, due to risk of dependence (in case of amphetamines and LSD) or side-effects. A safe method is the use of 5% solution of sodium amobarbital (amytal) or thiopentone sodium (pentothal), i.e. 500 mg dissolved in 10 cc. of normal saline. It is infused at a rate no faster than 1 cc/min to prevent sleep as well as respiratory depression.

The abreactive procedure is begun with neutral topics at first, gradually approaching area(s) of conflicts. Usually about 150-350 mg (3-7 cc.) of amytal is sufficient for the purpose. In elderly and patients with organic brain disorder, even 75 mg of amytal may produce excessive drowsiness.

The indications of *amytal interview* include:

i. Abreaction (mainly) e.g. in hysteria.
ii. Interview with a mute patient.
iii. Diagnostic test in catatonic syndrome.
iv. Differentiating test in stupor (for differential diagnosis of depression, schizophrenia, hysteria and organic brain disorder).

There are certain *contraindications* for the use of amytal interview:

i. Airway disease including upper respiratory tract infection.
ii. Severe renal or hepatic disease.
iii. History of porphyria.
iv. Hypotension.
v. Dependence on barbiturates.
vi. Psychosis (except for catatonia or stupor).

This is a contraindication for performing abreaction but not for amytal interview.

The other medications which can be used successfully for abreaction are diazepam (15-40 mg parenterally) and ketamine (30-90 mg parenterally; especially for mute patients).

10. Relaxation Therapies

The aim is to induce profound muscular relaxation. Since anxiety produces muscular tension which in turn reinforces (and thus increases) anxiety, any relaxation technique would decrease anxiety and muscular tension both.

Relaxation techniques are an integral part of a majority of behavior therapies, e.g. systematic desensitization.

There are many methods which can be used to induce relaxation and these include:

A. *Jacobson's progressive muscular relaxation*: This is the most frequently used technique. Patient first tenses and then relaxes major muscle groups of the body in a prefixed and systematic order, usually beginning at the top of the body and progressing downwards.

B. *Hypnosis*

C. *Transcendental meditation (TM)* or *Yoga*

D. *'Shavasna'* ('The corpse posture'): Similar to progressive relaxation but the sequence of progression is below upwards.

E. *Yog Nindra, Pranayama* and *Vipasna* are other Indian methods.

F. *Biofeedback.*

11. Biofeedback

Biofeedback (introduced for the first time in 1969) is the use of an instrument (usually electronic) which provides immediate feedback to the patient regarding his physiological activities normally not available to the conscious mind, e.g. EKG, EEG, pulse rate, blood pressure, EMG, galvanic skin response (GSR).

The feedback helps the patient, apparently to control these responses. Relaxation is easily achieved by this method.

A simpler form ('relaxometer') uses only one parameter, the GSR.

Other uses of biofeedback include treatment of enuresis, migraine headaches, tension headache, idiopathic hypertension, incontinence, cardiac arrhythmias, uncontrolled generalized tonic clonic seizures and also for neuromuscular rehabilitation.

12. Rehabilitation

Psychiatric rehabilitation is defined as restoration of the fullest physical, mental, social, vocational, and economic usefulness of which the person suffering from psychiatric disorder is capable.

A large number of patients with psychiatric disorders (e.g. schizophrenia) have a poor quality of life, residual symptoms, and long term disability. Although early recognition and treatment is the cornerstone of preventing long term disability, a substantial number of patients need rehabilitation.

There are several components and methods available for rehabilitation, depending on the type and/or stage of disorder and the type of support available to the patient. Necessarily, a complete assessment is needed before deciding on the individualized rehabilitation for a particular patient.

Some of the methods used for psychiatric rehabilitation include *housing placement* (e.g. half way homes, supervised housing), *vocational training and rehabilitation* (e.g. activity therapy, sheltered workshop, transitional/supported employment, vocational guidance, occupational therapy), and *treatment* (e.g. ensuring compliance with medication, social skills therapy, family therapy, cognitive remediation).

There is an acute shortage of psychiatric rehabilitation facilities in most parts of India. The *Persons with Disabilities (Equal Opportunities, Protection of Rights, and Full Participation) Act (PDA), 1995* is a step forward, as it includes psychiatric disorders and mental retardation.

13. Indian Perspective

Just about the time Freud was practicing psychoanalysis, Girindra Shekhar Bose was using his own version of psychoanalysis in Calcutta. However, currently psychoanalysis is not widely used in India.

It is believed by some that most Indian patients, as compared to patients in Western, developed countries, are not psychologically minded and are unable to introspect. They lack verbal fluency and have more physical symptoms.

The Indian patients have difficulty in maintaining one-to-one relationship with the physician-psychiatrist, as they believe him to be a healer who is of higher status than them (something like a Guru; Guru-Chela relationship, a concept given by J.S. Neki).

Psychoanalysis (which avoids giving direct advice) is difficult, as patients expect the therapist to guide them and make decisions for them. They are also fatalistic ('This had to happen'; 'it is the result of destiny and past *karma*') and often have magical expectations of cure.

Most psychotherapists in India agree that the western models of psychotherapy can not be directly transplanted in Indian setting. Psychotherapy in a majority of Indian patients should be preferably brief, direct, crisis-oriented, with the therapist playing an active role.

However, in psychologically minded and educated Indian patients, the western models can be used with or without modification.

The commonest type of psychotherapy used in India is supportive psychotherapy.

19 Emergency Psychiatry

An *emergency* is defined as an unforeseen combination of circumstances which calls for an immediate action.

A *medical emergency* is defined as a medical condition which endangers life and/or causes great suffering to the individual.

A *psychiatric emergency* is a disturbance in thought, mood and/or action which causes sud-den distress to the individual (or to significant others) and/or sudden disability, thus requiring immediate management.

A similar term *crisis* means a situation that presents a challenge to the patient, the family and/or the community.

TYPES OF PSYCHIATRIC EMERGENCIES

A psychiatric emergency can be one or more of the following:

1. A new psychiatric disorder with acute onset.
2. A chronic psychiatric disorder with relapse.
3. An organic psychiatric disorder.
4. An abnormal response to stressful situation.
5. Iatrogenic emergencies.
   i. Side-effects or toxicity of psychotropic medication.
   ii. Psychiatric symptomatology as a side-effect or toxicity of other medications.
6. Alcohol or drug dependence.
   i. Withdrawal syndrome.
   ii. Overdose.
   iii. Complications.
7. Deliberate harm to self or others.

EXAMINATION

When faced with a psychiatric emergency, it is important to combine speed with obtaining of complete/adequate information. A scheme for an emergency psychiatric evaluation is presented here:

I. Psychiatric History

Always obtain history from both the patient and the informant(s). Informant(s) may be more coherent and may provide more relevant information.

i. *Chief complaint*: elaborate, with emphasis on dating of onset and progression.
ii. *Recent life-changes*: like any losses (real or imaginary), any physical illnesses.
iii. *Level of adjustment* prior to the psychiatric emergency.
iv. *Past history* (briefly) of any physical or psychiatric disorder.
v. *Family history* (briefly) of any physical or psychiatric disorder.
vi. *Drug and alcohol history*: prescription drugs, street drugs and alcohol dependence or abuse.

II. Detailed General Physical and Neurological Examination

It is essential to rule out (or diagnose) secondary psychiatric disorders, with particular emphasis on presence of any head injury.

III. Mental Status Examination

i. Screen for *organicity* (most important). Test for consciousness, orientation, attention, concentration, memory, intelligence, abstract thinking, insight and judgement.
   Also test for aphasias, apraxias, alexias, agraphias, dysarthrias and anomias.
ii. Brief mental status examination to diagnose or rule out any psychiatric disorder.
iii. Particular emphasis should be placed on the presence of suicidal or homicidal ideation.

COMMON PSYCHIATRIC EMERGENCIES

I. Suicide

Suicide is the model of psychiatric emergencies and is also the commonest cause of death among psychiatric patients.

Suicide is a type of *deliberate self harm* (DSH) and is defined as a human act of self-intentioned and self-inflicted cessation (death). It ends with a fatal outcome.

An *attempted suicide* is an unsuccessful suicidal act with a non-fatal outcome. It is believed that 2-10% of all persons who attempt suicide, eventually complete suicide in the next 10 years.

A *suicidal gesture*, on the other hand, is an *attempted suicide* where the person performing the action never intends to die by the act. However, some of these persons may accidentally die during the act. Attempted suicide is more common in women while completed suicide is 2-4 times commoner in men.

Epidemiology

Suicide is among the top 10 causes of death in India and most other countries. The official suicide rate in India is 9.9/lakh population/year (1994 figures). However, as there is considerable under-reporting of the suicidal behavior, the probable suicide rate per year in India would be around 10-15/lakh population.

TABLE 19.1. COMMON THEMES IN SUICIDE

1. It is a crisis that causes intense suffering and feelings of hopelessness and helplessness.
2. There is a conflict between survival and unbearable stress.
3. There is a narrowing of the person's perceived options.
4. There is a wish to escape (it is an escape, rather than a going-towards).
5. There is often a wish to punish self and/or punish significant others with guilt.

The comparable period prevalence rate for suicide throughout the world ranges from 5-30/lakh population/year. The World Health Report, 2001, estimates that every year one million people worldwide commit suicide, while 10-20 million people attempt suicide.

Thus the ratio of attempted suicide to completed suicide is 10-20:1. In India, the highest suicide rate is in the age group of 18-30 years. Some of the highest rates of suicide in India are reported from Pondicherry, West Bengal, Madras and Bangalore.

Etiology

Some of the common causes of suicide are:

I. Psychiatric Disorders

Psychiatric disorders are a major cause of suicide. Some common causes are:

1. Depression
   i. Major depression.
   ii. Depression secondary to serious physical illness.
   iii. Reactive depression, secondary to life stressors, e.g. family and/or marital disputes, failure in goal achievement, occupational and financial difficulties, and death of significant others.

2. Alcoholism and drug dependence.
3. Schizophrenia.

Genetic factors (a concordance rate of 18% in monozygotic twins) and biochemical factors (low levels of 5-HIAA) are important in some cases of suicide.

II. Physical Disorders

Patients with incurable or painful physical disorders, like cancer and AIDS, often commit suicide (up to 13.5% of all suicides in some studies from India).

III. Psychosocial Factors

Psychosocial factors are a very important cause of suicide. Some examples are failure in examination, failure in love, dowry difficulties, marital difficulties, illegitimate pregnancy, family dispute or psychopathology, loss of a loved object by death or other means, occupational and financial difficulties, and social isolation.

Methods Used

In India, the commonest mode of committing suicide is by ingestion of poisons (about 35%) followed by hanging (about 23%), drowning (about 9%), jumping in front of a train (4%), and burning (12%).

TABLE 19.2. RISK FACTORS FOR SUICIDE

The presence of the following factors increases the risk of completed suicide:

1. Age > 40 years
2. Male sex
3. Staying single
4. Previous suicidal attempt(s)
5. Depression (risk about 25 times more than normal)
   i. Presence of guilt, self-accusation, agitation, nihilistic ideation, worthlessness, hypochondriacal delusions and/or severe insomnia
   ii. More at the beginning or towards the end of a depressive episode
6. Suicidal preoccupation (e.g. a 'suicide note' is written or detailed plans are made for committing suicide)
7. Alcohol or drug dependence
8. Severe, disabling, painful or untreatable physical illness
9. Recent serious loss or major stressful life event
10. Social isolation.

Men often use more violent methods for suicide as compared with women.

Medico-Legal Aspects

Under the Indian law, suicide and attempted suicide were till very recently punishable offenses.

TABLE 19.3. COMMON MISCONCEPTIONS ABOUT SUICIDE
(Modified from Shneidman and Farberow, 1961)

Misconceptions	Facts
1. People who talk about suicide, don't commit suicide. 2. Suicide happens without warning.	Nearly 80% of persons who commit suicide, give definite warnings and/or clues about their suicidal intentions.
3. Suicidal persons are fully intent on dying.	Most suicidal persons are undecided about dying or living.
nce a person is suicidal, he is suicidal rever.	Suicidal person is suicidal only for a limited period of time.
suicidal persons are mentally ill or ychotic.	Although the suicidal person is often extremely unhappy, he is not necessarily mentally ill.

Section 309 of IPC states that "whoever attempts to commit suicide and does any act towards the commission of such offense, shall be punishable with simple imprisonment for a term which may extend to one year and shall also be liable to fine".

It was argued that the law esteems the lives of men as not only valuable to their own possessors but also valuable to the State which protects them and for the protection of which the State exists. The State therefore had the right to prevent persons from taking their own lives. However, it compounded the sufferings of a person who survived after a suicide attempt by making him/her a punishable offender.

Section 309 of IPC was repealed by the Supreme Court of India in 1994. However, in March 1996, a five judge Constitution Bench of the Supreme Court again made 'attempt to suicide' a punishable offense. So, the Section 309 IPC continues to be valid at present.

Management

Once suicide is committed, it is no longer treatable. The management obviously lies in preventing the act.

This can be done at suicide prevention centers, crisis intervention centers (both of these are not available as yet on a large scale in India), psychiatric emergency services, medical emergency services, social welfare centers (like Samaritans, Sanjivini, Maitri, Sumaitri, Befrienders International) or even at home (of the patient).

The important steps for preventing suicide are:

1. Take all suicidal threats, gestures and/or attempts seriously and notify a psychiatrist.
2. Psychiatrist should quantify the seriousness of the situation and take remedial precautionary measures.
   i. Inspect physical surroundings and remove all means of committing suicide, like sharp objects, ropes, drugs, firearms etc. Also search the patient thoroughly.
   ii. Surveillance, depending on the severity of risk.
3. Acute psychiatric emergency interview.
4. Counseling and guidance
   i. to deal with the desire to attempt suicide.
   ii. to deal with ongoing life stressors, and teaching coping skills and interpersonal skills.
5. Treatment of psychiatric disorder with medication, psychotherapy and/or ECT. ECT is the treatment of choice for patients with major depression with suicidal risk. It should also be used for the treatment of suicidal risk associated with psychotic disorders.
6. Follow-up care is very important to prevent future suicidal attempts or suicide.

II. Stupor and Catatonic Syndrome

Stupor is a common condition which presents at the emergency services. It is defined as a clinical syndrome of *akinesis* and *mutism* but with relative preservation of conscious awareness. The term stupor, traditionally, has a psychiatric connotation, but a careful analysis of stuporous patients shows that a large majority has an underlying organic cerebral cause.

Stupor is often associated with catatonic signs and symptoms (catatonic withdrawal or *catatonic stupor*). Catatonic syndrome is any disorder which presents with at least two catatonic signs. Catatonia can be either excited or withdrawn. Only catatonic withdrawal is associated with stupor.

The various catatonic signs include mutism, negativism, stupor, ambitendency, echolalia, echopraxia, automatic obedience, posturing,

TABLE 19.4. CAUSES OF CATATONIC STUPOR

I. Neurological Disorders
- i. Post-encephalitic parkinsonism
- ii. Limbic encephalitis
- iii. Surgical procedures on basal ganglia
- iv. Neoplasms in diencephalon, frontal lobe and limbic system
- v. Subacute sclerosing panencephalitis (SSPE)
- vi. General paresis of insane (GPI)
- vii. Petit mal status
- viii. Post-ictal phase of epilepsy
- ix. Subdural hematoma
- x. Cerebral malaria
- xi. Cortical venous thrombosis

II. Systemic and Metabolic Disorders
- i. Diabetic ketoacidosis
- ii. Acute intermittent porphyria
- iii. Hyperparathyroidism causing hypercalcemia
- iv. Pellagra
- v. Hepatic encephalopathy
- vi. Systemic lupus erythematosis
- vii. Homocystinuria
- viii. Membranous glomerulonephritis

III. Drugs and Poisoning
- i. Organic alkaloids
- ii. Antipsychotics
- iii. ACTH (therapeutic doses)
- iv. Aspirin
- v. Illuminating gas
- vi. Ethyl alcohol (large doses)
- vii. Levodopa
- viii. Disulfiram
- ix. CO poisoning
- x. Lithium toxicity
- xi. Methylphenidate
- xii. Phencyclidine (large doses)
- xiii. Mescaline

IV. Psychiatric Disorders
- i. Catatonic schizophrenia
- ii. Depressive stupor
- iii. Manic stupor
- iv. Periodic catatonia
- v. Conversion & dissociative disorder
- vi. Reactive psychosis
- vii. During hypnosis.

mannerisms, stereotypies; excitement (not goal directed), impulsiveness, combativeness or nudism.

Etiology

A wide variety of disorders can cause catatonic stupor. The important causes are listed in Table 19.4.

Differential Diagnosis

It is of foremost importance to differentiate between organic stupor and psychogenic (or so called 'functional') stupor. This can be done on the basis of antecedent medial and psychiatric history, the mode of onset, and detailed physical and neurological examination.

The important differentiating points between organic and psychogenic stupor are tabulated in Table 19.5.

If a diagnosis of organic catatonic stupor is made, a search for underlying cause should be made. On the other hand, if pentothal/amytal interview reveals psychopathology, appropriate treatment can be instituted.

Examination

The examination consists of the following steps:

1. History and physical examination, with special emphasis on neurological examination.
2. Level of consciousness should ideally be rated on the Glasgow Coma Scale. This scale consists of three main categories of activity, namely eye opening (1-4), motor response (1-5) and verbal response (1-5). The rating is done on a scale of 3 to 14.
3. Pentothal/amytal interview is sometimes very helpful in differentiating organic and psychogenic catatonic stupor.
4. Investigations: Blood glucose, blood urea, serum creatinine, serum electrolytes, blood (arterial) gas analysis, EKG, blood and urine examination for drugs and poisons, blood and urine culture, peripheral smear for malarial parasite.

TABLE 19.5. ORGANIC AND PSYCHOGENIC STUPOR

	Organic Stupor	Psychogenic Stupor
1. Previous psychiatric illness	Usually absent	Usually present
2. Previous medical illness	Usually present	Usually absent
3. Previous history of stupor	10%	24-33%
4. Precipitating stressor	Usually absent	Usually present
5. Frequency	Much more common	Not so common (3-5% of all stupor cases)
6. Onset	Sudden or insidious	Often sudden
7. Course	Longer	Shorter. Recovery usually within 7 days
8. Protective reflexes (Blepharospasm, menace reflex, protective response)	Absent	Present
9. Resistance to eye opening	Absent	Usually present
10. Doll's head eye phenomenon (Oculocephalic reflex)	Usually present	Absent (avoids the gaze of examiner)
11. Meaningful posture and/or facial expressions	Absent	May be present
12. Urinary/fecal incontinence	Usually present	Unlikely
13. Neurological signs and deficits	May be present	Absent
14. Abnormal EEG	More often	Less often
15. Oculovestibular reflex	Absent	Present
16. Pentothal/amytal interview	Low dose (100-150 mg) increases stupor and neurological signs develop or increase	High dose (300-400 mg) increases alertness and a mental status examination can often be done
17. Mortality	35%	0-3%

Also hemoglobin, total leucocyte count (TLC), differential leucocyte count (DC), ESR, urine (routine and microscopic) examination, thyroid and adrenal functions, liver function tests, CSF examination, gastric lavage with examination of aspirate, EEG and CT scan/MRI scan brain (if indicated).

Management

Since psychogenic stupor may easily be mistaken for organic stupor and coma, certain steps must be taken even before detailed examination is done, to prevent irreversible brain damage and death which may otherwise occur. These steps should be taken in management of any unconscious patient.

1. Ensure patency of airway; and provide ventilatory support with oxygen (for possible hypoxia).
2. Check cardiac rhythm and stabilize it.
3. Maintain circulation; insert IV (Intravenous) line and give fluids (for possible fluid and electrolyte imbalance).

4. Investigations; withdraw blood, CSF and urine samples, before instituting any treatment.
5. 50 ml. of 50% dextrose (2 ml/kg body weight for a child) should be given IV (for possible hypoglycemia).
6. Administer:
   Naloxone 0.4 mg IV (if morphine poisoning is suspected);
   Physostigmine 1-2 mg IV (if anticholinergic poisoning is suspected);
   Thiamin 100 mg IV (if Wernicke's encephalopathy or delirium tremens is suspected);
   Hydrocortisone 100 mg IV (if adrenal crisis is suspected);
   L-Thyroxin 200-500 μg IV (if myxedemic coma is suspected);
   Flumazenil 0.2 mg IV (if benzodiazepine overdose is suspected).

This should be followed by a detailed workup. The underlying medical or psychiatric cause of stupor should be searched for and treated. The importance of supportive care during the period of stupor can not be overemphasized.

III. Excited Behavior and Violence

Excitement is a common reason for a referral to a emergency psychiatry setting. Although, a large majority of psychiatric patients are not dangerously violent, some patients are indeed aggressive especially during the acute phase.

Etiology

Some common causes of excited behavior are listed below.

I. Organic psychiatric disorders
   1. Delirium (acute organic brain syndrome), e.g. delirium tremens.
   2. Dementia, e.g. catastrophic reaction, loss of control.
   3. Wernicke-Korsakoff's psychosis.

II. Non-organic psychiatric disorders
   1. Schizophrenia and other psychoses.
      i. Schizophreniform psychosis.
      ii. Catatonic (excited) schizophrenia.
      iii. Paranoid schizophrenia.
      iv. Acute psychotic disorder.
   2. Mania.
      Although excitement is common, violence occurs only when the patient is interfered with in his activities, or when he is irritable.
   3. Depression.
      Agitated depression may present with excitement. Occasionally aggressive, violent behavior may occur if the patient is irritable and agitated.
   4. Drug and alcohol dependence.
      Excitement and violence may occur in,
      i. Intoxication.
      ii. Withdrawal syndrome.
   5. Epilepsy.
      i. Complex partial seizures.
      ii. Post-ictal confusion.
      iii. Epileptic furor.
   6. Acute stress reaction.
   7. Neurotic disorders.
      i. Panic disorder.
      ii. Agoraphobia with panic attacks.
      Marked excitement occurs during panic attack but violent behavior does not occur.
   8. Impulsive violent behavior
      i. Borderline personality disorder
      ii. Intermittent explosive disorder.
   9. Reactive psychosis.

Management

The patient is examined according to the guidelines suggested earlier in this chapter. The physician or psychiatrist handling an excited patient must demonstrate an attitude of kindness but at the same time must be firm and should exude confidence.

The measures which can be adopted to handle excited or violent behavior include:

1. *Reassurance*: In case of emergency, it rarely works alone but must be tried first.

2. *Sedation*: Diazepam 10-20 mg IV slowly can be given. In the presence of psychosis, haloperidol (Serenace) 10-20 mg IV or IM, with or without 10 mg diazepam or 50 mg of promethazine (Phenergan) can be given. Chlorpromazine (Largactil) 50-100 mg IM can also be given but painful injection abscess at the injection site may develop. It should never be given IV, as severe hypotension can occur.
3. *Restraint*: Restraint should always be used as a last resort, but when needed it must not be delayed. Restraint should always be done in a humane way, after taking (preferably) written consent from the attendant relatives.

   Restraint is usually followed by compulsory hospitalization and parenteral medication. It is rarely ever necessary to continue restraint for more than a few hours and restraint should be removed at the earliest possible time.

Electroconvulsive therapy (ECT) is not a treatment for excitement or violence per se. When used, there should be a clear indication for the use of ECT, which should be clearly recorded in the case file.

IV. Other Psychiatric Emergencies

The list of possible psychiatric emergencies is long. A few psychiatric emergencies are listed below, some of which have already been discussed in the book.

1. *Severe depression* (Chapter 6): Apart from presenting as a suicide/suicidal attempt and/or agitation, the depressive patient may come to casualty because of refusal to eat and drink leading to dehydration or because of refusal to take medication (e.g. hopelessness - "I can not be cured").
2. *Hyperventilation syndrome* (Chapter 8).
3. *Side-effects of psychotropic medication*, e.g. acute dystonia (promptly relieved by promethazine 25-50 mg IV), akathisia, neuroleptic malignant syndrome (Chapter 15).
4. *Psychiatric complications of medical and surgical diseases*, procedures and medication (e.g. ICU syndrome, severe depression caused by reserpine).
5. *Insomnia* (Chapter 11).
6. *Pseudo-seizures* (conversion and/or dissociation hysteria) (Chapter 8).
7. *Anorexia nervosa* (usually presenting with dehydration and/or cachexia) (Chapter 12).
8. *Battered child syndrome* or *child abuse*.
9. *Grief and bereavement* (Chapter 12).
10. *Psychosocial crises* (e.g. marital conflict, occupational and financial difficulties).
11. *Drug or alcohol use disorders* (Chapter 4).
12. *Panic disorder* (Chapter 8).
13. Acute psychosis (Chapter 7).

Psychiatric patients, especially when excited or emotionally disturbed, often arouse anxiety in treating physicians as well as other patients in the casualty. So, it is necessary to have an 'emergency psychiatry room' or 'psychiatric holding area' near the casualty, where the patients can be interviewed and treated.

An ideal place for treating psychiatric emergencies is a separate 'psychiatric intensive care unit' (PICU) or 'crisis intervention center' (CIC) attached to a psychiatric unit in a general hospital or to a psychiatric hospital or nursing home.

20 Legal and Ethical Issues in Psychiatry

Forensic psychiatry deals with the legal aspects of psychiatry.

Law comes in contact with psychiatry at many points. For example: admission of a mentally ill person in a mental hospital; crime committed by a mentally ill person; validity of marriage, witness, will, consent; right to vote; drug dependence.

The various legal aspects of psychiatry are briefly discussed below.

CRIMINAL RESPONSIBILITY

In January 1843, a young Scotsman, Daniel McNaughten shot dead Edward Drummond, the secretary to the British Prime Minister Sir Robert Peel. He had intended to kill the Prime Minister but Drummond was assassinated by mistake.

The Jury, after testification by 9 physicians, found McNaughten 'not guilty by reasons of insanity'. Queen Victoria, Sir Robert Peel and other prominent persons were outraged. Following this, 15 prominent judges were invited by the House of Lords. They were asked to respond to a series of questions on criminal responsibility. The answers, which are immortalized in the history of forensic psychiatry, have now come to be known as *McNaughten Rule(s)*.

McNaughten Rule is used in a slightly modified form in many countries even now. In India, Section 84 of Indian Penal Code (Act 45 of 1860) states that 'nothing is an offense, which is done by a person, who at the time of doing it, by reason of unsoundness of mind, is incapable of knowing the nature of the act or that he is doing what is either wrong or contrary to law'.

So, a mentally ill person in not protected *ipso facto*. He must satisfy the above mentioned rule.

An 'idiot' (mentally retarded person) is not liable in criminal law.

Law classifies 'criminal lunatics' into 3 classes:

i. An undertrial, who can not stand trial because of mental illness.
ii. Guilty but insane.
iii. Criminals who later become mentally ill.

A Class II criminal lunatic is acquitted but is detained in a mental hospital (asylum) for treatment.

CIVIL RESPONSIBILITY

There is a presumption in favor of sanity and the contrary must be proved. This applies both to civil and criminal proceedings in the court of law.

I. Marriage

The *Hindu Marriage Act* (Act 25 of 1955) provides for conditions for a Hindu Marriage under Section 5. One of the conditions, Section 5 (ii) introduced by Act 68 of 1976, states that 'at the time of the marriage, neither party,

a. is incapable of giving a valid consent... (due to)...unsoundness of mind; or
b. though capable of giving consent, has been suffering from mental disorder of such a kind or to such an extent as to be unfit for marriage and the procreation of children; or
c. has been subject to recurrent attacks of insanity or epilepsy.'

Any marriage solemnized in contravention to this condition shall be voidable and may be *annulled* by a decree of nullity under Section 12 of the Act. Another ground of nullity under the same section is the fact that the consent for marriage was obtained by 'fraud'...'as to any material fact or circumstance concerning the respondent', for example, the fact of mental illness or treatment for the same.

Divorce can be granted under Section 13 of the Act on a petition presented by either spouse on the ground that the other party 'has been incurably of unsound mind, or has been suffering continuously or intermittently from mental disorder of such kind and to such an extent that the petitioner can not reasonably be expected to live with the respondent' (Section 13 (iii) inserted by Act 68 of 1976).

Here, the term mental disorder means 'mental illness, arrested or incomplete development of mind, psychopathic disorder or any other disorder or disability of mind and includes schizophrenia'. The term psychopathic disorder means 'a persistent disorder or disability of mind (whether or not including subnormality of intelligence) which results in abnormally aggressive or seriously irresponsible conduct on the part of the other party, and whether or not it requires or is susceptible to medical treatment'.

Under the *dissolution of Muslim Marriages Act 1939*, a woman married under Muslim law is entitled to obtain a decree for the dissolution of marriage on the ground of her husband being insane for a period of 2 years. The husband under the Muslim law has the power to pronounce divorce (*talak*) at any time, anywhere, and without assigning any reason.

Any married person may be granted divorce, under the *Parsi Marriage and Divorce Act 1936*, on the ground that the other party had been of unsound mind at the time of marriage (and the petitioner was ignorant of the fact) and has been habitually so till the date of petition, which should be within 3 years of the date of marriage.

II. Adoption

Under the Hindu Adoptions and Maintenance Act (Act 78 of 1956), any Hindu male 'who is of sound mind and is not a minor' can adopt a child, with the consent of his wife unless '...(she) has been declared by a court...to be of unsound mind' (Section 7).

Similarly, any Hindu female 'who is of sound mind', is not a minor, and is not married, can adopt a child. If she is married then her husband '...has been declared by a court...to be of unsound mind' (Section 8).

Also, the person capable of giving in adoption of a child should be of sound mind.

III. Witness

Under the Indian Evidence Act 1872, a lunatic is not competent to give evidence if he is prevented by virtue of his lunacy from understanding the questions put to him and giving rational answers to them (Section 118).

However, such a person can give evidence during a lucid interval on the discretion of the judge and the jury.

IV. Testamentary Capacity

Testamentary disposition is regulated by the Indian Succession Act (Act 39 of 1925). Some of the salient points regarding testamentary disposition are as follows:

1. A will must be in writing, though it need not be registered.
2. It must be signed by *testator* in the presence of at least two witnesses.
3. A legatee can not attest a will.
4. An executor(s) is appointed under the will by the testator to carry out its terms after his death.
5. A will can be revoked or modified any time before the death of the testator.
6. A will comes into effect after the death of the testator. It is said to speak from grave and to be 'ambulatory'.
7. The testator must be of a 'sound and disposing mind'. Section 59 of the Act states that 'every person of sound mind, not being a minor, may dispose of his property by will'.

Explanation 4 of this section states that 'no person can make a will while he is in such a state of mind, whether arising from intoxication or from illnesses or from any other cause, that he does not know what he is doing'.

If a medical practitioner is called to examine a testator as to his fitness to make a valid will, the following points must be kept in mind:

1. Testamentary capacity consists of:
   i. an understanding of the nature of the will,
   ii. a knowledge of the property to be disposed of, and
   iii. an ability to recognize those who may have justifiable claims on his property.
2. The testator should be tested on the above mentioned points by thorough questioning.
3. If the testator is seriously ill, he must be made to read out aloud the will in the presence of the doctor.
4. A will is invalid if it is executed under undue influence of any other person. If there is reason to suspect that such is the case, the testator should be questioned when he is alone.
5. A will is invalid under the following conditions (for example):
   i. imbecility arising from advanced age or by excessive drinking.
   ii. insane delusions making the testator incapable of rational views and judgement.
6. A will is valid under the following conditions (for example):
   i. deaf, dumb or blind persons who are not thereby incapacitated for making a will and are able to know what they do by it.
   ii. lucid intervals.
   iii. if testator commits suicide immediately after making the will, in the absence of evidence of mental disorder.
   iv. presence of delusions not affecting in any way the disposal of the property or the persons affected by the will.
7. A will may be declared invalid if the testator disposes his property in a way which he would not have done under normal conditions.

V. Transfer of Property

Under the Transfer of Property Act 1882 (Section 7), only persons competent to contract, are authorized to transfer property.

Suicide within one year of insurance policy vitiates a policy, but suicide by a lunatic does not.

VI. Contract

Under the Indian Contract Act 1872 (Section 11), every person to be competent to contract must be a major and of sound mind.

A person is said to be of sound mind for the purposes of a contract, if at the time of making a contract he is capable of understanding it and of forming a rational judgement as to its effect upon his interests.

INDIAN LUNACY ACT, 1912

The Indian laws related to mental disorders were based on British Acts. For example, the Indian Lunacy Act (ILA), Act 4 of 1912, was based largely on the earlier English Lunacy Act of 1890 and replaced the existing Indian Lunatic Asylums Act, Act 36 of 1858..

The ILA had 8 Chapters. Chapter 1 defined a *lunatic* as 'an idiot or person of unsound mind'. Defectiveness of reasoning, whether partial or complete, was considered unsoundness of mind. In Chapter 3, five categories of admission methods were mentioned, namely voluntary, reception order n petition, reception order without petition, inquisition (judicial), and as a criminal lunatic.

There was a 'board of visitors' appointed by the Government which had a role in admission of voluntary patients, interfering with ongoing care and treatment and discharge (except in criminal cases). IG prisons was an ex-officio member of this board.

In 1950, three eminent psychiatrists appointed by the Indian Psychiatric Society prepared a draft 'Indian Mental Health Act' and forwarded it to Government of India. There was no action taken on the draft for next ten years and it was only in 1978 that the Mental Health Bill was introduced in Parliament. The bill had to be reintroduced in Lok Sabha in 1981 and was passed by Rajya Sabha in November 1986.

THE MENTAL HEALTH ACT, 1987

The Mental Health Bill became the Act 14 of 1987 on 22nd May 1987. Later, the Government of India issued orders that the Act came in force with effect from April 1, 1993 in all the states and Union territories of India.

The Act is divided into 10 chapters consisting of 98 sections. Chapter I (Preliminary) deals with the various definitions. The Act uses the term '*mentally ill person*' instead of 'lunatic' and defines it as 'a person who is in need of treatment by reason of any mental disorder other than mental retardation'.

The term 'mentally ill prisoner' is used instead of 'criminal lunatic'. Other new terms, which are defined in the Chapter 1, are psychiatric hospital (instead of mental hospital), psychiatric nursing home and psychiatrist.

Chapter II provides for establishment of Mental Health Authorities at Centre and State levels. These authorities will regulate and coordinate mental health services under Central and State Government, respectively.

Chapter III lays down the guidelines for establishment and maintenance of psychiatric hospitals and nursing homes. Also, there is a provision for a Licensing Authority who will process applications for licenses. No private psychiatric hospital or nursing home will be allowed to function without a valid license which has to be renewed every 5 years.

There is also a provision for an Inspecting Officer who will inspect the psychiatric hospitals and nursing homes to prevent any irregularities.

There is a provision for separate hospitals for:

1. Those under the age of 16 years,
2. Those addicted to alcohol or other drugs which lead to behavioral changes,
3. Mentally ill prisoners, and
4. Any other prescribed class or category.

Chapter IV deals with the procedures of admission and detention in psychiatric hospitals or nursing homes. In addition to the 5 methods allowed by the Indian lunacy Act of 1912, one more method has been incorporated.

Hence, the admission in a psychiatric hospital or nursing home can be made in one of the following manners:

1. Voluntary Admission.
   i. By the patient's request, if he is a major.
   ii. By the guardian, if a minor (a new provision).
2. Admission Under Special Circumstances. This is an involuntary hospitalization when the mentally ill person does not or can not express his willingness for admission. Admission is made, if a relative or a friend of the mentally ill person applies in writing for admission and the medical officer incharge of the hospital is satisfied that the admission will be in the interest of the mentally ill person.
   The duration of admission can not exceed 90 days.
3. Reception order on application.
4. Reception order without application, on production of mentally ill person (e.g. wandering, dangerous, ill-treated or neglected mentally-ill person) before Magistrate.
5. Admission as inpatient after judicial inquisition.
6. Admission as a mentally ill prisoner.

In addition, the Magistrate can order detention of an alleged mentally ill person for short periods pending report by medical officer (for a period not exceeding 10 days in aggregate) or pending his removal to psychiatric hospital or psychiatric nursing home (for a period not exceeding 30 days).

Chapter V deals with the inspection, discharge, leave of absence and removal of mentally ill persons.

Chapter VI deals with the judicial inquisition regarding alleged mentally ill person possessing property, custody of his person and management of his property.

If the court feels that the alleged mentally ill person is incapable of looking after both himself and his property, an order can be issued for the appointment of a Guardian. If, however, it is felt that the person is only incapable of looking after his property but can look after himself, a Manager can be appointed.

Chapter VII deals with the liability to meet the cost of maintenance of mentally ill persons detained in psychiatric hospitals or nursing homes.

Chapter VIII is aimed at the protection of human rights of mentally ill persons. This is a new chapter in the Act. It provides that:

1. No mentally ill person shall be subjected, during treatment, to any indignity (whether physical or mental) or cruelty.
2. No mentally ill person, under treatment, shall be used for the purposes of research, unless
   i. Such research is of direct benefit to him.
   ii. A consent has been obtained in writing from the person (if a voluntary patient) or from the guardian/relative (if admitted involuntarily).
3. No letters or communications sent by or to a mentally ill person shall be intercepted, detained or destroyed.

Chapter IX deals with the penalties and the procedure, while Chapter X provides for miscellaneous sections.

In addition, the State Mental Health Rules, 1990 (which also contains the nine important forms required by the Mental Health Act, 1987) and the Central Mental Health Authority Rules, 1990, have also been passed by the Government of India on December 29, 1990.

THE NARCOTIC DRUGS AND PSYCHOTROPIC SUBSTANCES ACT (NDPSA), 1985

The first Act for drug abuse and dependence in India was The Opium Act of 1857. This was revised first in 1878 (The Opium Act, 1878) and then in 1950 (The Opium and Revenue Laws Act, 1950). Another relevant Act was the Dangerous Drug Act of 1930, which included among other drugs, Opium and its alkaloids and Cocaine. This Act provided for a maximum punishment of 3 years.

With the coming in force of the NDPSA, Act 61 of 1985, on 16th September 1985, the above mentioned acts have been repealed.

The Act includes *narcotic drugs* (cannabis, cocaine, coca leaf, opium, poppy straw and all manufactured 'drugs') and *psychotropic substan-ces* (76 drugs and their derivatives are listed in the schedule' e.g. diazepam, pentazocine, pheno-barbital).

The authorities and officers have been suggested in Chapter 2.

If any person produces, possesses, transports, imports, exports, sells, purchases, or uses any narcotic drug or psychotropic substance (except 'ganja'), he shall be punishable with,

1. Rigorous imprisonment (RI) for not less than 10 years (which may extend to 20 years), *and*
2. A fine of not less than 1 Lakh rupees (which may extend to 2 Lakh rupees).

Punishment for a repeat offense is a RI for not less than 15 years (which may extend to 30 years) *and* a fine of not less than 1.5 Lakh rupees (which may extend to 3 Lakh rupees).

Punishment for ganja handling is a RI for 5 years and/or a fine of 0.5 Lakh rupees. For a repeat offense, the imprisonment may extend to 10 years and the fine to 1 Lakh rupees.

However, if a person is carrying 'small quantities' (e.g. 250 mg of heroin, 5 g of Charas, 5 g of opium, 125 mg of cocaine) which were later specified, then the punishment is a simple imprisonment which may extend to 1 year or a fine (unspecified) or both. For ganja (<500 g), imprisonment is up to 6 months.

There is also a provision for detoxification under court order.

A later enactment, the Prevention of Illicit Traffic in NDPS Act, 1988 has also been passed (Act 46 of 1988).

There is now a provision for preventive detention and seizure of property. The maximum punishment is death penalty, if a person is found to be trafficking more than or equal to 1 kg of pure heroin (for example), twice (despite conviction and warning on the first attempt).

CODE OF ETHICS FOR PSYCHIATRISTS

The Indian Psychiatric Society has recommended a code of ethics for psychiatrists (1989) which is summarized here:

Principles

1. A psychiatrist has a clear social *responsibility*.
2. A psychiatrist must maintain high standards of professional *competence* and ensure continuing self-education.
3. *Benevolence* and patient interest precede self interest.
4. A psychiatrist must maintain high *moral standards*.
5. *Patient welfare* is of paramount concern to a psychiatrist. It includes not to treat cases which are not in his domain, terminating treatment when can not help the patient, and treating with the best of the ability.
6. *Confidentiality* of the patient records must be meticulously maintained.

Recommendations

1. Treatment should be given with patient's *consent*. Every person who is a major and does not appear to have lost ability of reason is capable of consent.

   If the patient can not give consent due to mental illness, consent should be taken from a person close to the patient who appears to be clearly interested in patient's welfare. However treatment can be given without consent in an emergency situation involving immediate threat to the life or health of patient or others.

   For research purposes, consent should be entirely voluntary. The patient can withdraw consent at any stage, without this affecting patient's interest.
2. *Hospitalization* should be for patient's welfare, keeping in view the legal and administrative constraints, and social appropriateness.
3. *Psychiatric treatment* should be started only on clinical consideration for patient welfare and should be humane and never punitive.

   No psychiatrist should refuse to treat in an emergency.
4. No *gifts* and *gratifications* should be accep-ted from patients under treatment.
5. Any *sexual advance* towards any patient is unethical.
6. In case of doubt and/or unconventional treatment procedures a *second opinion* must be obtained.
7. It is unethical to force a *contract* on a patient during treatment.
8. Even if the patient is referred by legal or administrative authority, *patient's welfare* is paramount and patient should be informed of the purpose for which he is to be examined.
9. The basic *human rights* of mentally retarded should not be unethically abridged.
10. In the interest of the patient and the society, drug abusers who refuse to give consent may be treated with the consent of the their relatives. Effort has to be made to motivate them for accepting treatment voluntarily.

ICMR GUIDELINES FOR RESEARCH, 2000

Recently, in the year 2000, Indian Council of Medical Research (ICMR) has released '*Ethical guidelines for biomedical research in human subjects*'. The guidelines are similar to the GCP (Good Clinical Practice) guidelines and the prevalent international guidelines. These guidelines regulate all biomedical research in human subjects in India.

MCI CODE OF MEDICAL ETHICS, 2002

All psychiatrists as doctors are also bound by the Code of medical ethics of Medical Council of India (MCI).

Named as the *Indian Medical Council (Professional conduct, Etiquette and Ethics) Regulations, 2002,* the code came in to effect from 6th April, 2002. The full code is available at the web-site of MCI, at http://mohfw.nic.in/code.htm.

21 Community Psychiatry

Born in 1963, the community psychiatry movement has been hailed as *the third psychiatric revolution*. The first revolution was the age of enlightenment following the middle ages, when mental illness was viewed as a consequence of sin and witchcraft. The second revolution was the development of psychoanalysis which offered hope for a causative explanation of psychiatric disorders. However, the community psychiatry movement was made possible by another revolution, the one ushered by the advent of psychopharmacology. Therefore it may be more appropriate to refer to community psychiatry as the *fourth* psychiatric revolution.

The 'community psychiatry' concept has its antecedents in Clifford Beers' (1908) mental hygiene movement and Adolf Meyer's recommendation (1913) of establishment of treatment centers in the community. The period between 1955 to 1980 was an era of de-institutionalization in USA and other Western countries, consisting of discharging mentally ill patients from mental hospitals, to be cared for in community mental health centers. This provided an impetus to the development of community psychiatry.

In 1975, the World Health Organization strongly recommended the delivery of mental health services through primary health care system as a policy for the developing countries. In India, attempts to develop models of psychiatric services in the PHC (primary health center) setting were made nearly simultaneously at PGI, Chandigarh in 1975 (Raipur Rani block of Ambala district, Haryana) and NIMHANS, Bangalore in 1976 (Sakalwara, in Karnataka).

The basic model of community mental health was defined by Gerald Caplan in 1967. The predominant characteristics of community psychiatry are:

1. Responsibility to a population for mental health care delivery.
2. Treatment close to the patient in community based centers.
3. Provision of comprehensive services.
4. Multi-disciplinary team approach.
5. Providing continuity of care.
6. Emphasis on prevention as well as treatment.
7. Avoidance of unnecessary hospitalization.

NATIONAL MENTAL HEALTH PROGRAM

Mental health is an integral component of health, which is defined as a positive state of well being (physical, mental and social) and not merely an absence of illness. With this aim in mind, an expert group was formed in 1980. The final draft was submitted to the Central Council of Health and Family Welfare (the highest policy making body for health in the country) on 18-20 August 1982, which recommended its implementation. The NMHP appeared almost simultaneously with the National Health Policy (1993).

TABLE 21.1. EXTENT OF THE PROBLEM AND FACILITIES AVAILABLE IN INDIA

THE PROBLEM

Population = 1027 million (2001)
Prevalence of psychiatric disorders = 58/1000
Severe mental illness
Point prevalence = 10-20/1000 population
Incidence = 35/100,000 population
Neuroses and psychosomatic disorders
Point prevalence = 2-3%
Mental retardation
Point prevalence = 0.5-1.0% of all children
Psychiatric disorders in children
Point prevalence = 1-2% of all children
Psychiatric OPD attendance in (1990 data)
Govt. hospitals = 3.63 million/year
Private practice = 2.63 million/year
Total OPD attendance = 6.29 million/year
(~1% of population)
Additionally, 15-20% of all help-seekers in general health services do so for emotional & psychosocial problems.

EXISTING MENTAL HEALTH SERVICES

No. of govt. mental hospitals = 37
No. of mental hospital beds = ~19000
Private psychiatric hospital beds = 2000-3000
General hospital psychiatry units beds (GHPU beds) = 4000-5000
Total health beds in India = 8,70,161 (1994-95)
Psychiatric beds in India
Per 10,000 population = 0.3 (World = 4.36)*

MANPOWER AVAILABLE IN INDIA

Psychiatrists (qualified) in India
Numbers= ~3500
Per 100,000 population = 0.3 (World = 3.96)
Total qualified doctors in India = 503,900 (1999)
Clinical psychologists in India
Numbers = ~1000
Per 100,000 population < 0.1 (World = 6.43)*
Psychiatric social workers
Numbers = ~1000
Per 100,000 population < 0.1 (World = 8.64)*
Psychiatric nurses in India
Numbers = 800-900
Per 100,000 population < 0.1 (World = 12.6)*
Total nurses in India = 7,37,000 (1999)
PG centres = ~40 (very few of 140 medical colleges have a psychiatry department)
MD/DPM seats (Psychiatrists/year) = ~200 (For comparison: Doctors/year = 13,000) (1990)

* *Source: Atlas: Mental Health Resources in the World, 2001, WHO*

The objectives of National Mental Health Program (NMHP) are:

1. To ensure availability and accessibility of *minimum mental health care for all* in the foreseeable future, particularly to the most vulnerable and underprivileged sections of population.
2. To encourage *application of mental health knowledge* in general health care and in social development.
3. To promote *community participation* in the mental health service development and to stimulate efforts towards self-help in the community.

Three aims are specified in the NMHP in planning mental health services for the country:

1. Prevention and treatment of mental and neurological disorders and their associated disabilities.
2. Use of mental health technology to improve general health services.
3. Application of mental health principles in total national development to improve quality of life.

Two strategies, complementary to each other, were planned for immediate action:

1. *Center to periphery strategy:* Establishment and strengthening of psychiatric units in all district hospitals, with outpatient clinics and mobile teams reaching the population for mental health services.
2. *Periphery to center strategy*: Training of an increasing number of different

categories of health personnel in basic mental health skills, with primary emphasis towards the poor and the underprivileged, directly benefiting about 200 million people.

The mental health care service was envisaged to include three components or subprograms: treatment, rehabilitation and prevention.

1. Treatment Subprogram

Multiple levels were planned.

A. *Village and subcentre level:* Multi-purpose workers (MPW) and health supervisors (HS), under the supervision of medical officer (MO), to be trained for:
   - i. management of psychiatric emergencies.
   - ii. administration and supervision of maintenance treatment for chronic psychiatric disorders.
   - iii. diagnosis and management of grand mal epilepsy, especially in children.
   - iv. liaison with local school teacher and parents regarding mental retardation and behavior problems in children.
   - v. counseling in problems related to alcohol and drug abuse.

B. *Primary health center (PHC)*: MO, aided by HS, to be trained for:
   - i. supervision of MPW's performance
   - ii. elementary diagnosis
   - iii. treatment of functional psychosis
   - iv. treatment of uncomplicated cases of psychiatric disorders associated with physical diseases
   - v. management of uncomplicated psychosocial problems
   - vi. epidemiological surveillance of mental morbidity.

C. *District hospital:* It was recognized that there should be at least 1 psychiatrist attached to every district hospital as an integral part of the district health services. The district hospital should have 30-50 psychiatric beds. The psychiatrist in a district hospital was envisaged to devote only a part of his time in clinical care and greater part in training and supervision of non-specialist health workers.

D. *Mental hospitals and teaching psychiatric units:* The major activities of these higher centers of psychiatric care include:
   - i. Help in care of 'difficult' cases.
   - ii. Teaching.
   - iii. Specialized facilities like occupational therapy units, psychotherapy, counseling and behavior therapy.

2. Rehabilitation Subprogram

The components of this subprogram include maintenance treatment of epileptics and psychotics at the community levels and development of rehabilitation centers at both the district level and the higher referral centers.

3. Prevention Subprogram

The prevention component is to be community-based, with the initial focus on prevention and control of alcohol-related problems. Later, problems like addictions, juvenile delinquency and acute adjustment problems like suicidal attempts are to be addressed.

The other approaches designed to achieve the objectives of the NMHP include:

1. Integration of basic mental health care into general health services.
2. Mental health training of general medical doctors and paramedical health workers.

A plan of action was outlined in 1982, with the first opportunity to develop it in the 7th Five-year plan starting from 1985, with a plan allocation of Rs. 100 lacs. A National Mental

Health Advisory Group (NMHAG) was formed in August 1988 and a Mental Health Cell was opened in the Ministry of Health and Family Welfare under a Central Mental Health Authority (MHA).

Various activities were planned under action plan for implementation of national mental health program in the 7th Five-year plan, like community mental health programs at primary health care level in states and union territories; training of existing PHC personnel for mental health care delivery; development of a state level Mental Health Advisory Committee and state level program officer; establishment of Regional Centers of community mental health; formation of National Advisory Group on Mental Health; development of task forces for mental hospitals and mental health education for undergraduate medical students; involvement of voluntary agencies in mental health care; identification of priority areas (child mental health, public mental health education and drug dependence); mental health training of at least 1 doctor at every district hospital during the next 5 years; establishment of a department of psychiatry in all medical colleges and strengthening the existing ones; and provision of at least 3-4 essential psychotropic drugs in adequate quantity, at the PHC level.

District Mental Health Program (DMHP) was started in 1995 as a component of NMHP. The prototype of the District Mental Health Program was the Bellary district program (in Karnataka, ~320 km from Bangalore). Started in 1985, it caters to a population of 1.5 million. District hospital psychiatry units have been opened in every district of Kerala and Tamil Nadu.

Following the implementation of National Mental Health Program in India 1982, other neighboring countries soon followed the example by drawing national programs for mental health (Sri Lanka 1982; Bangla Desh 1982; Pakistan 1986; Nepal 1987).

The revised National Health Policy (NHP-2002) is soon being released. Its focus on mental health "envisages a network of decentralized mental health services for ameliorating the more common categories of disorders".

At the same time the NMHP draft proposal for the 10th five year plan is also being prepared, with a plan to extend the DMHP to 100 districts. It also emphasizes the need to broaden the scope of existing curriculum for undergraduate training in psychiatry and to give more exposure to psychiatry in undergraduate years and internship. An essential list of psychotropic drugs is also being prepared.

The emphasis of NMHP-1982 was primarily on the rural sector. It is being realized that the urban mental health needs also need to be addressed under the ambit of NMHP.

WORLD (MENTAL) HEALTH REPORT 2001

This landmark publication of the WHO was published in 2001 (Editor-in-Chief: RS Murthy). The 2001 World Health Report focused on mental health (*Mental Health: New Understanding, New Hope*), with a slogan, "*Stop Exclusion: Dare to Care*".

The report identified that "one person in every four will be affected by a mental disorder at some stage of life". It points out that the psychiatric disorders are estimated to account for 12% of the global burden of disease, yet the mental health budgets of the majority of countries constitute <1% of their total health expenditures.

The WHR-2001 appears along with the "Atlas", a unique publication of WHO giving a comparative account of the mental health resources in the world. The report identifies that "mental disorders affect all people in all countries", but the "people do not get the care they need...because of lack of resources,...because of fear of seeking help, ...and because of lack of (mental health) policies". The WHR-2001 makes ten recommendations for action:

1. Provide treatment in primary care
2. Make psychotropic drugs available
3. Give care in the community.
4. Educate the public
5. Involve communities, families and consumers
6. Establish national policies, programs and legislation
7. Develop human resources
8. Link with other sectors
9. Monitor community mental health
10. Support more research.

Appendix I

Nobel Prizes in Psychiatry and Allied Disciplines

	Nobel Laureates	Major Contributions	Year of Award
1.	**Ivan Petrovich Pavlov** (1849-1936; Russia)	• Classical conditioning Physiology of digestion	1904
2.	**Camillo Golgi** (1843-1926; Italy) **Santiago Ramon y Cajal** (1852-1934; Spain)	• Structure of CNS	1906
3.	**Julius Wagner von Jauregg** (1857-1940; US)	• Malarial treatment for GPI (First successful treatment of a major psychosis)	1927 (First psychiatrist to receive a Nobel Prize)
4.	**Antonio Caetano de Abreu Freire Egas Moniz (Egas Moniz)** (1874-1955; Portugal) **Walter Rudolf Hess** (1881-1973)	• Psychosurgery (prefrontal leucotomy) • Cerebral angiography	1949
5.	**Konrad Lorenz** (1903-1989; Austria) **Karl Von Frisch** (1886-1982; Germany) **Nikolaas Tinbergen** (1907-1988; UK)	• Ethology	1973
6.	**Sir Godfrey Newbold Hounsfield** (1919-; UK) **Allan M Cormack** (1924-1998; US)	• CT Scan	1979
7.	**Stanley B. Prusiner** (1942-; US)	• Discovery of *Prions*	1997
8.	**Eric R. Kandel** (1929-; US) **Arvid Carlsson** (1923-; Sweden) **Paul Greengard** (1925-; US)	• Signal Tranduction in CNS	2000

Appendix II

Some Important Contributors in Psychiatry

Contibutor	*Coined the term*	*Special Mention*
Adler, Alfred (1870-1937)	Life style Inferiority complex Will to power Creative self	Founder of the school of individual psychology
Alexander, Franz (1891-1964)	—	Sometimes known as the father of psychosomatic medicine
Ayurveda (< 4000 BC)	—	Five types of constitution and 3 main types of personality were described. Modernistic descriptions of mental disorders were given.
Beard, George Miller (1839-1883)	Neurasthenia	—
Berne, Eric (1910-1970)	Games Transactions	Founder of transactional analysis (TA). Wrote the book 'Games People Play'
Binet, Alfred (1857-1911)	—	Gave the 1st formal scale of intelligence
Bleuler, Eugen (1857-1939)	Schizophrenia	Described 'cardinal' symptoms of schizophrenia
Braid, James (1795-1860)	Hypnosis	—
Cicero (106-43 BC)	Libido	—
Cullen, William (1710-1790)	Neurosis	—
Delay, Jean PL (b 1907)	Neuroleptic Neuroleptic malignant syndrome (NMS)	1st antipsychotic treatment (chlorpromazine) of psychoses

Contd

Contibutor	Coined the term	Special Mention
Dendy, Walter Cooper (1794-1871)	Psychotherapy (Psychotherapeia)	—
Deniker, Pierre (b 1917)	'Hibernotherapie'	—
Erikson, Erik H (1902-1994)	Psychohistory Identity crisis	— Described the stages of life
Esquirol, Jean ED (1772-1840)	Hallucination Monomania	—
Falret, Jean-Pierre (1794-1870)	Mental alienation	Thus, psychiatrists came to be known as alienists
Fechner, Gustav Theodore (1801-1887)	Psychophysics	Founder of experimental & physiological psychology
Feuchtersleben, Ernst von (1806-1849)	Psychosis	—
Freud, Sigmund (1856-1939)	Free association Psychoanalysis Psychodynamics Oedipus complex Electra complex Penis envy Primal scene Ego defense mechanisms Repression Psychological determinism Pleasure principle Reality principle	Founder of psychoanalysis; some of the significant contributions include: interpretation of dreams, theory of infantile sexuality, structural and topographical model of mind, theory of instincts, psychopathology of everyday life and stages of psychosexual development
Gall, Franz Joseph (1758-1828)	—	Founder of phrenology
Gita Bhagavad (~4th Century BC)	—	Probably the 1st recorded evidence of crisis-intervention psychotherapy
Gockel (1547-1628)	Psychology	—
Griesinger, Wilhelm (1817-1868)	Unitary psychosis	Founder of the speciality of neuropsychiatry; 1st full time academic psychiatrist with a medical orientation

Contd

Contibutor	*Coined the term*	*Special Mention*
Hecker, Ewald (1843-1909)	Hebephrenia	—
Heinroth, Johann C (1773-1843)	Psychosomatic	—
Horney, Karen (1885-1952)	—	American psychoanalyst; Neo-Freudian; Described a theory of neurosis
Janet, Pierre (1859-1947)	Psychasthenia	—
Jones, Maxwell (b 1907)	Therapeutic community	—
Jung, Carl Gustav (1875-1961)	Collective and personal unconscious Complex Introvert and extrovert Archetypes Persona Anima and animus	Founder of the school of of analytical psychology
Kahlbaum, Karl (1828-1899)	Catatonia Symptom complex Cyclothymia	—
Kanner, Leo (1894-1981)	—	Described infantile autism
Klein, Melanie (1882-1960)	Basic trust	Child psychoanalyst
Kraepelin, Emil (1856-1926)	Dementia precox	Important work on psychiatric nosology and classification
Krafft-Ebing, B Richard von (1840-1902)	Sadism Masochism	Classic description of sexual perversions
Maslow, Abraham (1908-1970)	Self-actualization Self-realization	Humanistic psychology; Described hierarchy of needs
Mesmer, Franz Anton (1734-1815)	Animal magnetism	—
Meyer, Adolf (1866-1950)	—	Founder of psychobiology; Famous for 'common sense psychiatry'

Contd...

Contibutor	*Coined the term*	*Special Mention*
Morel, Benedict-Augustin (1809-1873)	Demence' precoce'	—
Pavlov, Ivan Petrovich (1849-1936)	Classical conditioning	Animal studies on conditioned reflexes
Piaget, Jean (1897-1980)	—	Extensive studies on the nature of children's intellectual development
Pinel, Philippe (1745-1826)	—	Famous for humane and 'moral' treatment of mentally ill
Prichard, James (1786-1848)	Moral insanity	—
Rado, Sandor (1890-1972)	Adaptational psychodynamics	Hungarian psychoanalyst
Rank, Otto (1884-1939)	Birth trauma Will therapy	—
Ray, Issac (1807-1881)	—	Father of American forensic psychiatry
Reil, Johann Christian (1759-1820)	Psychiatry	Founded the 1st psychiatric journal
Rogers, Carl (1902-1987)	Client-centred psychotherapy	American psychologist; Non-directive psychotherapist
Rush, Benjamin (1745-1828)	—	Father of American psychiatry
Skinner, Burrhus Frederic (1904-1990)	—	Founder of operant conditioning model of learning
Sullivan, Harry Stack (1892-1949)	—	Founder of interpersonal school of psychiatry
Tissot, Simon Andre (1728-1797)	Onanism	1st medical description of masturbation
Vives, Juan Louis (1492-1540)	—	Wrote the 1st 'modern' textbook of psychology
Watson, John Broadus (1878-1958)	—	Founder of behaviorism
Weyer, Johann (1515-1588)	—	Sometimes known as the father of modern psychiatry.
Zacchia, Paolo (1584-1659)	—	Probably the 1st forensic psychiatrist

Appendix III

Glossary of Some Important Terms in Psychiatry

Abstract thinking: Abstract thinking is the ability to assume a mental set voluntarily, shift voluntarily from one aspect of a situation to another, keep in mind simultaneously the various aspects of a situation, grasp the essentials of a 'whole' (e.g. situation or concept), and to break a 'whole' into its parts.

Affect: The outward expression of the immediate (*cross-sectional)* experience of emotion at a given time.

Agitation: Presence of anxiety with severe motor restlessness.

Alexithymia: Inability to verbally describe one's emotionally feelings.

Ambitendency: Due to ambivalence, tenta-tive actions are made, but no goal directed action occurs.

Ambivalence: Inability to decide for or against, due to co-existence of two opposing impulses for the same thing at the same time in the same person.

Anergia: Lack of energy for day-to-day activities.

Anhedonia: Inability to experience pleasure in previously pleasurable activities.

Anxiety: An unpleasurable emotional state, associated with psycho-physiological changes in response to an intrapsychic conflict.

Blunted affect: Severe reduction in the intensity of affect.

Catalepsy: The person maintains body posture in to which it is placed. Also see *waxy flexibility*.

Cataplexy: Abrupt loss of muscle tone without impairment of conciousness. Often seen in Narcolepsy.

Circumstantiality: Digression in to unnecessary details that distract from the central theme; however, the patient returns back to the original theme after digression (unlike in tangentiality).

Confabulation: A false memory that the patient believes to be true.

Deja entendu: A false sense of familiarity when hearing something new.

Deja vu: A false sense of familiarity with unfamiliar circumstances or scenes.

Delusion: A false, unshakable belief which is not amenable to reasoning, and is not in keeping with the patient's socio-cultural and educational background.

Delusional Perception: Normal perception has a private and illogical meaning.

Depersonalization: An alteration in the perception of self, so that the feeling of one's reality is (*as if*) temporarily changed or lost.

Derealization: An alteration in the perception of external world, so that the feeling of the reality of external world is (*as if*) temporarily changed or lost.

Disorientation: A disturbance in orientation in time, place and/or person.

Distractibility: Inability to concentrate or focus attention.

Echolalia: Repetition, echo or mimicking of phrases or words heard

Echopraxia: Repetition, echo or mimicking of actions observed.

Ecstasy: Very severe elevation of mood (seen in delirious or stuporous mania); Intense sense of rapture or blissfulness.

Elation: Moderate elevation of mood (seen in mania; Stage II); Feeling of confidence and enjoyment along with increased psychomotor activity.

Euphoria: Mild elevation of mood (seen in hypomania); Increased sense of psychological well-being and happiness, not in keeping with ongoing events.

Euthymia: Normal range of mood, with absence of depressed or elevated mood.

Exaltation: Severe elevation of mood (seen in severe mania; Stage III); Intense elation with delusions of grandeur.

Flight of Ideas: Rapid speech with sudden shifts in ideas, without loosing logical connection.

Folie å deux: Delusions shared between two closely connected persons. Also known are folie å trios, folie å quatre, and folie å famille.

Formication: A false sense of insects crawling on one's skin.

Fugue: Physical and psychological flight (wandering) from one's usual place.

Grandiosity: Excessive and exaggerated feeling of one's importance.

Hallucination: A perception that occurs in the absence of a stimulus.

Illusion: A misinterpretation of stimuli arising from external object(s).

Incoherence: Thought process that is disconnected, disorganized, or incomprehensible.

Insight: The ability to understand one's own behavior and emotions. In the context of psychiatric disorders, it implies the degree of awareness and understanding that the patient has regarding his/her illness.

Intelligence: The ability to think logically, act rationally, and deal effectively with the environment.

Jamais entendu: A sense of unfamiliarity when hearing something familiar.

Jamais vu: A sense of unfamiliarity with familiar circumstances or scenes.

Judgement: An ability to assess a situation correctly and act appropriately with in that situation.

Labile Affect: Rapid and abrupt changes in affect, unrelated to external stimuli.

Loosening of Associations: Thought process characterized by a series of ideas without apparent logical connections.

Mood: The pervasive feeling tone which is *sustained* (lasts for some length of time) and colors the total experience of the person.

Mutism: Complete absence of speech.

Negativism: An apparently motiveless resistance to all commands and attempts to be moved, or doing just the opposite.

Neologisms: These are idiosyncratically formed new words whose derivation can not be understood easily.

Panic: An acute, intense, overwhelming episode of anxiety, often associated with feelings of impending doom.

Perseveration: Persistent repetition of words or themes beyond the point of relevance.

Phobia: An irrational fear of an object, situation or activity.

Posturing: Voluntary assumption of an inappropriate and often bizarre posture for long periods of time

Poverty of Speech: Decreased speech production.

Poverty of Content of Speech: The speech production is adequate, but the content conveys little information.

Pressure of Speech: Rapid production of speech output, with a subjective feeling of racing thoughts.

Rigidity (Catatonic): Maintenance of a rigid posture against efforts to be moved.

Somatic Passivity: Bodily sensations, especially sensory symptoms, are experienced as imposed on body by some external force.

Somnolence: Inability to maintain a state of alertness without constant stimulation.

Stereotypy: A fixed pattern of purposeless behavior, verbal or motor.

Stupor: A clinical syndrome of akinesis (no movement) and mutism, with relative preservation of conscious awareness.

Suicide: A human act of self-intentioned and self-inflicted cessation (death).

Tangentiality: Sudden and oblique digression in to unnecessary details that completely distract from the central theme; however, the patient never returns back to the original theme after digression (unlike in circumstantiality).

Thinking: Normal thinking is a goal directed flow of ideas, symbols and associations initiated by a problem or a task, characterized by rational connections between successive ideas or thoughts, and leading towards a reality oriented conclusion.

Thought Diffusion or Broadcasting: Subject experiences that his thoughts are escaping the confines of his self and are being experienced by others around.

Thought Echo: Voices speaking out thoughts aloud; also called as *echo de la pense*.

Thought Insertion: Subject experiences thoughts imposed by some external force on his passive mind.

Thought Withdrawal: Thoughts cease and subject experiences them as removed by external force.

Trance: A sleep like state of reduced consciousness and suggestibility.

Verbigeration: Senseless repetition of same words or phrases over and over again.

Waxy Flexibility: Parts of body can be placed in positions that will be maintained for long periods of time, even if very uncomfortable; flexible like wax. The process is called as *waxy flexibility*, while the end result is called as *catalepsy*.

Suggested Further Reading

1. Abse DW. Hysteria and Related Mental Disorders: An Approach to Psychological Medicine. II Ed. John Wright. Bristol, 1987.
2. American Psychiatric Association. Diagnostic and Statistical Manual of Mental Disorders. IV Ed. Text Revision. American Psychiatric Association. Washington DC, 2000.
3. American Psychiatric Association. Task Force Report on Electroconvulsive Therapy. Washington DC. APA, 1990.
4. Arieti S. Interpretation of Schizophrenia. II Ed. Basic Books. New York, 1974.
5. Bancroft J. Human Sexuality and Its Problems. Churchill Livingstone. Edinburgh, 1985.
6. Barlett J, Bridges P, Kelly D. Contemporary indications for psychosurgery. British Journal of Psychiatry. 138:507, 1981.
7. Beck AT, Rush AJ, Shaw BI, et. al. Cognitive Therapy of Depression. Guilford. New York, 1979.
8. Beck AT. Cognitive Therapy and the Emotional Disorders. International Universities Press. New York, 1976.
9. Bellack AS, Hersen M, Kazdin AE. International Handbook of Behavior Modification and Therapy. Plenum Press. New York, 1982.
10. Benson DF, Blumer D. Eds. Psychiatric Aspects of Neurologic Disease. Grune and Stratton. New York. Vol. I, 1975. Vol. II, 1982.
11. Benson FD. Aphasia, Alexia and Agraphia. Churchill Livingstone. New York, 1979.
12. Bleuler E. Dementia Precox: The Group of Schizophrenias. International Universities Press. New York, 1950.
13. Brown GW, Birley JLT, Wing JK. Influence of family life on the course of schizophrenic disorders: A replication. British Journal of Psychiatry. 121:241, 1972.
14. Brown JAC. Freud and the Post-Freudians. Penguin. New York, 1978.
15. Cavenar JO, Brodie HKH. Eds. Signs and Symptoms in Psychiatry. JB Lippincott. Philadelphia, 1983.
16. Chapman JP. The early symptoms of schizophrenia. British Journal of Psychiatry. 112:225, 1966.
17. Cleckley H. The Mask of Sanity. IV Ed. Mosby. St. Louis, 1964.
18. Dement WC. Some Must Watch While Some Must Sleep. WH Freeman & Co. San Francisco, 1974.
19. Fenichel O. The Psychoanalytic Theory of Neurosis. Norton. New York, 1945.
20. Fink M. Convulsive Therapy: Theory and Practice. Raven Press. New York, 1979.
21. Folstein MF, Folstein SE, McHugh PR. Mini-Mental State: A practical method for grading the cognitive state of patients for the clinician. Journal of Psychiatric Research. 12:189, 1975.
22. Freud A. The Ego and the Mechanisms of Defense. Hogarth Press. London, 1937.
23. Freud S. The Psychopathology of Everyday Life. In: Strachey J. ed. The Standard Edition of the Complete Psychological Works of Sigmund Freud. Hogarth Press. London, 1960;6.
24. Gelder M, Mayou R, Cowen P. Shorter Oxford Textbook of Psychiatry. IV Ed. Oxford University Press. New York, 2001.
25. Gelenberg AJ. The catatonic syndrome. Lancet. 1:1339, 1976.
26. Gottesman II, Shields J. Schizophrenia: The Epigenetic Puzzle. Cambridge University Press. New York, 1982.
27. Govt. of India. The Mental Health Act. Act 14 of 1987, 1987.
28. Govt. of India. The Narcotic Drugs and Psychotropic Substances Act. Act 61 of 1985, 1985. (Amended in 1989, Act 2 of 1989).
29. Hall CS. A Primer of Freudian Psychology. World Publishing. Cleveland, 1954.
30. Hamilton M. Fish's Clinical Psychopathology. III Ed. John Wright. Bristol, 1983.
31. Hamilton M. Fish's Schizophrenia. III Ed. John Wright. Bristol, 1986.
32. Heilman KM, Valenstein E. Eds. Clinical Neuropsychology. II Ed. Oxford University Press. New York, 1985.
33. Hinsie LE, Campbell RJ. Psychiatric Dictionary. V Ed. Oxford University Press. New York, 1981.
34. Indian Council of Medical Research, Manual of Mental Health for Medical Officers. NIMHANS. Bangalore, 1983.
35. Jefferson JW, Griest JH, Ackerman DL. Lithium Encyclopedia for Clinical Practice. American Psychiatric Press. Washington DC, 1983.
36. Jellinek EM. The Disease Concept of Alcoholism. College and University Press. New Haven, 1960.
37. Jones E. The life and Work of Sigmund Freud. Basic Books, New York, 1957.
38. Kaplan HI, Sadock BJ, Grebb JA. Synopsis of Psychiatry. VIII Ed. Williams and Wilkins, 1998.
39. Kraepelin E. Dementia Praecox and Paraphrenia. Ed. GM Robertson. Huntington. NY: Krieger, 1971.

40. Kraepelin E. Manic-Depressive Insanity and Paranoia. Livingstone. Edinburgh, 1921.
41. Leff JP, Issacs AD. Psychiatric Examination in Clinical Practice. II Ed. Blackwell. Oxford, 1981.
42. Lerer B, Weiner RD, Belmaker RH. ECT: Basic Mechanisms. John Libbey. London, 1984.
43. Lishman WA. Organic Psychiatry: The Psychological Consequences of Cerebral Disorder. III Ed. Blackwell. Oxford, 1998.
44. Marks IM. Fears, Phobias and Rituals. Academic Press. New York, 1988.
45. Masters WH, Johnson VE. Human Sexual Inadequacy. Little Brown. Boston, 1966.
46. Masters WH, Johnson VE. Human Sexual Response. Little Brown. Boston, 1966.
47. Mellor CS. First rank symptoms of schizophrenia. British Journal of Psychiatry. 117:15, 1970.
48. Merksey H. The Analysis of Hysteria. Bailliére Tindall. London, 1979.
49. Ministry of Health and Family Welfare. National Mental Health Programme Booklet. DGHS. New Delhi, 1982.
50. Murthy RS, Wig NN. The WHO collaborative study on strategies for extending mental health care. American Journal of Psychiatry. 140:1486, 1983.
51. Murthy RS. National Mental Health Programme in India (1982-1989): Mid-point appraisal. Indian Journal of Psychiatry. 31:267, 1989.
52. Noshpitz JD Sr. Ed. Basic Handbook of Child Psychiatry. Vol I-IV. Basic Books. New York, 1979.
53. Paykel ES. Ed. Handbook of Affective Disorders. II Ed. Churchill Livingstone. New York, 1992.
54. Perry JC, Jacobs D. Overview: Clinical applications of the amytal interview in psychiatric emergency settings. American Journal of Psychiatry. 139:552, 1982.
55. Pincus J, Tucker GJ. Behavioral Neurology. III Ed. Oxford University Press. New York, 1985.
56. Plum F, Posner C. The Diagnosis of Stupor and Coma. III Ed. FA Davis. Philadelphia, 1980.
57. Sadock BJ, Sadock VA. Eds. Comprehensive Textbook of Psychiatry. VII Ed. Williams and Wilkins,
58. Sharma SD. Mental Hospitals in India. DGHS. New Delhi, 1990.
59. Shneidman ES, Farberow NL. Some Facts About Suicide. PHS Publication No. 852, US Govt. Printing Office. Washington DC, 1961.
60. Slater E, Roth M. Clinical Psychiatry (Mayer-Gross). III Ed. JPB Publishers. New Delhi, 1986.
61. Strub RL, Black FW. The Mental Status Examination in Neurology. II Ed. FA Davis. Philadelphia, 1985, reprinted by JPB Publishers. New Delhi, 1991.
62. Vyas JN, Ahuja Niraj. Editors. Textbook of Post-graduate Psychiatry. II Ed. JPB Publishers. New Delhi, 1999.
63. Walsh K. Neuropsychology: A Clinical Approach. III Ed. BI Churchill Livingstone. New Delhi, 1994.
64. Wolberg LR. The Technique of Psychotherapy. Vol. I & II. Secker & Warburg with Heinemann. London, 1989.
65. World Health Organization. The ICD-10 Classification of Mental and Behavioural Disorders: Clinical descriptions and diagnostic guidelines. World Health Organization. Geneva, 1992.
66. World Health Organization. The World health report: 2001. Mental Health: New Understanding, New Hope, World Health Organization, Geneva, 2001.
67. World Health Organization. Atlas: Mental Health Resources in the World. 2001. World Health Organization, Geneva, 2001.
68. Zilboorg GA, Henry GW. A History of Medical Psychology. Norton, 1941.

Index

B

C

F

G

H

I

N

O

P

Q

R

S

READER SUGGESTIONS SHEET

Please help us to improve the quality of our publications by completing and returning this sheet to us.

Author/Title: **A Short Textbook of Psychiatry, 5th edn, by Niraj Ahuja**

Your name and address:

E-mail address,
Phone and Fax:

How did you hear about this book? [please tick appropriate box (es)]

☐ Direct mail from publisher ☐ Conference ☐ Bookshop
☐ Book review ☐ Lecturer recommendation ☐ Friends
☐ Other (please specify) ☐ Website

Type of purchase: ☐ Direct purchase ☐ Bookshop ☐ Friends

Do you have any brief comments on the book?

Please return this sheet to the name and address given below.

JAYPEE BROTHERS
MEDICAL PUBLISHERS (P) LTD
EMCA House, 23/23B Ansari Road, Daryaganj
New Delhi 110 002, India